T0228999

Endocrine Surgery

Guest Editor

MARTHA A. ZEIGER, MD, FACS, FACE

SURGICAL CLINICS
OF NORTH AMERICA

www.surgical.theclinics.com

Consulting Editor
RONALD F. MARTIN, MD

October 2009 • Volume 89 • Number 5

SAUNDERS an imprint of ELSEVIER, Inc.

W.B. SAUNDERS COMPANY
A Division of Elsevier Inc.
1600 John F. Kennedy Blvd., Suite 1800, Philadelphia, PA 19103-2899
http://www.theclinics.com
SURGICAL CLINICS OF NORTH AMERICA Volume 89, Number 5
October 2009 ISSN 0039–6109, ISBN-10: 1-4377-1388-2, ISBN-13: 978-1-4377-1388-6
Editor: Catherine Bewick
Developmental Editor: Donald Mumford

Photocopying

Single photocopies of single articles may be made for personal use as allowed by national copyright laws. Permission of the Publisher and payment of a fee is required for all other photocopying, including multiple or systematic copying, copying for advertising or promotional purposes, resale, and all forms of document delivery. Special rates are available for educational institutions that wish to make photocopies for non-profit educational classroom use. For information on how to seek permission visit www.elsevier.com/permissions or call: (+44) 1865 843830 (UK)/(+1) 215 239 3804 (USA).

Derivative Works

Subscribers may reproduce tables of contents or prepare lists of articles including abstracts for internal circulation within their institutions. Permission of the Publisher is required for resale or distribution outside the institution. Permission of the Publisher is required for all other derivative works, including compilations and translations (please consult www.elsevier.com/permissions).

Electronic Storage or Usage

Permission of the Publisher is required to store or use electronically any material contained in this journal, including any article or part of an article (please consult www.elsevier.com/permissions). Except as outlined above, no part of this publication may be reproduced, stored in a retrieval system or transmitted in any form or by any means, electronic, mechanical, photocopying, recording or otherwise, without prior written permission of the Publisher.

Notice

No responsibility is assumed by the Publisher for any injury and/or damage to persons or property as a matter of products liability, negligence or otherwise, or from any use or operation of any methods, products, instructions or ideas contained in the material herein. Because of rapid advances in the medical sciences, in particular, independent verification of diagnoses and drug dosages should be made.

Although all advertising material is expected to conform to ethical (medical) standards, inclusion in this publication does not constitute a guarantee or endorsement of the quality or value of such product or of the claims made of it by its manufacturer.

Surgical Clinics of North America (ISSN 0039–6109) is published bimonthly by Elsevier Inc., 360 Park Avenue South, New York, NY 10010-1710. Months of publication are February, April, June, August, October, and December. Business and Editorial Offices: 1600 John F. Kennedy Blvd., Suite 1800, Philadelphia, PA 19103-2899. Periodicals postage paid at New York, NY and additional mailing offices. Subscription prices are $269.00 per year for US individuals, $432.00 per year for US institutions, $134.00 per year for US students and residents, $330.00 per year for Canadian individuals, $537.00 per year for Canadian institutions, $371.00 for international individuals, $537.00 per year for international institutions and $185.00 per year for Canadian and foreign students/residents. To receive student/resident rate, orders must be accompanied by name of affiliated institution, date of term, and the *signature* of program/residency coordinator on institution letterhead. Orders will be billed at individual rate until proof of status is received. Foreign air speed delivery is included in all *Clinics* subscription prices. All prices are subject to change without notice. POSTMASTER: Send address changes to *Surgical Clinics*, Elsevier Health Sciences Division, Subscription Customer Service, 3251 Riverport Lane, Maryland Heights, MO 63043. **Customer Service (orders, claims, online, change of address): Telephone: 1-800-654-2452 (U.S. and Canada); 314-447-8871 (outside U.S. and Canada). Fax: 314-447-8029. E-mail: journalscustomerservice-usa@elsevier.com (for print support); journalsonlinesupport-usa@elsevier.com (for online support).**

Reprints. For copies of 100 or more, of articles in this publication, please contact the Commercial Reprints Department, Elsevier Inc., 360 Park Avenue South, New York, New York 10010-1710. Tel. (212) 633-3812, Fax: (212) 462-1935, e-mail: reprints@elsevier.com.

The Surgical Clinics of North America is also published in Spanish by McGraw-Hill Interamericana Editores S.A., P.O. Box 5-237 06500 Mexico D.F. Mexico; and in Portuguese by Interlivros Edicoes Ltda., Rua Comandante Coelho 1085, CEP 21250, Rio de Janeiro, Brazil; and in Greek by Paschalidis Medical Publications, Athens Greece.

The Surgical Clinics of North America is covered in *MEDLINE/PubMed (Index Medicus)*, *EMBASE/Excerpta Medica*, *Current Contents/Clinical Medicine*, *Current Contents/Life Sciences*, *Science Citation Index*, and *ISI/BIOMED*.

Printed and bound by CPI Group (UK) Ltd, Croydon, CR0 4YY

Transferred to Digital Print 2011

Contributors

CONSULTING EDITOR

RONALD F. MARTIN, MD
Staff Surgeon, Marshfield Clinic, Marshfield; and Clinical Associate Professor, University of Wisconsin School of Medicine and Public Health, Madison, Wisconsin; Colonel, Medical Corps, United States Army Reserve

GUEST EDITOR

MARTHA A. ZEIGER, MD, FACS, FACE
Chief of Endocrine Surgery, Professor of Surgery, Oncology, Cellular and Molecular Medicine, Co-Director of Basic and Translational Research, Department of Surgery, Johns Hopkins University School of Medicine, Baltimore, Maryland

AUTHORS

GÖRAN ÅKERSTRÖM, MD, PhD
Professor, Department of Surgery, University Hospital, Uppsala, Sweden

PETER ANGELOS, MD, PhD, FACS
Professor and Chief of Endocrine Surgery; Associate Director, Section of General Surgery and Surgical Oncology, MacLean Center for Clinical Medical Ethics, University of Chicago, Chicago, Illinois

KIMBERLY J. BUSSEY, PhD
Associate Investigator, Translational Genomics Research Institute, Phoenix, Arizona

HERBERT CHEN, MD
Professor of Surgery and Vice Chairman, Department of Surgery; Chief of Endocrine Surgery, University of Wisconsin, Madison, Wisconsin

LEIGH DELBRIDGE, MD, FRACS
University of Sydney Endocrine Surgical Unit, Royal North Shore Hospital, Sydney, NSW, Australia

MICHAEL J. DEMEURE, MD, MBA
Senior Investigator, Translational Genomics Research Institute, Phoenix, Arizona; Director of Endocrine Tumors Center, Scottsdale Healthcare Shea Medical Center, Virginia G. Piper Cancer Center, Scottsdale, Arizona

THOMAS J. FAHEY III, MD
Division of Endocrine Surgery, Department of Surgery, New York Presbyterian Hospital, Weill Cornell Medical Center, New York, New York

PHILIP GORDEN, MD
Clinical Endocrinology Branch-NIDDK, National Institutes of Health, Bethesda, Maryland

MEREDITH A. KATO, MD
Division of Endocrine Surgery, Department of Surgery, New York Presbyterian Hospital, Weill Cornell Medical Center, New York, New York

CHRISTINE S. LANDRY, MD
Surgical Oncology Fellow, Department of Surgical Oncology, The University of Texas M. D. Anderson Cancer Center, Houston, Texas

JOHN I. LEW, MD, FACS
Assistant Professor of Surgery, Division of Endocrine Surgery, DeWitt Daughtry Family Department of Surgery, University of Miami Leonard M. Miller School of Medicine; Director, Fellowship in Endocrine Surgery, Jackson Memorial Hospital, University of Miami Health System, Miami, Florida

STEVEN K. LIBUTTI, MD, FACS
Director, Montefiore-Einstein Center for Cancer Care; Associate Director, Albert Einstein Cancer Center; Professor and Vice-Chairman, Department of Surgery Montefiore Medical Center/Albert Einstein College of Medicine, Bronx, New York

JOSEPH B. LILLEGARD, MD, PhD
Department of Surgery, Mayo Clinic, Rochester, Minnesota

AARTI MATHUR, MD
Surgery Branch, National Cancer Institute, National Institutes of Health, Bethesda, Maryland

TRAVIS J. McKENZIE, MD
Department of Surgery, Mayo Clinic, Rochester, Minnesota

JEFFREY F. MOLEY, MD
Professor of Surgery, Endocrine and Oncologic Surgery, Department of Surgery, Washington University School of Medicine; St Louis Veterans Administration Medical Center, St Louis, Missouri

TRICIA A. MOO-YOUNG, MD
Resident in General Surgery, Department of Surgery, Washington University School of Medicine, St Louis, Missouri

ELLEN H. MORROW, MD
Resident of Surgery, Division of General Surgery, Department of Surgery, Stanford University School of Medicine, Stanford, California

JEFFREY A. NORTON, MD
Professor and Chief, Division of General Surgery, Department of Surgery, Stanford University School of Medicine, Stanford, California

JANICE L. PASIEKA, MD, FRCSC, FACS
Clinical Professor of Surgery and Oncology, Divisions of Surgical Oncology and General Surgery, Department of Surgery, Faculty of Medicine, University of Calgary, Calgary, Alberta Canada

NANCY D. PERRIER, MD
Professor, Department of Surgical Oncology, The University of Texas M. D. Anderson
Cancer Center, Houston, Texas

SUSAN C. PITT, MD
Endocrine Surgery Research Fellow, Department of Surgery, University of Wisconsin,
Madison, Wisconsin

REBECCA S. SIPPEL, MD
Assistant Professor of Surgery, Department of Surgery, University of Wisconsin,
Madison, Wisconsin

CARMEN C. SOLORZANO, MD, FACS
Associate Professor of Surgery, Division of Endocrine Surgery, DeWitt Daughtry
Family Department of Surgery, University of Miami Leonard M. Miller School of Medicine;
Chief, Division of Endocrine Surgery, University of Miami Health System, Miami, Florida

PETER STÅLBERG, MD, PhD
Associate Professor, Department of Surgery, University Hospital, Uppsala, Sweden

JAMES SULIBURK, MD
Michael E. DeBakey Department of Surgery, Baylor College of Medicine, Houston, Texas

GEOFFREY B. THOMPSON, MD
Professor of Surgery, Department of Surgery, Mayo Clinic, Rochester, Minnesota

AMBER L. TRAUGOTT, MD
Resident in General Surgery, Department of Surgery, Washington University School
of Medicine, St Louis, Missouri

STEVEN G. WAGUESPACK, MD
Associate Professor, Department of Endocrine, Neoplasia and Hormonal Disorders,
The University of Texas M. D. Anderson Cancer Center, Houston, Texas

MELISSA WANDOLOSKI, BS
Research Associate, Translational Genomics Research Institute, Phoenix, Arizona

WILLIAM F. YOUNG Jr, MD
Professor of Medicine, Division of Endocrinology, Mayo Clinic, Rochester, Minnesota

Contents

Multiple endocrine neoplasia syndrome type 1 (MEN-1) consists of endocrine tumors of the parathyroid, the endocrine pancreas-duodenum, and
the pituitary. Surveillance and screening for the endocrinopathies is recommended in gene carriers. Surgery for MEN-1–related hyperparathyroidism is generally performed as radical subtotal parathyroidectomy,
because less surgery is likely to result in persistent or recurrent disease.
Multiple endocrine neoplasia syndrome type 2 (MEN-2) consists of medullary thyroid carcinoma, pheochromocytoma, and hyperparathyroidism.
Prophylactic thyroidectomy based on DNA testing in the MEN-2 syndrome
is considered one of the greater achievements in cancer treatment, because it may be performed before thyroid carcinoma development and
provides cure for the patient.

The development of genetic testing has given patients with familial endocrine diseases the opportunity to be identified earlier in life. The importance of this technological advancement cannot be underestimated, as
some of these heritable diseases have significant potential for malignancy.
This article focuses on the identification and surgical management of
familial endocrinopathies of the thyroid, parathyroid, adrenal glands, and
pancreas. Familial endocrinopathies discussed include hereditary nonmedullary carcinoma of the thyroid, Cowden disease, familial adenomatous
polyposis, Carney complex, Werner syndrome, familial medullary thyroid
carcinoma, Pendred syndrome, hereditary hyperparathyroidism jaw-tumor
syndrome, familial isolated hyperparathyroidism, Beckwith- Wiedemann
syndrome, Li-Fraumeni syndrome, neurofibromatosis I, von Hippel-Lindau
disease, and tuberous sclerosis.

Much has been learned about the diagnosis and treatment of Zollinger-Ellison Syndrome (ZES), and certain questions require further investigation. Delay in diagnosis of ZES is still a significant problem, and clinical suspicion should be elevated. The single best imaging modality for localization and staging of ZES is somatostatin receptor scintigraphy. Goals of surgical treatment for ZES differ between sporadic and MEN-1–related cases. All sporadic cases of ZES should be surgically explored (including duodenotomy) even with negative imaging results, because of the high likelihood of finding and removing a tumor for potential cure. Surgery for MEN-1–related cases should be focused on prevention of metastatic disease, with surgery being recommended when pancreatic tumors are greater than 2 cm. The role of Whipple procedure, especially for MEN-1 cases, should be explored further. Laparoscopic and endoscopic treatments are more experimental, but may have a role.

Insulinoma is a rare neuroendocrine tumor with an incidence of 4 per 1 million persons per year, which may occur as a unifocal sporadic event in patients without an inherited syndrome or as a part of multiple endocrine neoplasia type 1. Key neuroglycopenic and hypoglycemic symptoms in conjunction with biochemical proof establish the diagnosis. Once the diagnosis is established, the insulinoma is preoperatively localized within the pancreas with the goal of surgical excision for cure. This review discusses the historical background, diagnosis, and management of sporadic insulinoma.

Carcinoid tumors, which arise from the enterochromaffin cells of the gastrointestinal tract, encompass a diverse group of neoplasms. Once thought to be "carcinoma-like," these neoplasms exhibit a biologic behavior that varies from an indolent, benign course to an aggressive, rapidly progressive, and deadly disease. Today the term carcinoid is reserved for neuroendocrine tumors arising from the small bowel or neuroendocrine tumors that can cause carcinoid syndrome. This newer terminology has yet to be universally adopted, adding to the confusion in the literature. For the general surgeon there are several "carcinoid" tumors that he or she must be familiar with because many of these lesions are encountered during emergency laparotomies or incidentally discovered during investigation for vague abdominal pain. This review focuses on the gastrointestinal neuroendocrine tumors that general surgeons are likely to encounter during their career.

it is usually associated with a palpable mass and the presence of nodal metastases. Surgery is standard treatment for any patient presenting with resectable MTC. Further studies are needed to investigate the role of radiation therapy in the palliation and local control of postresection and advanced-stage MTC. New systemic therapies for metastatic disease are being investigated. Targeted molecular therapies, based on knowledge of the pathways affected by RET mutations, are being tested in multiple clinical trials.

Melissa Wandoloski, Kimberly J. Bussey, and Michael J. Demeure

Adrenocortical carcinoma (ACC) is a rare endocrine malignancy causing up to 0.2% of all cancer deaths This article reviews the incidence, presentation, and pathology of ACC. Particular attention is paid to the molecular oncogenesis of this disease, and the surgical and therapeutic options available for its cure.

ISSUE OF RELATED INTEREST

Endocrinology and Metabolism Clinics of North America, June 2008
Volume 37 Issue 2
Thyroid Tumors
Shereen Ezzat, MD and Sylvia L. Asa, MD, PhD, *Guest Editors*

THE CLINICS ARE NOW AVAILABLE ONLINE!

Access your subscription at:
www.theclinics.com

Foreword

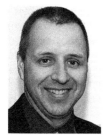

Ronald F. Martin, MD
Consulting Editor

As we complete production of this issue we are entering a new academic year. New residents enter our program and we all reassess our tasks. Our new residents integrate themselves into the academic conferences and one asks innocently, as one always does, during a colloquy about an illustrative patient, "has she had any previous *surgeries*?" The face of each resident of PG2 or greater rank simultaneously contorts into a bemused grimace as they know that I shall reply as I always do. I explain that "surgery" is a discipline, a state of mind, a way of life—occasionally a passion. "Operations" are procedures performed by surgeons in operating rooms. And that generally sets the tone for another year. That said, if one turns to most complete dictionaries one will find that the dictionaries actually side with the resident on this matter and I am factually incorrect. Also, the use of "surgery" to describe operating rooms, clinics, and other environments is also acceptable to professional wordsmiths. Still, I think there is good reason to maintain the distinction for surgeons between "surgery" and "operation." The discipline of surgery is far more encompassing than its technical operative subcomponent. And perhaps nowhere is that better illustrated than in endocrine surgery.

Some of the great clinics of this country were built on their adeptness at endocrine surgery; at least in part. The Mayo brothers were famed for their ability to safely perform thryroidectomy among other things. My alma mater, Lahey Clinic, was also largely founded on expertise in thyroid surgery. Success of a surgeon in the early days of endocrine surgery, particularly for operations performed in the neck, was judged by one's ability to avoid catastrophic postoperative technical complication. And the discussion and literature of the field largely focused on the technical aspects of surgical care.

In the decades since the Lahey and Mayo brothers made their large-volume referral centers based largely on technical expertise, the amount of discussion over the technical aspects has largely subsided in favor of concentration on the biochemical, molecular, and genetic aspects of endocrine care. A partial resurgence of technical interest has blossomed following Dr Gagner's (another Lahey Clinic alumnus) introduction of minimally invasive approaches to endocrine operation of the neck and retroperitoneum. These discussions have been fruitful and fascinating—especially to surgeons.

Surg Clin N Am 89 (2009) xiii–xiv
doi:10.1016/j.suc.2009.08.001
surgical.theclinics.com

The larger endocrine community, however, is more likely to be enthralled with the nonoperative features of the expanding literature.

As one reads this issue one will find a significant amount of material addressing operative techniques. One will also find an expanse of material relating to the molecular, biochemical, imaging, genetic, genomic, and proteomic aspects of what is known about endocrinology. I can think of few other areas of study where we have advanced as much in our ability to more fully understand the physiologic and structural aspects of pathologic target organs preoperatively as we now can in endocrine surgery. These advances have in some cases allowed us to significantly and reliably reduce our need to dissect and explore at the time of operation. Conversely, we may decide to reliably expand our initial operative plans based on gene analysis.

It has been quoted (multiple times in just this issue) that the most important localizing study in endocrine surgery is to localize a competent endocrine surgeon. The corollary for that could be that the surgeon who desires becoming facile and well-employed as an endocrine surgeon must localize an endocrinologist (or preferably group) with whom he or she can work well. Part of this relationship will likely depend on having an excellent working knowledge of the nonoperative aspects of endocrinology.

Despite the desires of the American Board of Surgery to claim that all general surgeons who are board certified have demonstrated expertise in endocrine surgery, the reality of the practice place is that these operations are almost always performed by persons with additional training and defined focus in one or more subsets of endocrine surgery. To be sure, there is overlap with otorhinolaryngologists, surgical oncologists, and hepatopancreatobiliary surgeons in the management of these patients but the reality that "specialty-" and "subspecialty"-trained surgeons perform the lion's share of these procedures is inescapable.

General surgeons will still maintain a need for knowledge in these areas. If for no other reason, endocrinopathies—both recognized and unrecognized—may be encountered in other patients and must be understood to safely manage their care. Also, we remain in a highly dynamic state regarding the delivery of health care. As events unfold, there may be a need to shift workforce supply and care distribution. Given the relative distribution of general surgeons compared with subspecialists, it is not inconceivable that some aspect of care previously relegated by degrees by some general surgeons may need to be reconsidered. A more important reason to be familiar with the larger breadth of material is because that is what is required for mastery of the topic. In an age where more people are looking for "just-in-time" information about small topics, mastery is becoming rarer. For those whom surgery is a passion, mastery is imperative.

Dr Zeiger and her colleagues have assembled an excellent group of reviews that should be informative and enlightening to any interested student of endocrine surgery. We appreciate her excellent work and professionalism on this project.

Ronald F. Martin, MD
Department of Surgery
Marshfield Clinic
1000 North Oak Avenue
Marshfield, WI 54449, USA

E-mail address:
martin.ronald@marshfieldclinic.org

Preface

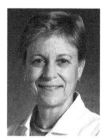

Martha A. Zeiger, MD, FACS, FACE
Guest Editor

Every endocrine surgeon is familiar with the quotation by the late Dr John Doppman, who said that the best localization study for primary hyperparathyroidism is to localize a good endocrine surgeon. And, we all know the story of the Indian rhinoceros and the discovery of the first parathyroid gland by the anatomist, Sir Richard Owen; of Albert, the trolley car conductor, who underwent one of the first successful parathyroidectomies by Felix Mandl; and of the sea captain, Charles Martell, who underwent seven parathyroidectomies only to die of hypocalcemic complications when a mediastinal parathyroid adenoma was removed. We are aware of the discovery of gastrinoma and the Zollinger-Ellison syndrome by Drs Robert M. Zollinger and Edwin H. Ellison in 1955; of the discovery of the *RET* proto-oncogene and its role in multiple endocrine neoplasia syndromes II and menin in multiple endocrine neoplasia syndromes I; and, most recently, of George Irvin III's contributions with the use of intraoperative parathyroid hormone measurement and the minimally invasive parathyroidectomy.

I chose "Multiple Endocrine Neoplasia Syndromes I and II" by Dr Göran Åkerström as the lead article because its subject so beautifully captures the richness of endocrine surgery, the discovery of syndromes and their responsible genetic abnormalities, the fascinating medical histories, the complex case presentations, and the interplay of hormonal and physiologic abnormalities. Not only are these medical histories fascinating regarding the quest for understanding and unraveling the keys to them but also the for the potential of as-yet unrecognized, unnamed syndromes for all who participate in this exciting discipline.

Furthermore, endocrine surgeons not only are united by the intellectual pursuit in evaluating complicated patients, solving a common clinical problem through research, identifying that genetic abnormality, or naming a syndrome but also they are all bound by friendships, collegiality, and mentorship. Call an endocrine surgeon anywhere in the world about a clinical problem, ask for a recommendation or an article written, and you will be called back that same day, most assuredly receive an excellent recommendation, and, at times, receive even two articles.

It is a great honor to have served as a guest editor for this issue of *Surgical Clinics of North America*. The articles herein represent those clinical syndromes that have associated controversy in clinical management, have had exciting recent developments or

Surg Clin N Am 89 (2009) xv–xvi
doi:10.1016/j.suc.2009.08.002
surgical.theclinics.com

discoveries, or are simply complex in their presentation and management. The nationally and internationally acclaimed authors chosen are expert in their field and have written extensively on the topic. I hope you enjoy reading these superbly written articles and in the process are brought up to date with regard to the rich discipline of endocrine surgery.

Martha A. Zeiger, MD, FACS, FACE
Department of Surgery
Johns Hopkins University School of Medicine
Blalock 606
600 N. Wolfe Street
Baltimore, MD 21287, USA

E-mail address:
mzeiger@jhmi.edu

Surgical Management of MEN-1 and -2: State of the Art

Göran Åkerström, MD, PhD*, Peter Stålberg, MD, PhD

KEYWORDS

- Multiple endocrine neoplasia type 1
- Multiple endocrine neoplasia type 2
- Surgical treatment • Genetic diagnosis
- Surveillance

MEN TYPE 1

MEN-1 is an autosomal-dominant syndrome comprising endocrine tumors of the parathyroid, the endocrine pancreas-duodenum, and the anterior pituitary. In addition to these classical lesions there is increased incidence of foregut carcinoids (in the thymus, bronchial tree, and the stomach); adrenocortical hyperplasia; and nonendocrine tumors, such as meningioma, ependymoma, leiomyoma, lipoma, facial angiofibroma, and collagenoma.

MEN-1 occurs as a result of inactivating mutations of the *MEN-1* tumor suppressor gene on chromosome 11q13 encoding for menin.[1] Menin has a role for DNA replication and repair, and is involved in transcriptional regulation and histone modification. MEN-1 is relatively rare, with a prevalence of 2 to 3 per 100 000, and is equally common in males and females. The MEN-1 gene is a complex gene, with more than 1000 mutations identified in different families, without strong genotype-phenotype correlations.[2] The disease expression is variable even within families. Complete *MEN-1* gene sequencing is the best method of diagnosis, and can reveal mutations in 70% to 90% of typical MEN-1 cases. A multiplex ligation-dependent probe amplification (MLPA) assay is recently used for detection of large deletions occurring in 4% of MEN-1 cases.[3] Because genetic diagnosis is difficult negative genetic testing cannot exclude the syndrome, unless mutation is known in the family. In absence of genetic diagnosis MEN-1 can be diagnosed if a patient has tumors in two of the three classical endocrine organs (parathyroid, pancreas-duodenum, or pituitary) or has family history of MEN-1 and one such tumor.[4]

Surveillance and screening for MEN-1 endocrine tumors is recommended in presymptomatic gene carriers, because biochemical abnormalities can be detected decades before clinical symptoms become overt.[4,5] Delaying screening until

Department of Surgery, University Hospital, Uppsala, 751 85 Sweden
* Corresponding author.
E-mail address: goran.akerstrom@surgsci.uu.se (G. Åkerström).

Surg Clin N Am 89 (2009) 1047–1068
doi:10.1016/j.suc.2009.06.016
0039-6109/09/$ – see front matter © 2009 Elsevier Inc. All rights reserved.

clinical symptoms develop can be associated with morbidity and mortality from MEN-1–related neuroendocrine pancreatic and thymic tumors.[4–6] Screening is done by a combination of biochemical tests and imaging studies aimed to reveal presence of any of the three classical endocrinopathies (**Table 1**), and is initiated in children during the first decade of life.[7]

Primary HPT

Primary HPT (pHPT) is the most common and generally first detected endocrinopathy in MEN-1, often possible to diagnose at approximately 20 years of age, and affecting more than 95% of patients by the age of 40 years.[4–7] MEN-1 pHPT accounts for 2% to 4% of all pHPT cases, and affects approximately 10% of patients with hyperplasia and multiglandular parathyroid disease. MEN-1 has been the most common of the familial pHPT syndromes, and the most important to exclude, and should be suspected in all cases with multiglandular involvement, or recurrent HPT. Younger patients may frequently (approximately 10%) be index cases for MEN-1 kindreds.[4–9] Screening with serum calcium may reveal MEN-1 in patients with pancreatic or pituitary tumors, or foregut carcinoids.

Symptoms are similar as in sporadic pHPT, with decrease in bone mineral density, nephrolithiasis in some patients, common fatigue, muscle weakness, asthenia, mild depression, and typical concentration difficulty. Bone mineral density decrease may be detected already at around 40 years of age.[10] Because hypercalcemia stimulates gastrin, early parathyroid surgery has been recommended in patients with MEN-1–associated Zollinger-Ellison syndrome (ZES), although similar effect is obtained by proton pump inhibitors.[11,12]

The diagnosis of pHPT is made by demonstration of raised ionized or total-albumin corrected serum calcium together with inappropriately raised serum parathyroid hormone (PTH).

Surgical Management

MEN-1 cases have markedly asymmetric nodular hyperplasia, where multiple mono-clonal tumors develop from polyclonal hyperplasia (**Fig. 1**).[11,13] Lesions may occur asynchronously, and normal glands can especially in younger patients coexist with enlarged ones. Some patients initially have single gland enlargement, easily misinterpreted as adenoma, when associated glands have normal size and histology.

MEN-1 patients have aggressive HPT, with high recurrence rate. The authors routinely use surgeon-performed preoperative ultrasound to have glandular localization depicted before surgery, although bilateral neck exploration is required for primary explorations.[11,14] Surgery is regarded as palliative, and aims to map the location of four parathyroid glands, also for forthcoming reoperations. To ensure removal of the largest, most severely diseased glands it is crucial to refrain from glandular excision until both sides of the neck have been explored.[11] The surgeon should then remove the largest glands in radical parathyroidectomy, and explore common ectopic sites, possibly harboring supernumerary glands, occurring normally in up to 15%.[14–16] Cervical thymectomy and clearance of perithyroid fat is performed to remove supernumerary glands and parathyroid cell clusters, which may grow as a result of the genetic stimulation.[15]

Resections less than subtotal parathyroidectomy are associated with high frequency of persistent or recurrent HPT in MEN-1.[14,16–20] Subtotal parathyroidectomy implying 3 to 3.5 gland resection (combined with cervical thymectomy) is now the commonly recommended operation.[14] The smallest, most normal gland is

Table 1 MEN-1 screening			
Tumor	**Age to Begin Screening (y)**	**Biochemical Tests (Annually)**	**Imaging (Every 3 y)**
Parathyroid	10	Serum calcium, (parathyroid hormone)	None
Gastrinoma	20	Serum gastrin	None
Insulinoma	5	Fasting serum glucose and insulin	None
Nonfunctioning pancreaticoduodenal tumors	20	Pancreatic polypeptide, proinsulin, insulin, glucagon, vasoactive intestinal polypeptide, chromogranin A	Endoscopic ultrasound (Octreoscan, CT)
Anterior pituitary	5	Prolactin, insulinlike growth factor-1	Brain MRI
Foregut carcinoid	20	None	CT

Data from Brandi ML, Gagel RF, Angeli A, et al. Guidelines for diagnosis and therapy of MEN type1 and type2. J Clin Endocrinol Metab 2001;86:5658–71.

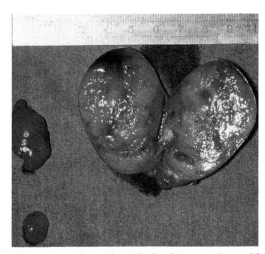

Fig. 1. Asymmetric enlargement of parathyroid glands in a patient with MEN 1–associated HPT and multiglandular parathyroid hyperplasia. The larger gland may be easily mistaken to represent a single adenoma. (*From* Åkerström G, Juhlin C. Surgical management of multiglandular parathyroid disease. In: Randolph GW, editor. Surgery of the thyroid and parathyroid glands. Philadelphia: WB Saunders; 2003. p. 529–48; with permission.)

selected as remnant, with circulation verified before removing other glands, by showing bleeding after transection (**Fig. 2**). When preparing the remnant cell seeding should be avoided to reduce risk for recurrence by implantation.

Total parathyroidectomy with forearm autotransplantation (or autotransplantation to subcutaneous fat on the thorax or abdomen) is less commonly performed. This procedure has higher risk for hypoparathyroidism, but may be required in presence of four markedly enlarged glands, or often at reoperation.[14,21] It is important to select tissue

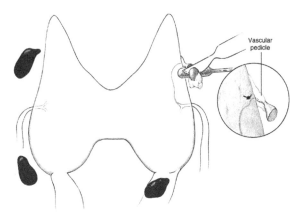

Fig. 2. Subtotal parathyroidectomy. After all four parathyroid glands have been visualized, the smallest gland is selected as remnant and resected to approximately 50 mg. When viability of the remnant is ensured (by verifying that it is bleeding after transection), the other glands are removed. The remnant location is marked with suture or clip. (*From* Åkerström G, Juhlin C. Surgical management of multiglandular parathyroid disease. In: Randolph GW, editor. Surgery of the thyroid and parathyroid glands. Philadelphia: WB Saunders; 2003. p. 529–48; with permission.)

for grafting from the smallest, least diseased gland. The patients experience long periods of postoperative hypocalcemia, and in contrast to what was initially thought, this procedure has not simplified treatment of recurrence.[22]

Intraoperative PTH determination is of reported value in MEN-1 patients, but requires special criteria to avoid false results, implying evaluation 20 minutes after glandular removal and that an end point value within the assay limits is reached.[14,23–25]

Because of risk for remnant ischemia and permanent hypoparathyroidism, cryo-preservation of parathyroid tissue is recommended if facilities are available.[14] Needle biopsy aspiration with rapid PTH determination has more or less replaced the use of frozen sections for parathyroid tissue verification in resected specimens.

Series of reoperative pHPT patients have emphasized that MEN-1 HPT is a common cause of failed parathyroid surgery.[12,22,23,25–27] Persistent HPT is common if the syndrome is not recognized at the primary operation and all glands have not been visualized, or if one has not searched for ectopic glands. Recurrence is encountered in MEN-1 patients because it is genetically determined, but can with appropriate surgery be minimized to around 30% during 10 years, but with markedly higher rate (>50%), and earlier recurrence with less than subtotal parathyroidectomy.[16,20,23,27]

Reoperation in MEN-1 is undertaken only after careful localization studies, comprising percutaneous ultrasound, sestamibi scintigraphy, CT with contrast enhancement, occasionally positron emission tomography with methionine tracer, ultrasound-guided fine-needle biopsy with PTH measurement, and in selected cases selective venous sampling with rapid PTH determination.[26,27] Concordant results of two investigations are generally required. Four-dimensional contrast-enhanced dynamic CT scan seems to provide improved parathyroid localization, but is not yet generally available.[28] The reoperative surgery is often done as focused operation with guidance from results of the preoperative localization diagnosis, and with results approaching that of primary operations, but to markedly higher costs and with increased complication risks.[25–27]

Endocrine Pancreatic and Duodenal Tumors

Like the other MEN-1 endocrinopathies pancreatic involvement is multicentric. Minute, numerous microadenomas, with possible origin in pancreatic duct precursor cells, are typically spread in the entire pancreas, and sometimes in the duodenum.[4,29] The microtumors express immunoreactivity for pancreatic polypeptide, glucagon, insulin, proinsulin, somatostatin, or only chromogranin A.[30] Duodenal microtumors, identified in 50% of patients with MEN-1 pancreaticoduodenal tumors (PETs), stain for serotonin, gastrin, and somatostatin.[31] Presence of the endocrinopathy can be demonstrated by serum measurements, most often showing raised values of pancre-atic polypeptide and chromogranin A, sometimes gastrin, insulin, and proinsulin.[4,5] A minority of the microtumors grow to clinically relevant lesions, because each patient during lifetime experiences rather few large tumors. Total pancreaticoduodenectomy is only rarely considered because of the risks associated with resulting severe diabetes. MEN-1 PETs have been claimed to have favorable prognosis compared with the corresponding sporadic tumors. Earlier diagnosis of MEN-1 tumors, or dispa-rate survival for patients with pancreatic and duodenal gastrinomas, however, may explain this difference. Recent review of 324 patients with PETs treated in Uppsala, Sweden, revealed no survival difference for MEN-1 PETs compared with sporadic tumors.[32] Survival was related to TNM stage and Ki67 proliferation index. Nonfunc-tioning tumors (57%) had worse survival than functioning tumors, and outcome was markedly better in operated patients.

Malignant progression of PETs has been identified as the most important cause of premature disease-related death in MEN-1.[4,5,33–36] Screening studies have revealed that endocrine symptoms of PETs occur late in MEN-1, and when a clinical syndrome of hormone excess is awaited up to 50% of patients already have metastases.[4,5,36] High prevalence of malignancy is also seen with PETs larger than 3 cm. The authors have proposed screening for PETs in MEN-1 carriers to achieve early diagnosis, and surgery before metastases occur, and suggested that this may limit the risk for progressive metastatic disease, although randomized evaluation is lacking.[4,36–39]

Surgery for Nonfunctioning Pancreaticoduodenal Tumors

Raised serum pancreatic polypeptide values in 75% of patients with nonfunctioning tumors are important for early detection of the endocrinopathy. The patients may also have raised insulin, proinsulin, or glucagon values without a syndrome of hormone excess. The policy is to admit MEN-1 patients to surgery when the diagnosis is established by biochemical markers and radiologic studies detect tumors of appreciable size. From studies of nonfunctioning MEN-1 PETs in the French GTE register Triponez and coworkers[40,41] recommended surgery for nonfunctioning MEN-1 tumors greater than or equal to 2 cm, but revealed 4% metastases for tumors less than or equal to 10 mm and markedly higher metastases rate (15%–52%) for larger tumors. The present authors recommend surgery for nonfunctioning tumors around or greater than 10 mm, because they consider that the metastases rate is otherwise unacceptably high, and in their experience larger tumors may have distinct malignant features **(Fig. 3)**.[42,43]

Contrast-enhanced CT is used to provide anatomy and reveal liver metastases, and is often used together with ^{11}C-5-hydroxytryptophane positron emission tomography, which may efficiently reveal smaller tumors. Endoscopic ultrasound has become the most important method for early detection of MEN-1 PETs and is now used for routine follow-up.[42–44]

The generally applied operative procedure consists of tumor enucleation in the pancreatic head, and concomitant distal 80% subtotal pancreatic resection. Few

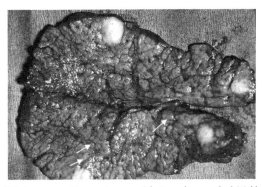

Fig. 3. Transected distal pancreatic specimen with two larger (*whitish*) and three smaller (*arrows*) tumors. All tumors in this case were clinically nonfunctioning. The larger tumors often have apparent malignant features and often occur in patients with syndromes of hormone excess, such as ZES (where the functioning tumor is commonly in the duodenum), and may easily be mistaken to represent the functional lesion. (*From* Åkerström G, Hessman O, Hellman P, et al. Pancreatic tumors as part of the MEN-I syndrome. Best Pract Res Clin Gastroenterol 2005;19:819–30; with permission.)

patients develop diabetes with this resection (**Fig. 4**). Larger or multiple tumors may require more extensive procedures (**Fig. 5**). Minimal tumors (<5 mm) deep in the pancreatic head may be left if enucleation is risky. Duodenotomy is not done unless the patient has a rise in gastrin.

Surgery for Pancreaticoduodenal Tumors with Syndromes of Hormone Excess

ZES has been the most common hormone syndrome in MEN-1, ultimately present in 50% of patients; the hypoglycemia syndrome has been revealed in less than 10%, vipoma in 3% to 5%, and symptomatic glucagonoma has occurred exceptionally (<1%).[4,42]

Surgery for Insulinomas, Vipomas, and Glucagonomas

It is generally agreed that MEN-1 patients with hypoglycemia syndrome and patients with vipoma and glucagonoma should be subjected to surgery after biochemical diagnosis irrespective of tumor size.[42,43,45,46]

Malignancy rate is higher with MEN-1 associated than with sporadic insulinoma. A single tumor greater than or equal to 5 mm in size is expected to cause the hyperinsulinism, and can often be revealed by endoscopic ultrasound. Concomitant nonfunctioning tumors are common, however, and if multiple tumors are revealed by radiology, source of insulin (or proinsulin) excess may be determined by selective intra-arterial calcium-injection test, which may regionalize the hypersecretion and identify unusual multifocal insulinoma.[46-48] Cure rate after surgery has been favorable in MEN-1 insulinomas, but concomitant distal (80%) pancreatic resection is recommended to minimize the risk for recurrence.[45,46] Tumor enucleation has also been done, but with higher risk for recurrence of nonfunctioning tumors or new insulinoma.

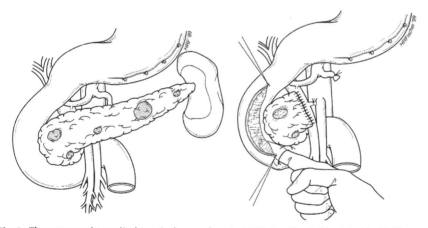

Fig. 4. The commonly applied surgical procedure in MEN-1 patients (depicted by N. Thompson). The pancreas is scanned with intraoperative ultrasound; identified lesions in the pancreatic head are enucleated, and distal tumors are removed with approximately 80% distal pancreatic resection. Duodenotomy is performed in patients with raised gastrin levels, allowing palpation of the entire duodenal mucosa, to identify duodenal gastrinomas, which in 90% is the cause of gastrin excess in MEN-1 patients. (*From* Skogseid B, Rastad J, Åkerström G. Pancreatic endocrine tumors in multiple endocrine neoplasia type I. In: Doherty GM, Skogseid B, editors. Surgical endocrinology. Philadelphia: Lippincott Williams & Wilkins; 2001. p. 511–24; with permission.)

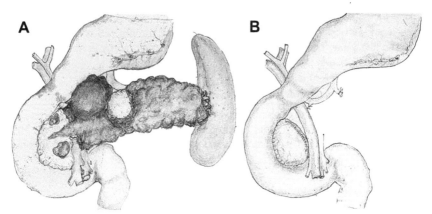

Fig. 5. (A) Operation for a large nonfunctioning PET, with dissection of deep extension into the pancreatic head, and enucleation of additional tumors within the opened pancreas. (B) Limited part of the pancreatic head remained without development of diabetes. (*From* Åkerström G, Hessman O, Hellman P, et al. Pancreatic tumors as part of the MEN-I syndrome. Best Pract Res Clin Gastroenterol 2005;19:819–30; with permission.)

MEN-1–associated vipoma, glucagonoma, or somatostatinoma syndromes are rare. Tumors causing these syndromes are usually large with high risk of malignancy, and should be treated with radical surgery.[49,50] Liver metastases from the pancreatic tumors should be considered for liver resection or radiofrequency ablation to alleviate severe hormone symptoms.[51]

Surgery for ZES

Surgery has been controversial for MEN-1 ZES patients because cure is rarely achieved. Some surgeons have advocated surgery if a tumor greater than 2 to 3 cm has been visualized, others when gastrin excess could be regionalized.[52–55] The authors have proposed surgery in absence of liver metastases also without preoperative tumor localization or regionalization, because most (90%) MEN-1 ZES patients have solitary, or typically multiple, small duodenal tumors causing the gastrin excess.[31,37,38,52,53] Despite sometimes inconspicuous size the duodenal tumors are frequently associated with conspicuously larger regional lymph gland metastases often mistaken to represent the primary tumor (**Fig. 6**).[56] Because of delay before liver metastases develop, there may be a favorable interval for surgical intervention where lymph gland metastases may be excised together with the primary lesion to prevent further spread.[57] Gastrin-secreting pancreatic tumors have been uncommon in MEN-1, but reported to be large and associated with early liver metastases.

Normalization of gastrin excess may be achieved by surgical excision of gastrinoma and lymph gland metastases, but most patients recur with hypergastrinemia, and surgery is done to reduce the risk for further progression.[53–55,58] ZES patients with liver metastases have significantly shorter survival, and liver metastases develop less frequently in operated patients.[55,58] The hypergastrinemia in ZES can be efficiently controlled by proton pump inhibitors, and surgery has the additional goal to delay malignant development also by removal of concomitant nonfunctioning tumors.[4,29]

MEN-1 patients with raised serum gastrin are subjected to duodenotomy, with excision of duodenal gastrinomas; enucleation of possible tumors in the head of the

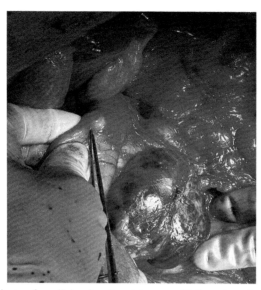

Fig. 6. Operation photo of small duodenal gastrinoma with large lymph gland metastases in a patient with MEN-1 ZES. (*From* Åkerström G, Hellman P, Stålberg P. Carcinoid: presentation and diagnosis, surgical management. In: Hubbard JGH, Inabnet WB, Lo C-Y, editors. Endocrine surgery (Springer Specialist Surgery Series). London: Springer-Verlag; 2008. Chapter 44; with permission.)

pancreas; dissection of regional metastases; and as in other MEN-1 patients, concomitant distal (80%) pancreatic resection (see **Fig. 4**).

Pancreaticoduodenectomy may offer prolonged postoperative eugastrinemia, perhaps even better than the excision of duodenal gastrinomas combined with subtotal pancreatic resection.[43,59] Common concomitant nonfunctioning tumors in ZES patients have, in the authors' experience, virtually always necessitated distal pancreatic resection (see **Fig. 3**).[38] Moreover, frequently required reoperation for recurrent tumor may be exceedingly difficult if pancreaticojejunostomy has been performed. After pancreaticoduodenectomy there is also a risk for ascending infection by the hepaticojejunostomy, making treatment of liver metastases with embolization or radiofrequency ablation hazardous.[51] Pancreaticoduodenectomy is still required in MEN-1 patients with large or recurrent pancreatic head or duodenal tumors. Pancreas-preserving duodenectomy has been reported to remove all duodenal gastrinomas, although this is a difficult procedure with the possible drawback to leave concomitant pancreatic tumors remaining.[60]

Patients with MEN-1 ZES may develop multiple gastric type 2 carcinoids, which may sometimes regress if eugastrinemia is achieved.[61] Remaining tumors should be locally excised. Some MEN-1 patients have died of malignant gastric carcinoids with spread metastases, and large gastric carcinoids may require gastrectomy.[61,62]

Operation

Pancreaticoduodenal exploration in MEN-1 patients is performed by bilateral subcostal incision. The head of the pancreas and the duodenum are mobilized to the aorta, and the ventral and dorsal surfaces of the pancreatic head are dissected. The pancreatic body and tail are explored by way of the lesser sack, with the retroperitoneum incised below the pancreas, allowing blunt dissection of the body and tail. The entire pancreas is bidigitally palpated and scanned with intraoperative ultrasonography, from anterior and posterior surfaces.[4,29] Intraoperative ultrasonography can reveal most lesions larger than 3 to 4 mm and also visualizes relations between tumors and pancreatic and bile ducts, facilitating safe enucleation. Metastatic lymph glands are mainly searched for by exploration and palpation around the splenic and celiac vessels, in the hepatoduodenal ligament, and at the posterior surface of the pancreatic head.

Any tumor in the head of the pancreas is enucleated by dissection from the surrounding pancreatic tissue, with careful ligation of vessels and pancreatic duct tributaries. A distal 80% body and tail resection is performed, transecting the neck of the pancreas just to the left of the superior mesenteric vein (see **Fig. 4**). An enucleated area in the pancreatic head is left open with carefully applied drainage.

Because most MEN-1 patients require prophylactic cancer operation with efficient removal of lymph node metastases, which have predilection site in the splenic hilum, splenectomy is recommended generally as part of the procedure rather than spleen preservation.

Duodenotomy

In patients with ZES routine duodenal exploration is undertaken by longitudinal duodenotomy in the descending part of the duodenum (see **Fig. 4**). Small tumors can be identified by palpation after digital inversion of proximal and distal parts of the duodenum. Duodenal tumors smaller than 5 mm can be enucleated with the overlying mucosa; larger tumors require excision of the duodenal wall.

Postoperative Follow-up and Reoperation

After primary surgery lifelong cure is uncommon with the MEN-1 pancreaticoduodenal endocrinopathy and recurrence should be anticipated.[58] The patients are followed with biochemical markers and radiologic investigations, including endoscopic ultrasonography. Reoperation is considered when a lesion of arbitrarily approximately 10 mm or larger is visualized concomitant with rise of biochemical markers. Reoperations have been performed with resection or enucleation of new tumors, and have been uncomplicated and compatible with long survival and preserved pancreatic function. Total pancreatectomy may be required for recurrent, rapidly growing, or unusually large tumors, and perhaps even initially in patients with a family history of especially malignant pancreatic tumors.[63] This is avoided or delayed as much as possible because of the generally severe diabetes that ensues. In patients with metastatic disease oncologic treatment is given, with common response to combinations of streptozotocin and 5-fluorouracil or doxorubicin in patients with low-proliferative lesions as determined with the Ki67 index. In addition, liver metastases is liberally treated with liver resection and radiofrequency ablation.

The active management strategy for MEN-1 PETs is supported by several patient series revealing apparently reduced death risk in operated patients.[64–67] Strong evidence for effects on survival is still lacking. Liberally applied pancreatic surgery has to be performed with minimal morbidity and virtually absent mortality, because long survival may be obtained also without surgery.[68,69]

MEN TYPE 2

MEN-2 is an autosomal-dominant hereditary syndrome caused by germline activating mutations of the *RET* proto-oncogene on chromosome 10q11.2, affecting 1 per

30,000 individuals.[70–74] MEN-2 comprises MEN-2A, MEN-2B, and familial MTC (FMTC). Uncommon variants include MEN-2A with cutaneous lichen amyloidosis (a pruritic lichenoid skin lesion usually on the upper back) and MEN-2A with Hirschsprung disease.[71,72,74]

In MEN-2A, originally described by Sipple in 1961, virtually all patients (more than 90%) have MTC, in combination with pheochromocytoma (in 40%–50%), and pHPT (in approximately 20%). This is the most common of MEN-2 syndromes (accounting for approximately 50%–60% of patients with hereditary MTC). MTC is generally the first manifestation of MEN-2A, developing most often between 5 and 25 years of age.

MEN-2B is the rarest subtype (approximately 5%–10% of MEN-2 cases), consisting of MTC in all cases; pheochromocytoma (50% of patients); ganglioneuromatosis; and typical features with marfanoid habitus, enlarged lips, and mucosal neuromas in the tongue, lips, and eyelids.[72,75,76] pHPT is not part of the MEN-2B syndrome. Ganglioneuromatosis of the gastrointestinal tract may frequently cause abdominal complaints, megacolon, obstipation, or diarrhea. Patients with MEN-2B have early disease onset and aggressive MTC, developing during the first year of life and associated with early dissemination and mortality. Most patients have spontaneous new RET mutations, as index cases without positive family history.[72] The patients often experience delay in diagnosis until mucosal neuromas or palpable thyroid tumors are obvious. The syndrome may be recognized in early childhood by characteristic neuromas and typical features (patients look different than other family members).[72,75,76]

FMTC (approximately 35%–40% of MEN-2 cases) is a generally milder variant of MEN-2, more frequently diagnosed in recent years.[72–74,77] MTC may have later onset, with better prognosis. Many cases have initially been thought to have sporadic MTC, but revealed by genetic screening. Identical germline mutations have been reported in MEN-2A and FMTC families, and some FMTC patients belong to MEN-2A kindreds, where pheochromocytoma or HPT have not been detected. Strict criteria are required to exclude MEN-2 with need of screening and follow-up of multiple members in a kindred.[72,73,78] Unclassified cases have few family members with too limited follow-up to exclude MEN-2A.[72]

MTC

MTC is a rare carcinoma developing from thyroid calcitonin-producing parafollicular C-cells, occurring most frequent in-between the upper and middle thirds of both thyroid lobes.[72,78] Hereditary MTC occurs at younger age than sporadic MTC; is associated with C-cell hyperplasia (CCH); and has multifocal, frequently bilateral tumors in contrast to solitary sporadic MTC tumors. Tumor cells have granulated cytoplasm and stain for calcitonin and amyloid (with Congo red reactive with calcitonin prohormone). CCH consists of C-cell clusters dispersed in-between the thyroid follicles, and is considered a premalignant condition preceding hereditary MTC, but occurs also in 20% to 30% of normal individuals. Time required for progression from CCH to microscopic carcinoma is variable.[72] Frequency of lymph node metastases relates to tumor size, being 20% and 30% for tumors greater than or equal to 1 cm, 50% for tumors measuring 1 to 4 cm, and up to 90% for tumors greater than 4 cm.[78] Distant metastases occur to liver, bone, and lung. Liver metastases are often initially small (1–3 mm) and easily missed by imaging with CT, MRI, or contrast-enhanced ultrasound, and may require visualization by laparoscopy.

Approximately 50% of index patients with MEN-2 present with palpable tumor and locally advanced disease, with regional lymph gland metastases.[78] Diagnosis of MTC is made by fine-needle aspiration and calcitonin staining. Basal serum calcitonin is virtually always high in patients with palpable MTC, and correlates with tumor burden. Raised calcitonin levels following surgical tumor removal indicate persistent or recurrent disease. Previously, family screening for hereditary MTC used pentagastrin (or calcium) to stimulate calcitonin secretion from malignant or hyperplastic C cells. Raised stimulated, but normal basal calcitonin occurs with CCH, but the stimulation test cannot distinguish between CCH and minimal MTC.[72] Occasionally, calcitonin release from nonfunctioning PETs may give suspicion of MTC, but values then fail to rise after stimulation as expected with MTC. Carcinoembryonic antigen can be used as additional tumor marker together with calcitonin, but is not specific for MTC.

Genetic Diagnosis

The *RET* proto-oncogene on chromosome 10q11.2 was identified by genetic linkage analysis in 1987, and the MEN-2 syndrome was demonstrated to result from missense germline mutations in this gene.[70–74,79–81] The *RET* proto-oncogene with 21 exons, encodes a tyrosine kinase receptor, with an extracellular domain containing a ligand-binding site; a cysteine-rich region (exons 10 and 11); a transmembrane domain; an intracellular part with two tyrosine kinase domains (exons 13–15); and an intracellular catalytic core (exon 16) (**Fig. 7**).[72,82,83] *RET* is expressed mainly in neuronal and neuroepithelial cells of neural crest origin, as thyroid C-cells, adrenomedullary chromaffin cells, and parathyroid cells. Gain-of-function mutations activate the *RET* receptor kinase causing thyroid CCH, adrenomedullary hyperplasia, and parathyroid hyperplasia. Alteration in the intracellular catalytic core (mutations in codon 918, classical MEN-2B genotype) has the highest transforming capacity; ligand-independent dimerization and cross-phosphorylation (mutations in codon 609, 611,

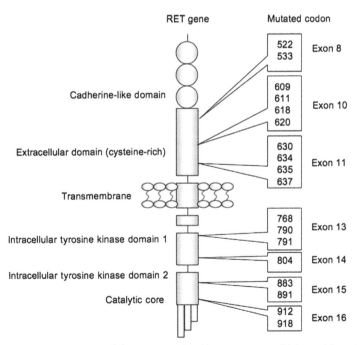

Fig. 7. The schematic structure of the *RET* tyrosine kinase receptor. (*Adapted from* Machens A, Dralle H. Genotype-phenotype based surgical concept of hereditary medullary thyroid carcinoma. World J Surg 2007;31:957–68; with permission.)

618, 630, and 634) has intermediate activity; and interference with ATP binding (mutations in codons 768, 790, 791, 804, and 891) has lower transforming activity.[82,83] Age-related progression from CCH to MTC, and development of pheochromocytoma and parathyroid nodular hyperplasia, correlates with transforming capacity of the *RET* mutations, but require also additional somatic second hits.[83] MTC is generally the first neoplastic manifestation because of higher susceptibility of C cells to the oncogenic *RET* activation.[73]

Somatic RET mutations are found in approximately 25% of patients with sporadic MTC. The most frequent mutations in codon 918 are associated with aggressive MTC.[72,84–87] Somatic *RET* mutations also occur in sporadic pheochromocytoma.[72,85] Somatic *RET* rearrangements are seen in papillary thyroid carcinoma.

MEN-2 accounts for approximately 25% of MTC cases and 7% to 25% of patients with "apparently sporadic" MTC.[74,88] Mutation testing has identified over 50 different missense *RET* gene mutations in MEN-2 families, and genetic testing detects approximately 98% of mutation carriers.[73] Only family members with germline missense mutations have the disease. *RET* gene testing should be performed before surgical intervention in all patients with diagnosed MTC, to provide risk assessment for family members, determine risk for associated endocrinopathies, and guide surgical management of MTC.[72,73] All members of MEN-2 and FMTC kindreds should undergo genetic testing and gene carriers should be offered prophylactic thyroidectomy during childhood. *RET* gene testing is recommended also as screening of patients with pheochromocytoma.

Genotype-phenotype Correlation

MEN-2A is most often caused by RET mutations in codons of exons 10 and 11, but also by more rare intracellular mutations (**Fig. 8**).[70–74,89] Codon 634 mutations (exon 11) are reported in approximately 40% of MEN-2A patients,[73] and also seen with MEN-2A and cutaneous lichen amyloidosis (in 12% of codon 634 mutations).[71,72,74] With codon 634 mutation MTC develops during the first decade of life, not influenced by the type of amino acid substitute at codon 634. Mutations in codons 609, 611, 618, and 620 (exon 10) cause 10% to 15% of MEN-2A and MEN-2A associated with

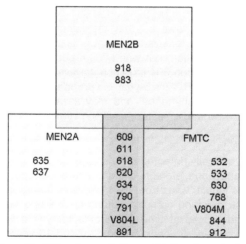

Fig. 8. Correlation of specific RET codon mutations with the phenotypic expression of hereditary MTC.

Hirschsprung disease.[72] Pheochromocytoma is less prevalent in these families, and MTC rarely presents before the age of 10 years. MEN-2A mutations also include codons 635 and 637 (exon 11); 790 and 791 (exon 13); 804 L (exon 14); and 891 (exon 15).[72] Mutations at codon 804 were initially believed to be associated with FMTC, although subsequent studies identified patients with late-onset pheochromocytoma, and HPT (associated with 804 L but not 804 M mutations).[90,91]

FMTC mutations are distributed throughout the *RET* gene including the codons causing MEN-2A at exons 10, 11, 13, 14, and 15.[72] Mutations at codon 532, 533, 768, 844, and 912 have only been identified in families with FMTC. FMTC rarely develops before the age of 20 years.

Codon 918 mutations (exon 16), revealed in 95% of MEN-2B cases, have aggressive MTC with metastases reported before the age of 12 months.[71,92] Few MEN-2B patients have mutations in codon 883 (exon 15).[93]

Risk Levels

A three-level risk stratification has been adopted by an international consensus panel, suggesting time for prophylactic thyroidectomy generally as close as possible to the earliest reported age of onset for each genotype.[7,72,94–97] For the highest-risk group, including MEN-2B carriers (mutations of codons 918 and 883), prophylactic thyroidectomy should be done within the first year of life, preferably by the age of 6 months. For the high-risk group (mutations of codons 609, 611, 618, 620, and 634), where most patients have MEN-2A, prophylactic thyroidectomy is recommended before the age of 5 years. For the least high-risk group, (mutations of codons 768, 790, 791, 804, and 891), the recommended age for thyroidectomy remains controversial, suggested at 5 to 10 years, or when a calcitonin stimulation test becomes abnormal.[7,72–74,91,94–97] Codon 609 was subsequently reclassified to the high-risk group, and codon 630 previously not classified was included as high-risk group.[74,95] Evidence-based evaluation has supported DNA-based evaluation as superior to calcitonin-based screening in asymptomatic *RET* carriers, and some centers consider this to have limited value because of poor specificity and tolerance.[95] If basal calcitonin values are raised thyroidectomy should be performed.[95] The outlined recommendations can result in undertreatment of codon 634 mutation carriers, where MTC has developed between 1 and 2 years of age, and some surgeons recommend testing during first year of life and thyroidectomy by age 2.[78,96] MTC in codon 634 mutation carriers younger than 5 years has been so rare, however, that thyroidectomy before age 5 is often accepted.[96] There is also risk for overtreatment of least high-risk mutation carriers, with variable disease penetration, but with MTC reported from the second to third decade. The exception is codon 804 mutation carriers with variable disease onset, and reported ultimately fatal MTC in a 6-year-old proband.[95,97,98] Codon 791 mutation carriers have low disease penetrance, and may as alternative to the age-related thyroidectomy be followed with repeated basal and stimulated calcitonin screening.[73]

Lymph Node Dissection

MEN-2 patients with clinically detected MTC should be subjected to total thyroidectomy with bilateral central and lateral neck compartment dissection, removing lymph nodes in-between the jugular veins from the hyoid bone to the innominate vein.

For the highest-risk mutation carriers bilateral central and lateral cervical lymph node dissection is advocated at time of thyroidectomy.[96] It is recommended for high-risk mutations from age 5 years (codon 634) and 10 years (codons 609, 611, 618, 620, and 630). Lymph node dissection is recommended from the age of 20 years for the least high-risk mutations, but data are inconclusive.[96]

Prophylactic thyroidectomy based on DNA testing in the MEN-2 syndrome is considered as one of the greater achievements in cancer treatment, because it may be performed before thyroid carcinoma development, and provides cure for the patient. The association between disease phenotype and *RET* mutation genotype also has important implications for the clinical management of MEN-2 patients and families. A patient's genotype can be used to decide intensity of screening for pheochromocytoma and HPT, which always need to be excluded before thyroidectomy for MTC.

Pheochromocytomas

Pheochromocytomas are most frequent with mutations in codons 634 and 918, but occur with germline mutations in all MEN-2–associated codons except 768.[7,72,89,90,98–100] The MEN-2 tumors are generally diagnosed at younger age than sporadic tumors, with mean age of diagnosis in MEN-2A approximately 35 years, MEN-2B approximately 25 years, and as early as age 5 years in codon 634 mutation carriers.[7,72,98,100–102] Screening for pheochromocytoma is recommended from age of 5 to 7 years, especially for codon 634 mutation carriers. Pheochromocytomas are rarely (approximately 15%) the initial manifestation of MEN-2, occur concomitant with MTC in 25%, but most often after MTC, with mean approximately 10 years delay.[70,72,99–101] The pheochromocytomas are often bilateral, but often develop asynchronously, with a contralateral new pheochromocytoma occurring after 4 years in approximately 30% of patients.[99,100,103]

The histologic pattern is similar in MEN-2A and -B, with single or multiple tumors in a background of micronodular or diffuse medullary hyperplasia.[104] Pheochromocytomas in MEN-2 are rarely extra-adrenal (<1%) or malignant (3%–4%).[99–102] Malignant pheochromocytomas are more likely with tumor size exceeding 5 cm. Histologic features are uncertain, and malignant diagnosis generally requires demonstration of metastases, or is sometimes evident after long follow-up.[99,104]

Diagnosis

MEN-2 pheochromocytomas have an adrenergic biochemical phenotype, with diagnosis based on measurements of plasma or 24-hour urinary fractionated metanephrine. Annual biochemical screening and CT is done to exclude development of pheochromocytoma in patients with MEN-2. Because of increased detection by screening approximately 50% or more of MEN-2 patients with pheochromocytoma have been asymptomatic at time of diagnosis.[99]

Surgical Management

A unilateral pheochromocytoma in MEN-2 patients is generally removed by total removal of this adrenal, most often by laparoscopy, and this leaves a macroscopically normal gland for follow-up.[99,100] Only few large or suspect malignant tumors require open surgery. The risk for recurrent contralateral pheochromocytoma has been approximately 30% during 5 years, and 50% during 11 years of follow-up.[99–101,103] Bilateral pheochromocytomas in MEN-2 patients may require bilateral adrenalectomy, and the patient needs lifelong substitution with glucocorticoid and mineralocorticoid replacement, with risk for development of Addison crisis.[99] To avoid adrenal insufficiency efforts have been made to preserve adrenal function by partial, cortical-sparing adrenalectomy in MEN-2A. This can be done as an open, laparoscopic, or retroperitoneoscopic operation, aided by intraoperative ultrasound.[99,105–107] For bilateral pheochromocytomas or subsequent operation of the contralateral gland after prior adrenalectomy, an adrenal cortical-sparing operation is generally recommended, unless a large tumor or unfavorable location precludes sparing of a significant amount of the adrenal. Recurrence has been reported in 10% to 20% of patients, subjected to long-term follow-up.[105,108] Also for recurrence in the remnant gland an additional subtotal adrenalectomy has been performed without morbidity.[107-109]

Hyperparathyroidism

pHPT occurs in 20% of patients with MEN-2A, most commonly associated with codon 634 mutations, less frequently with mutations in codons 609, 611, 618, 620, 790, and 791, and is not part of the MEN-2B syndrome.[11,70,72,74,110,111] Parathyroid disease in MEN-2A is generally mild, with only slight elevation of serum calcium.[11,110] Most patients (85%) have been asymptomatic, few patients have had renal stone disease or evident neuropsychiatric symptoms.[110,111] Most patients have presented with slight parathyroid enlargement discovered during prophylactic or therapeutic thyroidectomy, with normal serum calcium and PTH levels, and with diagnosis based on morphology.[11,110,111] Histologically, the predominant finding has been nodular parathyroid chief-cell hyperplasia, affecting more than one gland, but asymmetrically, implying that enlarged glands coexist with normal-sized ones.[111] Single and multiple adenomas have been described and it is suggested that adenomas may evolve from the nodular hyperplasia. The principal problem in patients with the MEN-2A syndrome has been to avoid hypoparathyroidism during thyroidectomy combined with extensive lymph node dissections, and the surgical management of pHPT should aim to preserve parathyroid function.[11,111] All parathyroids should be identified, but only enlarged glands should be removed, although this is recommended even if the patient is eucalcemic. In cases with four-gland enlargement subtotal parathyroidectomy is preferred to total parathyroidectomy with autotransplantation. The strategy during thyroidectomy is generally to leave normal parathyroids in situ, and perform autotransplantation of devascularized glands. If normal parathyroids are inadvertently removed or are at risk during lymph node dissection, they should be liberally autotransplanted to the forearm in MEN-2A cases (and to the sternocleidomastoid muscle in MEN-2B cases).[74]

Many cases of HPT develop several years after thyroidectomy, resulting from single adenoma or multiglandular disease, and can then be managed with conservative strategy, removing only enlarged parathyroid glands.[74,110]

Cure rate after a depicted conservative approach of parathyroid surgery in MEN-2A patients has been 97% and 100%, and recurrence rate low (3%–5%).[11,110,111]

REFERENCES

1. Chandrasekharappa SC, Guru SC, Manickam P, et al. Positional cloning of the gene for multiple endocrine neoplasia-type 1. Science 1997;276:404–7.
2. Lemos MC, Thakker RV. Multiple endocrine neoplasia type 1 (MEN 1): analysis of 1336 mutations reported in the first decade following identification of the gene. Hum Mutat 2008;29:22–32.
3. Tham E, Grandell U, Lindgren E, et al. Clinical testing for mutations in the MEN 1 gene in Sweden: a report on 200 unrelated cases. J Clin Endocrinol Metab 2007; 92:3389–95.
4. Skogseid B, Rastad J, Åkerström G. Pancreatic endocrine tumors in multiple endocrine neoplasia type I. In: Doherty GM, Skogseid B, editors. Surgical endocrinology. Philadelphia: Lippincott Williams & Wilkins; 2001. p. 511–24.

5. Skogseid B, Eriksson B, Lundquist G, et al. Multiple endocrine neoplasia type I: a 10-year prospective screening study in four kindreds. J Clin Endocrinol Metab 1991;73:281–7.

6. Lairmore TC, Piersall LD, DeBenedetti MK, et al. Clinical genetic testing and early surgical intervention in patients with multiple endocrine neoplasia type 1 (MEN 1). Ann Surg 2004;239:637–45.

7. Brandi ML, Gagel RF, Angeli A, et al. Guidelines for diagnosis and therapy of MEN type1 and type2. J Clin Endocrinol Metab 2001;86:5658–71.

8. Uchino S, Noguchi S, Sato M, et al. Screening of the MEN 1 gene and discovery of germ-line and somatic mutations in apparently sporadic parathyroid tumors. Cancer Res 2000;60:5553–7.

9. Langer P, Wild A, Hall A, et al. Prevalence of multiple endocrine neoplasia type 1 in young patients with apparently sporadic primary hyperparathyroidism or pancreaticoduodenal endocrine tumors. Br J Surg 2003;90:1599–603.

10. Burgess JR, David R, Greenway TM, et al. Osteoporosis in multiple endocrine neoplasia type 1: severity, clinical significance, relationship to primary hyperparathyroidism, and response to parathyroidectomy. Arch Surg 1999;134:1119–23.

11. Åkerström G, Juhlin C. Surgical management of multiglandular parathyroid disease. In: Randolph GW, editor. Surgery of the thyroid and parathyroid glands. Philadelphia: Saunders; 2003. p. 529–48.

12. Norton JA, Venzon DJ, Berna MJ, et al. Prospective study of surgery for primary hyperparathyroidism (HPT) in multiple endocrine neoplasia-type 1 and Zollinger-Ellison syndrome: long-term outcome of a more virulent form of HPT. Ann Surg 2008;247:501–10.

13. Harach HR, Jasani B. Parathyroid hyperplasia in multiple endocrine neoplasia type 1: a pathological and immunohistochemical reappraisal. Histopathology 1992;21:513–9.

14. Stålberg P, Carling T. Familial parathyroid tumors. In: Evidence Based Symposium on Hyperparathyroidism, World J Surg 2009 [epub ahead of print].

15. Åkerström G, Malmaeus J, Bergström R. Surgical anatomy of human parathyroid glands. Surgery 1984;95:14–21.

16. Hellman P, Skogseid B, Öberg K, et al. Primary and reoperative parathyroid operations in hyperparathyroidism of multiple endocrine neoplasia type 1. Surgery 1998;124:993–9.

17. O'Riordain DS, O'Brien T, Grant CS, et al. Surgical management of primary hyperparathyroidism in multiple endocrine neoplasia types 1 and 2. Surgery 1993;114:1031–7 [discussion: 1037–9].

18. Goudet P, Cougard P, Verges B, et al. Hyperparathyroidism in multiple endocrine neoplasia type I: surgical trends and results of a 256-patient series from Groupe D'etude des Neoplasies Endoccriniennes Multiples Study Group. World J Surg 2001;25:886–90.

19. Elaraj DM, Skarulis MC, Libutti SK, et al. Results of initial operation for hyperparathyroidism in patients with multiple endocrine neoplasia type 1. Surgery 2003;134:858–64 [discussion: 864–5].

20. Kraimps JL, Denizot A, Carnaille B, et al. Primary hyperparathyroidism in multiple endocrine neoplasia type IIa: retrospective French multicentric study. Groupe d'Etude des Tumeurs a Calcitonine (GETC, French Calcitonin Tumors Study Group), French Association of Endocrine Surgeons. World J Surg 1996; 20:808–12 [discussion: 812–3].

21. Wells SA, Farndon JR, Dale JK, et al. Long-term evaluation of patients with primary parathyroid hyperplasia managed by total parathyroidectomy and heterotopic autotransplantation. Ann Surg 1980;192:451–8.

22. Hubbard JGH, Sebag F, Maweja S, et al. Subtotal parathyroidectomy as an adequate treatment for primary hyperparathyroidism in multiple endocrine neoplasia type 1. Arch Surg 2006;141:235–9.
23. Kivlen M, Bartlett DL, Libutti SK, et al. Reoperation for hyperparathyroidism in multiple endocrine neoplasia type 1. Surgery 2001;130:991–8.
24. Clerici T, Brandle M, Lange J, et al. Impact of intraoperative parathyroid hormone monitoring on the prediction of multiglandular parathyroid disease. World J Surg 2004;28:187–92.
25. Thompson GB, Grant CS, Perrier ND, et al. Reoperative parathyroid surgery in the era of sestamibi scanning and intraoperative parathyroid hormone monitoring. Arch Surg 1999;134:699–705.
26. Udelsman R, Donovan PI. Remedial parathyroid surgery: changing trends in 130 consecutive cases. Ann Surg 2006;244:471–9.
27. Hessman O, Stålberg P, Sundin A, et al. High success rate of parathyroid reoperation may be achieved with improved localization diagnosis. World J Surg 2008;32:774–81 [discussion: 782–3].
28. Rodgers SE, Hunter GJ, Hamberg LM, et al. Improved preoperative planning for directed parathyroidectomy with 4-dimensional computed tomography. Surgery 2006;140:932–40.
29. Åkerström G, Hessman O, Hellman P, et al. Pancreatic tumours as part of the MEN-I syndrome. Best Pract Res Clin Gastroenterol 2005;19:819–30.
30. Klöppel G, Willemer S, Stamm B, et al. Pancreatic lesions and hormonal profile of pancreatic tumors in multiple endocrine neoplasia type I: an immunocytochemical study of nine patients. Cancer 1986;57:1824–32.
31. Pipellers-Marichal M, Somers G, Willems E, et al. Gastrinomas in the duodenums of patients with multiple endocrine neoplasia type I and the Zollinger-Ellison syndrome. N Engl J Med 1990;322:723–7.
32. Ekeblad S, Skogseid B, Dunder K, et al. Prognostic factors and survival in 324 patients with pancreatic endocrine tumor treated at a single institution. Clin Cancer Res 2008;14:7798–803.
33. Doherty GM, Olson JA, Frisella MM, et al. Lethality of multiple endocrine neoplasia type I. World J Surg 1998;22:581–7.
34. Dean PG, van Heerden JA, Farley DR, et al. Are patients with multiple endocrine neoplasia type I prone to premature death? World J Surg 2000;24:1437–41.
35. Lowney J, Frisella MM, Lairmore TC, et al. Islet cell tumor metastasis in multiple endocrine neoplasia type I: correlation with primary tumor size. Surgery 1998;124:1043–9.
36. Skogseid B, Öberg K, Eriksson B, et al. Surgery for asymptomatic pancreatic lesion in multiple endocrine neoplasia type I. World J Surg 1996;20:872–7.
37. Åkerström G, Johansson H, Grama G. Surgical treatment of endocrine pancreatic lesions in MEN-I. Acta Oncol 1991;30:541–5.
38. Grama D, Skogseid B, Wilander E, et al. Pancreatic tumors in multiple endocrine neoplasia type I: clinical presentation and surgical treatment. World J Surg 1992;16:611–9.
39. Skogseid B, Öberg K, Åkerström G. Limited tumor involvement found at multiple endocrine neoplasia type I pancreatic exploration: can it be predicted by preoperative tumor localization? World J Surg 1998;22:673–8.
40. Triponez F, Goudet P, Dosseh D, et al. Is surgery beneficial for MEN 1 patients with small (≤ 2 cm), nonfunctioning pancreaticoduodenal endocrine tumor? An analysis of 65 patients from the GTE. World J Surg 2006;30:654–62.

41. Triponez F, Dosseh D, Goudet P, et al. Epidemiology data on 108 MEN 1 patients from the GTE with isolated nonfunctioning tumors of the pancreas. Ann Surg 2006;243:265–72.
42. Doherty GM, Thompson NW. Multiple endocrine neoplasia type 1: duodeno-pancreatic tumours. J Intern Med 2003;253:590–8.
43. Bartsch DK, Fendrich V, Langer P, et al. Outcome of duodenopancreatic resections in patients with multiple endocrine neoplasia type 1. Ann Surg 2005;242: 757–66.
44. Hellman P, Hennings J, Åkerström G, et al. Endoscopic ultrasound for evaluation of pancreatic tumors in multiple endocrine neoplasia type 1. Br J Surg 2005;92:1508–12.
45. O'Riordian DS, O'Brian T, van Heerden JA, et al. Surgical management of insulinoma associated with multiple endocrine neoplasia type 1. World J Surg 1994; 18:488–94.
46. Demeure MJ, Klonoff CC, Karam JH, et al. Insulinomas associated with multiple endocrine neoplasia type 1: the need for a different surgical approach. Surgery 1991;110:998–1005.
47. Grant CS. Insulinoma. Best Pract Res Clin Gastroenterol 2005;19:783–98.
48. Kato M, Imamura M, Hosotani R, et al. Curative resection of microgastrinomas based on the intraoperative secretin test. World J Surg 2000;24:1425–30.
49. Levy-Bohbot N, Merie C, Goudet P, et al. Prevalence, characteristics and prognosis of MEN 1-associated glucagonomas, VIPomas, and somatostatinomas. Gastroenterol Clin Biol 2004;28:1075–81.
50. Bartsch D, Langer P, Wild A, et al. Pancreaticoduodenal endocrine tumors in multiple endocrine neoplasia type 1: surgery or surveillance? Surgery 2000; 128:958–66.
51. Hellman P, Ladjevardi S, Skogseid B, et al. Radiofrequency tissue ablation using coiled tip for liver metastases of endocrine tumors. World J Surg 2002;26: 1052–6.
52. Thompson NW, Vinik AI, Eckhauser F. Microgastrinomas of the duodenum: a cause of failed operations for the Zollinger-Ellison syndrome. Ann Surg 1989;168:396–404.
53. Thompson NW. Current concept in the surgical management of multiple endocrine neoplasia type 1 pancreaticoduodenal disease: results in the treatment of 40 patients with Zollinger-Ellison syndrome, hypoglycaemia or both. J Intern Med 1998;243:495–500.
54. Norton JA, Fraker DL, Alexander HR, et al. Surgery to cure the Zollinger-Ellison syndrome. N Engl J Med 1999;341:635–44.
55. Norton J, Jensen RT. Role of surgery in Zollinger-Ellison syndrome. J Am Coll Surg 2007;205(Suppl 4):S34–7.
56. Åkerström G, Hellman P, Stålberg P. Carcinoid: presentation and diagnosis, surgical management. In: Hubbard JGH, Inabnet WB, Lo C-Y, editors. Endocrine surgery (Springer Specialist Surgery Series). London: Springer-Verlag; 2008. Chapter 44.
57. Modlin IM, Lawton GP. Duodenal gastrinoma: the solution to the pancreatic paradox. J Clin Gastroenterol 1994;19:184–8.
58. Hausman MS Jr, Thompson NW, Gauger PG, et al. The surgical management of MEN-1 pancreatoduodenal neuroendocrine disease. Surgery 2004;136: 1205–11.
59. Tonelli F, Fratini G, Falchetti A, et al. Surgery for gastroenteropancreatic tumors in multiple endocrine neoplasia type 1: review and personal experience. J Intern Med 2005;257:38–49.

60. Imamura M, Komoto I, Doi R, et al. New pancreas-preserving total duodenectomy technique. World J Surg 2005;29:203–7.

61. Richards ML, Gauger P, Thompson NW, et al. Regression of type II gastric carcinoids. World J Surg 2004;28:652–8.

62. Norton JA, Melcher ML, Gibril F, et al. Gastric carcinoid tumors in multiple endocrine neoplasia-1 patients with Zollinger-Ellison syndrome can be symptomatic, demonstrate aggressive growth, and require surgical treatment. Surgery 2004; 136:1267–74.

63. Tisell LE, Ahlman H, Jansson S, et al. Total pancreatectomy in the MEN 1 syndrome. Br J Surg 1988;75:154–7.

64. You YN, Thompson GB, Young WF, et al. Pancreatoduodenal surgery in patients with multiple endocrine neoplasia type 1: operative outcomes, long-term function, and quality of life. Surgery 2007;142:829–36.

65. Kouvaraki MA, Shapiro SE, Cote GJ, et al. Management of pancreatic endocrine tumors in multiple endocrine neoplasia type 1. World J Surg 2006;30:643–53.

66. Tonelli F, Fratini G, Nesi G, et al. Pancreatectomy in multiple endocrine neoplasia type 1-related gastrinomas and pancreatic endocrine neoplasias. Ann Surg 2006;244:61–70.

67. Wilson SD, Krzywda EA, Zhu Y-r, et al. The influence of surgery in MEN-1 syndrome: observations over 150 years. Surgery 2008;144:695–702.

68. Norton JA, Jensen RT. Resolved and unresolved controversies in the surgical management of patients with Zollinger-Ellison syndrome. Ann Surg 2004;240: 757–73.

69. Lairmore TC, Chen VY, DeBenedetti MK, et al. Duodenopancreatic resections in patients with multiple endocrine neoplasia type I. Ann Surg 2000;231:909–18.

70. Mulligan LM, Eng C, Healey CS, et al. Specific mutations of the RET proto-oncogene are related to disease phenotype in MEN 2A and FMTC. Nat Genet 1994;6: 70–4.

71. Eng C, Clayton D, Schuffenecker I, et al. The relationship between specific RET proto-oncogene mutations and disease phenotype in multiple endocrine neoplasia type 2. International RET Mutation Consortium Analysis. JAMA 1996;276:1575–9.

72. Kouvaraki MA, Shapiro SE, Perrier ND, et al. *RET* proto-oncogene: a review and update of genotype-phenotype correlations in hereditary medullary thyroid cancer and associated endocrine tumors. Thyroid 2005;15:531–44.

73. Raue F, Frank-Raue K. Multiple endocrine neoplasia type 2: 2007 update. Horm Res 2007;68(Suppl 5):101–4.

74. Callender GG, Rich TA, Perrier ND. Multiple endocrine neoplasia syndromes. Surg Clin North Am 2008;88:863–95.

75. Schimke RN, Hartmann WH, Prout TE, et al. Syndrome of bilateral pheochromocytoma, medullary thyroid carcinoma and multiple neuromas: a possible regulatory defect in the differentiation of chromaffin tissue. N Engl J Med 1968;279:1–7.

76. Wray CJ, Rich TA, Waguespack SG, et al. Failure to recognize multiple endocrine neoplasia 2B: more common than we think? Ann Surg Oncol 2008;15: 293–301.

77. Farndon JR, Leight GS, Dilley WG, et al. Familial medullary thyroid carcinoma without associated endocrinopathies: a distinct clinical entity. Br J Surg 1986; 73:278–81.

78. Grant CS. Medullary thyroid carcinoma and associated multiple endocrine neoplasia type 2. In: Hay ID, Wass JAH, editors. Clinical endocrine oncology. 2nd edition. Singapore: Blackwell Publishing; 2008. p. 515–22.

79. Mulligan LM, Kwok JB, Healey CS, et al. Germ-line mutations of the RET proto-oncogene in multiple endocrine neoplasia type 2A. Nature 1993;363:458–60.
80. Donis-Keller H, Dou S, Chi D, et al. Mutations in the RET proto-oncogene are associated with MEN 2A and FMTC. Hum Mol Genet 1993;2:851–6.
81. Mulligan LM, Marsh DJ, Robinson BG, et al. Genotype-phenotype correlation in multiple endocrine neoplasia type 2: report of the International RET Mutation Consortium. J Intern Med 1995;238:343–6.
82. Eng C. Seminars in medicine of the Beth Israel Hospital, Boston. The RET proto-oncogene in multiple endocrine neoplasia type 2 and Hirschsprung's disease. N Engl J Med 1996;335:943–51.
83. Machens A, Dralle H. DNA-based window of opportunity for curative pre-emptive therapy of hereditary medullary thyroid cancer. Surgery 2006;139:279–82.
84. Hofstra RM, Landsvater RM, Ceccherini I, et al. A mutation in the RET proto-oncogene associated with multiple endocrine neoplasia type 2B and sporadic medullary thyroid carcinoma. Nature 1994;367:375–6.
85. Eng C, Smith DP, Mulligan LM, et al. Point mutation within the tyrosine kinase domain of the RET proto-oncogene in multiple endocrine neoplasia type 2B and related sporadic tumours. Hum Mol Genet 1994;3:237–41.
86. Zedenius J, Larsson C, Bergholm U, et al. Mutations of codon 918 in the RET proto-oncogene correlate to poor prognosis in sporadic medullary thyroid carcinomas. J Clin Endocrinol Metab 1995;80:3088–90.
87. Alemi M, Lucas SD, Sallstrom JF, et al. A complex nine base pair deletion in RET exon 11 common in sporadic medullary thyroid carcinoma. Oncogene 1997;14:2041–5.
88. Elisei R, Romei C, Cosci B, et al. RET genetic screening in patients with medullary thyroid cancer and their relatives: experience with 807 individuals at one center. J Clin Endocrinol Metab 2007;92:4725–9.
89. Yip L, Cote GL, Shapiro SE, et al. Multiple endocrine neoplasia type 2: evaluation of the genotype-phenotype relationship. Arch Surg 2003;138:409–16.
90. Nilsson O, Tisell LE, Jansson S, et al. Adrenal and extra-adrenal pheochromo-cytomas in a family with germline RET V804L mutation. JAMA 1999;281:1587–8.
91. Learoyd DL, Gosnell J, Elston MS, et al. Experience of prophylactic thyroidec-tomy in multiple endocrine neoplasia type 2A kindreds with *RET* codon 804 mutations. Clin Endocrinol (Oxf) 2005;63:636–41.
92. Vasen HF, van der Feltz M, Raue F, et al. The natural course of multiple endocrine neoplasia type 2b. Arch Intern Med 1992;152:1250–2.
93. Smith DP, Houghton C, Ponder BA. Germline mutation of RET codon 883 in two cases of de novo MEN 2B. Oncogene 1995;15:1213–7.
94. Gimm O, Ukkat J, Niederle BE, et al. Timing and extent of surgery in patients with familial medullary thyroid carcinoma/multiple endocrine neoplasia type 2A-related *RET* mutations not affecting codon 634. World J Surg 2004;28:1312–6.
95. Learoyd DL, Robinson BG. Do all patients with *RET* mutations associated with multiple endocrine neoplasia type 2 require surgery? Nat Clin Pract Endocrinol Metab 2005;1:60–1.
96. Machens A, Dralle H. Genotype-phenotype based surgical concept of heredi-tary medullary thyroid carcinoma. World J Surg 2007;31:957–68.
97. Frohnauer MK, Decker RA. Update on the MEN 2A c804 RET mutation: is prophylactic thyroidectomy indicated? Surgery 2000;128:1052–7 [discussion: 1057–8].

98. Webb TA, Sheps SG, Carney JA. Differences between sporadic pheochromocy-toma and pheochromocytoma in multiple endocrine neoplasia, type 2. Am J Surg Pathol 1980;4:121–6.
99. Yip L, Lee JE, Shapiro SE, et al. Surgical management of hereditary pheochro-mocytoma. J Am Coll Surg 2004;198:525–34 [discussion: 534–5].
100. Åkerström G, Hellman P. Genetic syndromes associated with adrenal tumors. In: Linos D, van Heerden JA, editors. Adrenal surgery. Heidelberg, Germany: Springer; 2005. p. 251–4.
101. Modigliani E, Vasen HM, Raue K, et al. Pheochromocytoma in multiple endocrine neoplasia type 2: European study. J Intern Med 1995;238:363–7.
102. Casanova S, Rosenberg-Bourgin M, Farkas D, et al. Phaeochromocytoma in multiple endocrine neoplasia type 2A: survey of 100 cases. Clin Endocrinol 1993;38:531–7.
103. Lairmore TC, Ball DW, Baylin SB, et al. Management of pheochromocytomas in patients with multiple endocrine neoplasia type 2 syndromes. Ann Surg 1993; 217:595–603.
104. Pomares FJ, Canas R, Rodriguez JM, et al. Differences between sporadic and multiple endocrine neoplasia type 2A phaeochromocytoma. Clin Endocrinol 1998;48:195–200.
105. Lee JE, Curley SA, Gagel RF, et al. Cortical-sparing adrenalectomy for patients with bilateral pheochromocytoma. Surgery 1996;120:1064–71.
106. Inabnet WB, Caragliano P, Pertsemlidis D. Pheochromocytoma, inherited asso-ciations, bilaterality, and cortex preservation. Surgery 2000;128:1007–12.
107. Walz MK, Peitgen K, Diesing D, et al. Partial versus total adrenalectomy by the posterior retroperitoneoscopic approach: early and long-term results of 325 consecutive procedures in primary adrenal neoplasia. World J Surg 2004;28: 1323–9.
108. Asari R, Scheuba C, Kaczirek K, et al. Estimated risk of pheochromocytoma recurrence after adrenal-sparing surgery in patients with multiple endocrine neoplasia type 2A. Arch Surg 2006;141:1199–205.
109. Brauckhoff M, Gimm O, Brauckhoff K, et al. Repeated adrenocortical-sparing adrenalectomy for recurrent hereditary pheochromocytoma. Surg Today 2004; 34:251–5.
110. Raue F, Kraimps JL, Dralle H, et al. Primary hyperparathyroidism in multiple endocrine neoplasia type 2A. J Intern Med 1995;238:369–73.
111. Snow KJ, Boyd AE. Management of individual tumor syndromes: medullary thyroid carcinoma and hyperparathyroidism. Endocrinol Metab Clin North Am 1994;23:157–66.

Surgical Management of Nonmultiple Endocrine Neoplasia Endocrinopathies: State-of-the-Art Review

Christine S. Landry, MD[a], Steven G. Waguespack, MD[b],
Nancy D. Perrier, MD[c],*

KEYWORDS

- Endocrinopathy • Familial • Adrenal • Pancreas
- Thyroid • Parathyroid

Endocrinopathy is defined as "a disorder in the function of an endocrine gland and the consequences thereof."[1] In many endocrinopathies, surgical intervention is a necessary part of the treatment algorithm to achieve cure. In fact, surgical treatment of endocrine organs is centuries old. Pierre-Joseph Desault of Paris performed the first documented successful thyroidectomy in 1791.[2] At that time, thyroidectomy had a 40% mortality rate from complications of bleeding and sepsis.[2]

As the development of general anesthesia, hemostasis, and antiseptic techniques transformed the discipline of surgery, systematic surgical intervention of endocrine glands emerged by the early 1900s as a treatment to control hypersecretion of hormones.[2] Theodor Kocher was awarded the Nobel Prize in Medicine in 1909 for his work on physiology, pathology, and surgery of the thyroid gland.[3] Endocrine surgery was further advanced when Charles Huggins discovered that certain malignancies are sensitive to specific hormones, and removal of these hormones can induce tumor regression; this discovery earned him the Nobel Prize in 1966.[4]

---

[a] Department of Surgical Oncology, Unit 444, The University of Texas M. D. Anderson Cancer Center, 1515 Holcombe Boulevard, Houston, TX 77030, USA
[b] Department of Endocrine Neoplasia and Hormonal Disorders, Unit 1461, The University of Texas M. D. Anderson Cancer Center, 1515 Holcombe Boulevard, Houston, TX 77030, USA
[c] Department of Surgical Oncology, Unit 444, The University of Texas M. D. Anderson Cancer Center, 1400 Holcombe Boulevard, Unit 444, Houston, TX 77230-1402, USA
* Corresponding author. Department of Surgical Oncology, Unit 444, M. D. Anderson Cancer Center, 1515 Holcombe Boulevard, Houston, TX 77030.
E-mail address: nperrier@mdanderson.org (N.D. Perrier).

Surg Clin N Am 89 (2009) 1069–1089
doi:10.1016/j.suc.2009.06.020
0039-6109/09/$ – see front matter © 2009 Elsevier Inc. All rights reserved.

Over the last 50 years, endocrine surgery has evolved even more with the development of genetic testing to help identify patients with familial disorders. The discovery of multiple endocrine neoplasia syndrome (MEN) had a profound impact on endocrine surgery. This article focuses on the identification and surgical management of non-MEN familial endocrinopathies (**Table 1**).

THYROID ENDOCRINOPATHIES
Hereditary Nonmedullary Carcinoma of the Thyroid

Hereditary nonmedullary thyroid cancer (HNMTC) accounts for 3% to 6% of all thyroid malignancies, and is transmitted in an autosomal dominant pattern with incomplete penetrance.[5,6] More than 90% of patients with HNMTC have papillary thyroid cancer, whereas the remainder have follicular thyroid cancer or Hurthle cell carcinoma.[6] No single causative gene has been identified, but linkages to 1q21, 2q21, and 19p13.2 have been reported.[5,6] Thyroid malignancies in patients with HNMTC are thought to be more aggressive and to have higher rates of multicentricity, lymph node metastasis, and invasion into adjacent tissues compared with thyroid malignancies in patients with sporadic disease.[6–9] HNMTC has also been associated with renal malignancies, benign thyroid tumors, and nonautoimmune hyperthyroidism.[6] According to statistical analyses of the incidence of thyroid cancer in the United States, there is a 94% chance of familial predisposition to nonmedullary thyroid cancer when 3 or more family members have the disease.[10] However, when only 2 family members are affected, 62% to 69% of nonmedullary thyroid cancer cases are sporadic rather than familial.[10] Screening recommendations for HNMTC have not been fully established, but it has been suggested that families with 2 or more affected members should be screened with physical examination, thyroid ultrasound, and serum thyroid-stimulating hormone levels.[6,11] Surgical management of patients with HNMTC is similar to patients with sporadic thyroid cancer.

Cowden Disease

Cowden disease, named after a patient's surname in 1962 by Llyod and Dennis, is an autosomal dominant disorder characterized by multiple hamartomas, and breast and thyroid malignancies.[12] Other manifestations include uterine leiomyoma, megacephaly, mucocutaneous lesions (eg, facial trichilemmoma, acral keratoses, and oral papillomatous papules), benign tumors of the breast and thyroid gland, Lhermitte-Duclos disease, and endometrial carcinoma (**Box 1**).[13] Eighty percent of patients diagnosed with Cowden disease have germ-line mutations of the *PTEN* gene, a tumor suppressor gene located on chromosome 10q23.3.[14–18] An additional 10% of patients have mutations in the *PTEN* promoter region, and there are likely other patients with deletions and rearrangements of the *PTEN* gene.[19] By 20 years of age, more than 90% of individuals with Cowden disease present with mucocutaneous lesions.[13,20] By age 29, more than 99% of affected patients show signs of the disease.[13]

Up to 10% of patients with Cowden disease develop follicular carcinoma, and 50% to 75% develop benign lesions of the thyroid gland.[20,21] There have been a few reports of papillary thyroid cancer, but the predominant histopathology associated with Cowden disease is follicular thyroid cancer.[20] Follicular adenomas, which are often multicentric, may progress to follicular carcinoma.[20,22] Patients with Cowden disease should undergo annual physical thyroid examinations beginning at age 18 years or 5 years younger than the age of first diagnosis of thyroid cancer in the family, whichever is earlier.[23] Likewise, a baseline thyroid ultrasound with repeat studies annually or biannually may be useful.[20]

Table 1
Non-MEN familial endocrinopathies

Familial Disease	Genetic Transmission	Affected Endocrine Organ(s)	Gene	Gene Function	Location
Beckwith-Wiedemann syndrome	Autosomal dominant	Adrenal, pancreas	Multiple	Not available	11p15
Carney complex	Autosomal dominant	Adrenal, thyroid	PRKAR1A, unknown	Tumor suppressor	17q22-24, 2p16
Cowden disease	Autosomal dominant	Breast, thyroid	PTEN	Tumor suppressor	10q23.3
Familial adenomatous polyposis	Autosomal dominant	Thyroid	APC	Tumor suppressor	5q21-22
Hereditary nonmedullary carcinoma of the thyroid	n/a	Thyroid	Unknown	n/a	1q21, 2q21, 19p13.2
Hereditary hyperparathyroidism jaw-tumor syndrome	Autosomal dominant	Parathyroid	HRPT2 [CDC73]	Tumor suppressor	1q25-32
Li-Fraumeni syndrome	Autosomal dominant	Breast, adrenal	P53	Tumor suppressor	17p13
Neurofibromatosis I	Autosomal dominant	Adrenal, GI tract	NF1	Tumor suppressor	17q11.2
Pendred syndrome	Autosomal recessive	Thyroid	PDS	Iodide and chloride transport	7q31
Tuberous sclerosis	Autosomal dominant	Adrenal, pancreas	TSC1 TSC2	Tumor suppressor	9q34 16p13.3
Von Hippel-Lindau disease	Autosomal dominant	Adrenal, pancreas	VHL	Tumor suppressor	3p25
Werner syndrome	Autosomal recessive	Thyroid	WRN	DNA repair	8p11-21

<table>
<tr><td>

Box 1
Cowden disease

Thyroid cancer

Breast cancer

Hamartomas

Uterine leiomyoma

Megacephaly

Thyroid adenoma

Benign breast disease

Mucocutaneous lesions

Endometrial carcinoma

Lhermitte-Duclos disease

</td></tr>
</table>

The percentage of patients with Cowden disease who develop breast cancer during their lifetime ranges from 25% to 50%, and 75% develop benign breast diseases, such as fibroadenoma or fibrocystic breast disease.[24] Patients with Cowden disease who develop breast cancer are diagnosed approximately 10 years younger than sporadic breast cancer counterparts.[25] Likewise, breast cancer in these patients is more likely to be multifocal and bilateral than in sporadic breast cancer patients.[25] The predominant histopathology for patients who develop breast cancer is ductal adenocarcinoma.[21] Screening of patients with Cowden disease should include monthly breast self-examinations with alternating mammograms and breast MRI every six months starting at age 30 years or 5 years younger than the earliest diagnosis of breast cancer in the family.[23]

Familial Adenomatous Polyposis

Familial adenomatous polyposis (FAP) is an autosomal dominant condition associated with multiple polyps in the colon that develop during early adulthood.[14,20,26] This disease has been linked to the *APC* gene on chromosome 5q21-22.[20,26] Other characteristics of the disease include desmoid tumors, osteomas, epidermal cysts, hepatoblastomas, congenital hypertrophy of retinal pigmented epithelium, nonfunctioning adrenal adenomas, and upper gastrointestinal tract polyps (**Box 2**).[20,26] Approximately 2% of patients with FAP are diagnosed with papillary carcinoma of the thyroid gland.[20] Females with FAP have a 160 times greater risk of developing papillary carcinoma than the general population.[26,27] The average age at diagnosis is 27 years.[20,28] Papillary thyroid carcinomas that are associated with FAP are usually multifocal, bilateral, and often have a rare cribriform-morular histologic subtype (**Fig. 1**).[20,27] Patients who are found to have a cribriform-morular histologic pattern should be screened for FAP, because 90% of patients with FAP and papillary thyroid carcinoma have this histology.[20] Furthermore, this histologic subtype comprises 0.1% to 0.2% of all papillary thyroid carcinoma cases.[26,29]

Screening recommendations for FAP-associated thyroid disease are not currently established, although many institutions recommend yearly thyroid physical and ultrasonographic examinations.[29] These screening techniques reportedly detected papillary thyroid carcinomas in 7% of patients at one center.[26] The treatment for patients with papillary thyroid carcinoma and FAP is the same as patients with sporadic papillary thyroid cancer.[20,27]

Box 2
Familial adenomatous polyposis

Papillary thyroid carcinoma

Adrenal adenomas

Colon polyps

Desmoid tumors

Osteomas

Hepatoblastomas

Retinal pigmented epithelial hypertrophy

Carney Complex

First described by Mayo Clinic pathologist J. Aidan Carney, Carney complex is an autosomal dominant disorder associated with spotty skin pigmentation, myxomas, endocrine disorders, and schwannomas (**Box 3**).[14,20,30] Patients with this disease commonly have multinodular thyroid glands and multiple follicular adenomas.[14,20,31] Approximately 15% of these patients are diagnosed with papillary or follicular carcinoma of the thyroid gland.[20] Annual cervical ultrasonographic examination is recommended as a primary screening tool. Surgical resection is the appropriate treatment when a malignancy or suspicious lesions are identified. Other endocrine findings associated with Carney complex are discussed later in this article.

Werner Syndrome

Werner syndrome, named after the German physician C.W. Otto Werner, is a rare autosomal recessive disease characterized by premature aging, skin atrophy, and bilateral cataracts (**Box 4**).[14,20] This condition has been linked to a gene, referred to as the *WS* gene, located at chromosome 8p11-21.[32] Patients with this disease have an increased incidence of papillary and follicular thyroid carcinoma, with a mean

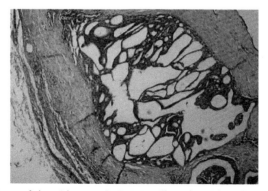

Fig. 1. Histopathology of thyroid cancer in FAP. Papillary thyroid carcinomas associated with FAP are usually multifocal and bilateral, and often have a rare cribriform-morular histologic subtype. Ninety percent of patients with FAP and papillary thyroid carcinoma have this histology.

Box 3
Carney complex

Thyroid cancer

Primary pigmented nodular adrenocortical disease

Multinodular thyroid

Spotty skin pigmentation

Myxomas

Schwannomas

---

age of 34 years at presentation.[14] Moreover, as many as 2% of patients with Werner syndrome develop anaplastic carcinoma of the thyroid.[20]

Familial Medullary Thyroid Carcinoma

Historically, medullary thyroid carcinoma (MTC) is thought to occur in both familial and sporadic forms, or as a part of MEN type 2. In 2009, the American Thyroid Association (ATA) Guidelines Task Force defined familial medullary thyroid carcinoma (FMTC) as "a clinical variant of MEN 2A in which MTC is the only manifestation."[33] For patients to be diagnosed with FMTC, they must have a RET mutation identified in kindreds with only FMTC, or demonstrate the absence of pheochromocytoma or primary hyperparathyroidism in two or more generations within a family.[33] Because this observation is a new development, and some individuals consider FMTC to be a distinct entity from MEN, we have included FMTC in this chapter. The remainder of this section outlines the guidelines from the most recent ATA Task Force. These guidelines are intended to assist physicians with the management of medullary thyroid cancer, but each patient should be treated on an individual basis.

FMTC is transmitted in an autosomal dominant pattern and typically presents with bilateral and multicentric disease at a later age than patients with MEN.[14,20] Thyroid glands in these patients are characterized by the presence of C-cell hyperplasia prior to the development of carcinoma.[20,34] Because 25% of MTCs are hereditary, all patients who are diagnosed with primary C cell hyperplasia, MTC, or MEN 2 should be offered RET (rearranged during transfection) genetic testing.[33] Similarly, because 88% of individuals with FMTC have an identifiable RET mutation, everyone who has a first-degree relative with FMTC or MEN 2A should be offered RET genetic testing during childhood.[33]

The biologic behavior of MTC can be predicted by the specific RET mutation and the patient's age when MTC becomes clinically apparent.[35–37] The ATA Task Force

---

Box 4
Werner syndrome

Papillary thyroid carcinoma

Follicular thyroid carcinoma

Anaplastic thyroid carcinoma

Premature aging

Skin atrophy

Bilateral cataracts

---

created a classification system of RET mutations based on the historical aggressiveness of MTC, allowing screening and surgical intervention to be optimized for the best overall outcome.[33] Patients with ATA level A RET mutations (codons 768, 790, 791, 804, 891) or ATA level B RET mutations (codons 609, 611, 618, 620, 630) have the lowest risk of aggressive MTC, and may undergo prophylactic thyroidectomy after 5 years of age if they have a normal annual serum calcitonin level, normal annual neck ultrasound, and a less aggressive family history.[33] However, if the calcitonin level is elevated, the family history is aggressive, or the ultrasound is abnormal, then prophylactic thyroidectomy is warranted.[33] Patients with ATA level C RET mutations (codon 634) have a higher risk of aggressive MTC, and should undergo prophylactic total thyroidectomy before 5 years of age.[33] Individuals with ATA level D (MEN 2B) RET mutations (codons 883, 918) have the youngest age of onset and the highest risk of metastatic disease.[33] These patients should undergo prophylactic total thyroidectomy within the first year of life.[33]

Preoperative calcitonin levels and cervical ultrasound may be considered in children who undergo prophylactic thyroidectomy after 3 years of age to rule out the possibility of metastatic MTC.[33] Caution should be used when interpreting calcitonin values in children less than 3 years old as preoperative testing in this age group has not been established.[33] In addition, patients who undergo prophylactic thyroidectomy before 5 years of age should have the surgery performed at an experienced tertiary care center to decrease the chance of recurrent laryngeal nerve or parathyroid injury.[33] According to the ATA guidelines, central neck dissection is not indicated for FMTC patients undergoing prophylactic thyroidectomy at any age unless there is evidence of lymph node metastasis, thyroid nodules greater than 5 mm, or a basal serum calcitonin greater than 40 pg/mL.[33]

Patients with suspected MTC should have a cervical neck ultrasound, serum CEA, serum calcium, and a serum calcitonin level preoperatively.[33] If there is no evidence of local invasion by the primary tumor, and there is no evidence of lymph node metastasis, then the ATA task force recommends total thyroidectomy with prophylactic central neck dissection.[33] If the serum calcitonin level is greater than 400 pg/mL or there is evidence of local lymph node metastasis, then a neck, chest, and three-phase liver computed tomography scan or MRI is indicated to rule out metastatic disease.[33] If distant metastasis is evident, the degree of surgical resection should be determined on an individual basis. Less aggressive neck surgery may be considered to control locoregional disease, while maintaining parathyroid, swallowing and speech function.[33]

If central neck disease is diagnosed or suspected in a FMTC patient with MTC, the patient should have a total thyroidectomy with central lymph node dissection. The role for prophylactic lateral neck dissection for patients without evidence of lateral neck disease is currently not established, and should be considered on an individual basis. However, if lateral neck disease is demonstrated preoperatively without evidence of distant metastasis, the task force recommends a central neck dissection and a compartment oriented lateral neck dissection (levels IIA, III, IV, V) on the affected side. If the parathyroid glands are removed or devascularized during surgery, they may be reimplanted in the neck if the genetic mutation is consistent with FMTC, or in the forearm in conjunction with cryopreservation, if the genetic defect is more consistent with MEN 2A.[33,35]

Two to three months postoperatively, calcitonin and CEA levels should be measured. These tumor markers may be obtained every 6-12 months initially, and then annually depending on the patient.[33] A neck ultrasound six months after surgical intervention may be used as a baseline. The ATA task force recommends thyroid replacement therapy rather than thyroid suppressive T4 therapy after thyroidectomy.[33] Radioactive iodine is not indicated for patients after thyroidectomy for MTC. If patients have undetectable serum tumor markers, they may be followed with serial laboratory testing.[33] Patients who have detectable calcitonin levels less than 150 pg/mL should have a neck ultrasound to evaluate for additional disease, and additional imaging may be considered.[33] Patients with calcitonin levels greater than 150 pg/mL should have additional imaging of the neck, chest, liver, and axial skeleton to rule out distant metastatic disease.[33] Adjuvant chemotherapy and external beam radiation may be beneficial in some patients, such as those with unresectable disease or positive margins, and the use of these modalities should be individualized.[33,38]

Pendred Syndrome

In 1896 Pendred syndrome was first described in an Irish family by Vaughan Pendred, an English physician.[39] This autosomal recessive disorder is characterized by nonreversible bilateral sensorineural hearing loss and thyroid goiter (**Box 5**).[40] In addition, this disease is thought to represent up to 10% of cases of hereditary deafness, which can be noted at birth or may progressively develop during childhood.[41] The most common gene associated with Pendred syndrome, located on 7q31, produces pendrin, a protein involved with chloride and iodide transport.[41] The loss of pendrin production leads to defective iodide organification, resulting in thyroid overgrowth and goiter.[42] The diagnosis of Pendred syndrome is supported with the perchlorate discharge test, whereby affected individuals have less than 10% of radioactive discharge after administration of radioactive iodine.[43] Affected individuals often develop thyroid goiters.[44] Patients who have adequate iodine intake typically are euthyroid. However, approximately one-third of patients actually develop overt hypothyroidism, especially those with iodine deficiency.[44] Treatment of Pendred syndrome consists of thyroid hormone replacement and surgery if the patient has compressive symptoms.[44]

Other Conditions Associated with Thyroid Goiter

Iodide transport deficiency disease and iodotyrosine deiodinase defect disease comprise some of the syndromes characterized by hypothyroidism and the development of a goiter. Even though no chromosome has been linked to these syndromes, both seem to be inherited in an autosomal-recessive fashion.[45,46] Like Pendred syndrome, these conditions should be treated with thyroid hormone replacement and surgery if patients have compressive symptoms.[44]

PARATHYROID ENDOCRINOPATHIES
Hereditary Hyperparathyroidism Jaw-Tumor Syndrome

Hereditary hyperparathyroidism jaw-tumor syndrome is a rare autosomal dominant disorder with incomplete penetrance associated with the gene *HRPT2* (also known as CDC73), which is thought to be a tumor suppressor gene located on 1q25-32.[44,47] This syndrome is characterized by renal cysts or solid tumors, ossifying fibromas of the mandible or maxilla (**Fig. 2**), uterine fibromas, and PTH-mediated

---

Box 5
Pendred syndrome

Thyroid goiter

Bilateral sensorineural hearing loss

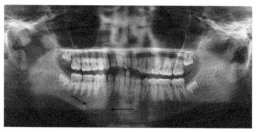

Fig. 2. Ossifying fibromas associated with hereditary hyperparathyroidism jaw-tumor syndrome. Hereditary hyperparathyroidism jaw-tumor syndrome is characterized by renal cysts or solid tumors, ossifying fibromas of the mandible or maxilla, uterine fibromas, and hypercalcemia.

hypercalcemia (**Box 6**).[44,46,48] Approximately 80% of patients with this disease develop hyperparathyroidism.[44] Moreover, 15% of patients may develop parathyroid carcinoma.[48] Patients with hereditary hyperparathyroidism jaw-tumor syndrome should be followed closely with annual screening of serum calcium and intact parathyroid hormone levels. If biochemical testing is elevated, cervical ultrasonography should be used.[48] Surgical resection should involve excision of enlarged parathyroid adenomas.[45] In the case of suspected parathyroid carcinoma, an *en bloc* resection should be performed with an ipsilateral thyroid lobectomy and any involved adjacent structures.[45]

Familial Isolated Hyperparathyroidism

It has been postulated that familial isolated hyperparathyroidism is a genetic variant of hereditary hyperparathyroidism jaw-tumor syndrome or MEN with incomplete penetrance.[49] However, currently the diagnosis of familial isolated hyperparathyroidism requires that the patient and at least one relative be diagnosed with primary hyperparathyroidism associated with abnormal histology, but without the clinical manifestations of MEN or hereditary hyperparathyroidism jaw-tumor syndrome.[50–52] To date, this disease has been linked to an area on chromosome 2p14, and it has been associated with mutations of the *HRPT2* (CDC73) gene, the *MEN1* gene, and the *CASR* gene.[48,49] Genetic testing should be considered to definitively rule out MEN, because patients may have incomplete penetrance.[53] However, genetic testing is low-yield for patients who do not have early-onset, multiglandular, cystic, atypical, or malignant parathyroid glands. Also, *CASR* testing is of little utility except to distinguish familial isolated hyperparathyroidism from primary hyperparathyroidism. The surgical management of familial hypercalcemic hypocalciuria should be the same as for

Box 6
Hereditary hyperparathyroidism jaw-tumor syndrome
Primary hyperparathyroidism
Parathyroid carcinoma
Ossifying fibromas of the jaw
Renal cysts
Renal solid tumors
Uterine fibromas

hyperparathyroidism: uniglandular resection for single-gland disease and subtotal parathyroidectomy for multiglandular disease.[48]

ADRENAL ENDOCRINOPATHIES
Adrenocortical Tumors

Beckwith-Wiedemann syndrome

Usually recognized at birth, Beckwith-Wiedemann syndrome is a congenital overgrowth syndrome that presents in an autosomal dominant pattern with variable expressivity (15% of cases) or in a sporadic form (85% of cases).[54] John Bruce Beckwith, an American pediatric pathologist, first reported this syndrome from autopsy findings of 3 affected children.[55] German pediatrician Hans-Rudolf Wiedemann further described this syndrome among 3 siblings in 1964.[56] Linked to the 11p15 chromosomal locus, this disorder is characterized by omphalocele, macroglossia, macrosomia, hemihypertrophy, hypoglycemia, visceromegaly, and renal abnormalities in the neonate (**Box 7**).[53,57] Multiple genes have been linked to this syndrome, such as *IGF-2*, *KCNQ10T1*, *H19*, *CDKN1C*, and *KCNQ1*.[58] Among patients with this syndrome, 5% to 10% develop childhood embryonal tumors, such as Wilms tumor (5%), adrenocortical tumors (3%), or less commonly, hepatoblastoma, neuroblastoma, pancreatoblastoma, and rhabdomyosarcoma.[59]

Most, but not all patients with Beckwith-Wiedemann syndrome who develop adrenocortical abnormalities have symptoms resulting from the overproduction of steroids associated with these tumors.[50] It is currently recommended that all patients with Beckwith-Wiedemann syndrome undergo routine screening with annual serum and urine cortisol levels, a-fetoprotein levels, and adrenal ultrasound until 9 years of age.[60] Laparoscopic adrenalectomy is contraindicated in the setting of suspected adrenal cortical carcinoma because of its association with peritoneal carcinomatosis.[61] Therefore, open adrenalectomy is the treatment of choice for adrenocortical carcinomas, even for patients with isolated metastatic disease.[57,61]

Li-Fraumeni syndrome

First described in 1969 by American cancer epidemiologist and internist Joseph F. Fraumeni, Li-Fraumeni syndrome is an autosomal dominant disorder classically characterized by multiple cancers, including sarcoma, breast cancer, leukemia, brain tumors, and adrenocortical tumors (**Box 8**).[62] This syndrome has been associated with germ-line mutations of the *p53* gene.[63,64] Three percent of patients with this disease actually develop adrenal cortical carcinoma, usually during childhood.[64,65] *En bloc* surgical resection is the treatment of choice for adrenocortical carcinomas,

Box 7
Beckwith-Wiedemann syndrome
Adrenocortical carcinoma
Omphalocele
Macroglossia
Macrosomia
Hemihypertrophy
Hypoglycemia
Visceromegaly
Renal abnormalities

Box 8
Li-Fraumeni syndrome

Adrenocortical carcinoma

Breast cancer

Leukemia

Sarcoma

Brain tumors

---

even when isolated metastatic disease is present.[61,66] Adjuvant chemotherapy with mitotane, one of the most commonly used chemotherapy drugs administered after radical resection for adrenal cortical carcinoma, has been reported to have different responses at different centers.[67] The authors' experience at The University of Texas M. D. Anderson Cancer Center has been that although adjuvant mitotane may not improve overall survival compared with other chemotherapy drugs, the time to progression of disease is prolonged with the use of mitotane alone.[68] The authors have also found that patients with recurrent disease who regress or have stable disease with the use of mitotane have a better overall prognosis.[69]

Pheochromocytoma

Neurofibromatosis 1 (von Recklinghausen disease)

Von Recklinghausen disease, also known as neurofibromatosis 1 (NF1), is the most common autosomal dominant disorder. Named after the German histopathologist Friedrich Daniel von Recklinghausen, von Recklinghausen disease affects 1 in 3000 to 4000 individuals, with variable presentation.[70] Identified in 1990, the *NF1* gene is a tumor suppressor gene located at the 17q11.2 chromosome locus that encodes neurofibrin, a GTPase-activating protein, which affects the production pathway of the Ras oncoprotein.[71,72] Approximately 50% of affected patients have de novo mutations.[73] This condition is characterized by neurofibromas, skin pigmentations (eg, café-au-lait macules, freckling in non-sun–exposed areas), optic gliomas, Lisch nodules, bony lesions, short stature, learning disabilities, and macrocephaly (**Box 9**).[73] Approximately 25% of patients with NF1 have intestinal fibromas that may result in bleeding.[73] NF1 is often identified during childhood when patients are noted to have 6 or more café-au-lait spots, or during the late teens and early twenties with the identification of Lisch nodules.[73]

Box 9
Neurofibromatosis I

Pheochromocytoma

Neurofibromas

Café-au-lait spots

Optic gliomas

Lisch nodules

Short stature

Learning disabilities

Macrocephaly

A 1999 literature review of 148 patients with NF1 found the incidence of pheochromocytomas to be 0.1% to 5.7%, with a mean age of 42 years at presentation.[73] Among these patients, 84% had unilateral disease, 9.6% had bilateral disease, and 6.1% had extra-adrenal paragangliomas.[64] The percentage of these patients who had tumors with metastatic disease or local invasion was 12%.[74,75] Moreover, 78% of patients had symptoms of hypertension.[66] Patients with a known diagnosis of NF1 may be followed with plasma metanephrine levels, especially if they have hypertension.[66]

The surgical management of patients with hereditary pheochromocytoma and NF1 is dependent on the presence of bilaterality. Patients who have uniglandular disease should undergo complete open or laparoscopic adrenalectomy.[76] When bilateral disease is involved, the potential morbidity of an acute Addisonian crisis associated with total bilateral adrenalectomy needs to be considered. The authors recommend bilateral cortical-sparing adrenalectomy for patients with bilateral pheochromocytoma associated with NF1, because the risk of metastatic and recurrent disease is low, and the necessity of lifelong steroid dependence is avoided.[76,77] However, when bilateral cortical-sparing adrenalectomy is performed, lifelong surveillance of the remnant glands and annual biochemical screening studies are imperative to monitor for recurrent disease.[76,77]

The preoperative management of patients with pheochromocytoma is important in minimizing complications in the perioperative setting. The primary goal is to control hypertension and heart rate, restore volume depletion, and prevent the patient from having a surgical catecholamine-induced storm.[78] Therapy should begin at least 1 to 2 weeks before surgery with α-adrenergic blockade to normalize blood pressure to 130/80 mm Hg while sitting and 100 mm Hg systolic when standing.[78] Likewise, the target heart rate should range from 60 to 70 beats per minute (bpm) while sitting and 70 to 80 bpm while standing.[78] Phenoxybenzamine, the most common α-antagonist used, can be started at a dose of 10 mg twice a day and increased until the clinical manifestations of the disease are controlled.[78] β-Blockers are indicated to help control catecholamine or α-blocker induced tachycardia.[78] β-Blockers must always be used in conjunction with an α-antagonist because the use of β-blockers alone could exacerbate hypertension in these patients. β-1 blockers are preferred, such as atenolol in doses of 12.5 or 25 mg 2 to 3 times a day or metoprolol in doses of 25 to 50 mg 3 to 4 times a day.[78] In addition, preoperative coordination with essential personnel, including a dedicated anesthesiologist, endocrinologist, surgeon, internist, and cardiologist, ensures the best preparation for surgery while minimizing the risks of complications in the perioperative setting.[78]

The surgical approach to pheochromocytoma or other benign adrenal tumors can be performed by open or laparoscopic surgery. The authors recommend the posterior retroperitoneoscopic adrenalectomy as a minimally invasive approach. Performed in the prone jackknife position, this technique avoids mobilization of intra-abdominal solid organs.[79] Trocars are placed in the retroperitoneal space, followed by separation of the adrenal gland from the kidney using blunt and sharp dissection. The adrenal vein is identified, clipped, and divided.[79] Next, the adrenal gland is completely mobilized and placed into an endocatch device.[79] Posterior retroperitoneoscopic adrenalectomy is useful for bilateral adrenalectomies because repositioning the patient is avoided.

Von Hippel-Lindau disease

Von Hippel-Lindau disease (VHL) occurs in approximately 1 in 36,000 births and is associated with hemangioblastomas of the nervous system, retinal angiomas, clear cell renal carcinoma, pheochromocytomas, pancreatic neuroendocrine cell tumors, and endolymphatic sac tumors (**Box 10**).[80] In 1895 Eugen von Hippel was the first to report retinal angiomas associated with this disease.[81] Many years later in 1926, Swedish pathologist, Arvid Lindau, recognized the coexistence of cerebellar tumors and other cystic tumors involved in VHL.[82] Other findings associated with this disease include pancreatic, renal, epididymal, and broad ligament cysts, and crystadenomas.[83,84] VHL has been associated with mutations of the von Hippel-Lindau gene (VHL gene, autosomal dominant), a tumor suppressor gene located on chromosome 3p25 that regulates hypoxia-induced cell proliferation and angiogenesis.[76,77] Type I VHL families have a low risk of developing a pheochromocytoma, and type II families have a high risk of pheochromocytoma.[77] Type II families can be further subdivided into type IIA (low risk of renal cell carcinoma), type IIB (high risk of renal cell carcinoma), and type IIC (pheochromocytoma with no other characteristics of VHL).[76] Screening for this disease should begin in childhood with a yearly eye examination to detect retinal angiomas, analysis of urinary or plasma metanephrine levels, abdominal ultrasound, and magnetic resonance imaging.[77] When plasma metanephrine levels are analyzed patients should withhold the use of acetaminophen, because this drug may cause a false-positive result.[85] In addition, tricyclic antidepressants, phenoxybenzamine, diuretics, and β-blockers also interfere with norepinephrine responses to the clonidine suppression test, another modality occasionally used in the diagnosis of pheochromocytoma.[85]

All patients who are diagnosed with familial, early-onset, or multiple pheochromocytomas should be offered genetic testing, because 5% to 11% of patients diagnosed with pheochromocytoma have germ-line mutations of the VHL gene.[86,87] Approximately 20% of patients with VHL develop a pheochromocytoma at a mean age at diagnosis of 20 years.[88] Cortical-sparing adrenalectomy is the favored approach for resection rather than total adrenalectomy because pheochromocytomas are malignant only 3.3% of the time, and are frequently bilateral.[76,77,87] The benefit of this approach lies in avoidance of long-term steroid dependence as well as the risk of an Addisonian crisis.[76,77,87] Furthermore, the risk of recurrence of pheochromocytomas for these patients is only 10%.[89] These patients also often require multiple treatments and surgical procedures whereby having adrenocortical function may be of substantial benefit.[89] Patients must be treated with α- and, possibly, β-blockade at least 2 weeks before surgery.[78]

Syndromes Associated with Cortisol Hypersecretion

Carney complex
The median age of diagnosis of patients with Carney complex is 20 years-old.[90–92] Cases are often associated with a mutation of the tumor suppressor gene, PRKAR1A

Box 10
Von Hippel-Lindau disease

Pheochromocytoma

Pancreatic neuroendocrine tumors

Pancreatic and renal cysts

Clear cell renal carcinoma

Retinal angiomas

Hemangioblastomas of the nervous system

Endolymphatic sac tumors of the inner ear

Cystadenomas of the pancreas, epididymis, and round ligament

on chromosome 17, or another gene at 2p16, with a 97% penetrance.[90,91] Patients with this disease have a shortened life span, most often because of cardiac problems associated with cardiac myxomas.[91,92]

Clinical manifestations of Carney complex begin during the first few years of life, with the identification of abnormal spotty skin pigmentation, and cardiac and cutaneous myxomas.[91] Testicular tumors, most commonly large-cell calcifying Sertoli cell tumors, and thyroid adenomas or carcinomas (discussed earlier), often develop within the first 10 years of life.[91] The characteristic lentigines, or spotty skin pigmentation, are often not apparent until puberty and may fade after the fourth decade of life.[91] Growth hormone secreting pituitary adenomas are most commonly identified during the third and fourth decades of life.[91] Additional manifestations include mammary myxoid fibroadenoma, epithelioid blue nevus, psammomatous melanotic schwannomas, and osteochondromyxoma.[91] Diagnosis requires that the patient have 2 or more manifestations of the disease, or 1 manifestation plus a first-degree relative with the diagnosis or an inactivating mutation of the *PRKAR1A* gene.[91]

Screening recommendations for postpubertal patients who are diagnosed with Carney complex include annual echocardiograms, urinary cortisol and serum IGF-I levels, and testicular ultrasound for men.[93] Thyroid ultrasound examinations should be obtained at the time of diagnosis and repeated as needed.[93] Pediatric patients should undergo annual echocardiograms as well as testicular ultrasound examinations.[93,94] Routine screening for endocrinopathies in the prepubescent population is not recommended because most of these conditions manifest later in life, although Cushing syndrome can present earlier.[93,94]

Approximately one-fourth of patients with Carney complex have been diagnosed with primary pigmented nodular adrenocortical disease (PPNAD) (**Fig. 3**) and can present with corticotrophin-independent Cushing syndrome.[95] This fraction could be an underestimation of the number of patients with PPNAD, as many have subclinical disease. Moreover, the histologic presence of PPNAD has been found in almost every autopsy of deceased patients.[96] Patients with subclinical or periodic forms of PPNAD can be identified with the dexamethasone stimulation test.[96] Symptomatic PPNAD can be cured with bilateral laparoscopic adrenalectomy, as previously described.[60]

PANCREATIC ENDOCRINOPATHIES
Beckwith-Weideman Syndrome

Fifty percent of children diagnosed with Beckwith-Wiedemann syndrome have hypoglycemia.[94,96] The hypoglycemia usually resolves after the first few days of life, but in 5% of patients it persists beyond the neonatal period.[96,97] Persistent hypoglycemia can be severe and may even result in brain damage.[96] Management primarily involves continuous feeding, but can involve partial pancreatectomy when hypoglycemia cannot be controlled medically.[96] The etiology of the hyperinsulinemia is unclear, but has been linked to overexpression of a mutated insulinlike growth factor (*IGF2*) gene.[96,98]

Tuberous Sclerosis

Tuberous sclerosis, an autosomal dominant disorder occurring in approximately 1 in 6700 births, is associated with hamartomas of any organ, but most commonly the brain, skin, kidney, and heart.[94,99] Other manifestations of the disease include kidney cysts and angiomyolipomas.[94] Fifty percent to 70% of patients present with sporadic forms of this disease, whereas the remaining 30% to 50% of cases are familial.

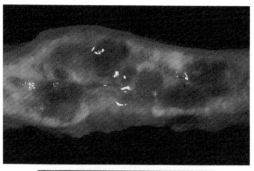

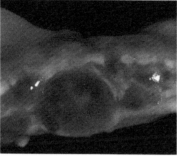

Fig. 3. PPNAD associated with Carney complex. Approximately one-fourth of patients with Carney complex have been diagnosed with PPNAD. Patients with subclinical or periodic forms of PPNAD can be identified with the dexamethasone stimulation test.

Tuberous sclerosis has been linked to the *TSC1* gene on the 9q34 chromosome and the *TSC2* gene on the16p13.3 chromosome.[99] Tuberin, a *TSC2* gene product associated with cell growth and proliferation, has been linked to the development of malignant pancreatic neuroendocrine tumors associated with tuberous sclerosis.[94,100] Pancreatic neuroendocrine tumors in these patients can be both nonfunctional and functional.[100] Because of the possible malignant potential of these tumors, surgical resection should be considered.[100]

Von Hippel-Lindau Disease

The percentage of patients with VHL who have pancreatic involvement is 20% to 75%.[83,87,89] Pancreatic lesions associated with VHL may be the only abdominal finding associated with the disease and may precede other manifestations by several years.[83,91] Most of the patients with pancreatic involvement have pancreatic cysts, and 10% to 17% of patients are diagnosed with pancreatic neuroendocrine tumors (PNET).[100] One study of 158 patients with VHL showed that among patients with pancreatic involvement 91% had pancreatic cysts, 12.3% had serous cystadenomas, 12.3% had PNET, and 11.5% had combined lesions.[90] Although pancreatic cysts are typically asymptomatic, these lesions can have local compressive effects, require treatment, and thus should be closely monitored.[83,91] Patients with VHL who are diagnosed with PNET are diagnosed at a younger age (mean, 29 to 38 years) than their sporadic counterparts.[91,100] In addition, PNETs among patients with VHL can be multiple in nature and are located throughout the pancreas.[91] As many as 60% of PNETs associated with VHL have a clear cell morphology.[91] Patients with PNET involvement require surgical resection because of the malignant potential of these tumors.[83,91,100]

Patients with VHL should be screened for pancreatic lesions starting at age 12 years.[101] Lesions should be resected if there is no evidence of metastatic disease, the lesion is larger than 2 cm if located in the head of the pancreas, and the lesion is larger than 3 cm when located elsewhere in the pancreas.[101] In addition, resecting PNETs should be carefully considered if the patient is having an exploratory laparotomy for another manifestation of VHL.[101]

Neurofibromatosis 1 (Von Recklinghausen Disease)

Even though pheochromocytomas are the most common endocrine malignancy associated with NF1, other tumors, such as pancreatic insulinomas (only a few case reports) and duodenal somatostatinomas, have been associated with NF1.[66] Patients with duodenal somatostatinomas may present with hyperglycemia, cholelithiasis, and malabsorption, but more commonly complain of nonspecific symptoms, such as weight loss, abdominal pain, or change in bowel habits.[75] To date, only 34 patients with both NF1 and duodenal somatostatinomas have been reported in the literature.[75] Among these patients, 56% of the tumors measured less than 2 cm.[74] Sixty percent of the patients underwent a pancreaticoduodenectomy, whereas the remaining patients had local excision.[102] The optimal surgical treatment of duodenal somatostatinomas is unclear at this time.[102] Some experts advocate local excision for tumors smaller than 2 cm, and total excision for tumors larger than 2 cm.[102] However, given that as many as 70% of surgical cases are associated with regional or portal metastasis, an aggressive surgical approach is indicated.[86,100]

SUMMARY

The development of genetic testing has allowed the identification of patients with familial endocrine diseases. The importance of this technological advancement cannot be underestimated, as some of these inheritable diseases have significant malignant potential. For instance, locating high-risk patients may improve overall survival when prophylactic surgery is warranted, as in familial medullary carcinoma of the thyroid. Similarly, appropriate screening in patients with inheritable diseases will help clinicians recognize specific malignancies early in their course in attempts to achieve the best potential cure. As technology continues to progress, the knowledge base of familial endocrinopathies will continue to expand.

ACKNOWLEDGMENTS

The authors thank Jack W. Martin, DDS, Professor of Dental Oncology at the University of Texas M. D. Anderson Cancer Center, Houston TX, for his contributions to this manuscript and Linda McGraw, surgical endocrinology program coordinator at the University of Texas M. D. Anderson Cancer Center, for her administrative assistance. The authors would also like to thank Roberto and Lucy Faith for their support of the surgical endocrinology education fund.

REFERENCES

1. Stedman TL. Stedman's medical dictionary. 28th edition. Philadelphia: Lippincott Williams & Wilkins; 2006.
2. Welbourn RB, Friesen SR, Johnston IDA, et al. The history of endocrine surgery. New York: Praeger Publishers; 1990.

3. Kocher T. Concerning pathological manifestations in low-grade thyroid diseases. Nobel lectures, physiology or medicine 1901-1921. Amsterdam: Elsevier; 1967.
4. Huggins C. Nobel Lectures, Physiology or Medicine 1963-1970. Endocrine-induced regression of cancers. Amsterdam: Elsevier; 1972.
5. Canzian F, et al. A gene predisposing to familial thyroid tumors with cell oxyphilia maps to chromosome 19p13.2. Am J Hum Genet 1998;63(6):1743–8.
6. Kebebew E. Hereditary non-medullary thyroid cancer. World J Surg 2008;32(5): 678–82.
7. Grossman RF, et al. Familial nonmedullary thyroid cancer. An emerging entity that warrants aggressive treatment. Arch Surg 1995;130(8):892–7 [discussion: 898–9].
8. Triponez F, et al. Does familial non-medullary thyroid cancer adversely affect survival? World J Surg 2006;30(5):787–93.
9. Alsanea O, et al. Is familial non-medullary thyroid carcinoma more aggressive than sporadic thyroid cancer? A multicenter series. Surgery 2000;128(6): 1043–50 [discussion: 1050–1].
10. Charkes ND. On the prevalence of familial nonmedullary thyroid cancer in multiply affected kindreds. Thyroid 2006;16(2):181–6.
11. Malchoff CD, Malchoff DM. Familial nonmedullary thyroid carcinoma. Cancer Control 2006;13(2):106–10.
12. Lloyd KM 2nd, Dennis M. Cowden's disease. A possible new symptom complex with multiple system involvement. Ann Intern Med 1963;58:136–42.
13. Eng C. PTEN: one gene, many syndromes. Hum Mutat 2003;22(3):183–98.
14. Dotto J, Nose V. Familial thyroid carcinoma: a diagnostic algorithm. Adv Anat Pathol 2008;15(6):332–49.
15. Xiao Y, et al. PTEN catalysis of phospholipid dephosphorylation reaction follows a two-step mechanism in which the conserved aspartate-92 does not function as the general acid-mechanistic analysis of a familial Cowden disease-associated PTEN mutation. Cell Signal 2007;19(7):1434–45.
16. Teresi RE, et al. Cowden syndrome-affected patients with PTEN promoter mutations demonstrate abnormal protein translation. Am J Hum Genet 2007;81(4):756–67.
17. Nelen MR, et al. Novel PTEN mutations in patients with Cowden disease: absence of clear genotype-phenotype correlations. Eur J Hum Genet 1999; 7(3):267–73.
18. Liaw D, et al. Germline mutations of the PTEN gene in Cowden disease, an inherited breast and thyroid cancer syndrome. Nat Genet 1997;16(1):64–7.
19. Zhou XP, et al. Germline PTEN promoter mutations and deletions in Cowden/Bannayan-Riley-Ruvalcaba syndrome result in aberrant PTEN protein and dys-regulation of the phosphoinositol-3-kinase/Akt pathway. Am J Hum Genet 2003;73(2):404–11.
20. Nose V. Familial non-medullary thyroid carcinoma: an update. Endocr Pathol 2008; 19(4):226–40.
21. Blumenthal GM, Dennis PA. PTEN hamartoma tumor syndromes. Eur J Hum Genet 2008;16(11):1289–300.
22. Harach HR, et al. Thyroid pathologic findings in patients with Cowden disease. Ann Diagn Pathol 1999;3(6):331–40.
23. Eng Charis, Parsons R. Cowden syndrome. In: Seils Andrea, Boyle Peter J, editors. The genetic basis of human cancer, SRN. New York: McGraw-Hill; 2002. p. 527–37.
24. Thull DL, Vogel VG. Recognition and management of hereditary breast cancer syndromes. Oncologist 2004;9(1):13–24.

25. Fackenthal JD, et al. Male breast cancer in Cowden syndrome patients with germline PTEN mutations. J Med Genet 2001;38(3):159–64.
26. Groen EJ, et al. Extra-intestinal manifestations of familial adenomatous polyposis. Ann Surg Oncol 2008;15(9):2439–50.
27. Perrier ND, et al. Thyroid cancer in patients with familial adenomatous polyposis. World J Surg 1998;22(7):738–42 [discussion: 743].
28. Uchino S, et al. Mutational analysis of the APC gene in cribriform-morula variant of papillary thyroid carcinoma. World J Surg 2006;30(5):775–9.
29. Herraiz M, et al. Prevalence of thyroid cancer in familial adenomatous polyposis syndrome and the role of screening ultrasound examinations. Clin Gastroenterol Hepatol 2007;5(3):367–73.
30. Carney JA, et al. The complex of myxomas, spotty pigmentation, and endocrine overactivity. Medicine (Baltimore) 1985;64(4):270–83.
31. Boikos SA, Stratakis CA. Carney complex: pathology and molecular genetics. Neuroendocrinology 2006;83(3-4):189–99.
32. Ishikawa Y, et al. Unusual features of thyroid carcinomas in Japanese patients with Werner syndrome and possible genotype-phenotype relations to cell type and race. Cancer 1999;85(6):1345–52.
33. Kloos RT, et al. Medullary thyroid cancer: management guidelines of the American Thyroid Association. Thyroid 2009;19(6):565–612.
34. Etit D, et al. Histopathologic and clinical features of medullary microcarcinoma and C-cell hyperplasia in prophylactic thyroidectomies for medullary carcinoma: a study of 42 cases. Arch Pathol Lab Med 2008;132(11):1767–73.
35. Evans DB, Shapiro SE, Cote GJ. Invited commentary: medullary thyroid cancer: the importance of RET testing. Surgery 2007;141(1):96–9.
36. Brandi ML, et al. Guidelines for diagnosis and therapy of MEN type 1 and type 2. J Clin Endocrinol Metab 2001;86(12):5658–71.
37. Kouvaraki MA, et al. RET proto-oncogene: a review and update of genotype-phenotype correlations in hereditary medullary thyroid cancer and associated endocrine tumors. Thyroid 2005;15(6):531–44.
38. Schwartz DL, et al. Postoperative radiotherapy for advanced medullary thyroid cancer—local disease control in the modern era. Head Neck 2008;30(7):883–8.
39. Pendred V. Deaf-mutism and goitre. Lancet 1896;148(3808):532.
40. Everett LA, et al. Pendred syndrome is caused by mutations in a putative sulphate transporter gene (PDS). Nat Genet 1997;17(4):411–22.
41. Banghova K, et al. Pendred syndrome among patients with congenital hypothyroidism detected by neonatal screening: identification of two novel PDS/SLC26A4 mutations. Eur J Pediatr 2008;167(7):777–83.
42. Lai CC, et al. Analysis of the SLC26A4 gene in patients with Pendred syndrome in Taiwan. Metabolism 2007;56(9):1279–84.
43. Kopp P, Pesce L, Solis SJ. Pendred syndrome and iodide transport in the thyroid. Trends Endocrinol Metab 2008;19(7):260–8.
44. DeVita Vincent T Jr, Lawrence TS, Rosenburg Steven A. Devita, Hellman & Rosenberg's cancer: principles & practice of oncology. Philadelphia: Lippincott Williams & Wilkins; 2008.
45. Masi G, et al. Clinical, genetic, and histopathologic investigation of HRPT2-related familial hyperparathyroidism. Endocr Relat Cancer 2008;15(4):1115–26.
46. Guarnieri V, et al. Diagnosis of parathyroid tumors in familial isolated hyperparathyroidism with HRPT2 mutation: implications for cancer surveillance. J Clin Endocrinol Metab 2006;91(8):2827–32.

47. Villablanca A, et al. Germline and de novo mutations in the HRPT2 tumour suppressor gene in familial isolated hyperparathyroidism (FIHP). J Med Genet 2004;41(3):e32.
48. Carling T, Udelsman R. Parathyroid surgery in familial hyperparathyroid disorders. J Intern Med 2005;257(1):27–37.
49. Masi G, et al. Clinical, genetic, and histopathologic investigation of CDC73-related familial hyperparathyroidism. Endocr Relat Cancer 2008;15(4):1115–26.
50. Kjellman M, Larsson C, Backdahl M. Genetic background of adrenocortical tumor development. World J Surg 2001;25(7):948–56.
51. Soon PS, et al. Molecular markers and the pathogenesis of adrenocortical cancer. Oncologist 2008;13(5):548–61.
52. Maher ER, Reik W. Beckwith-Wiedemann syndrome: imprinting in clusters revisited. J Clin Invest 2000;105(3):247–52.
53. Alsultan A, et al. Simultaneous occurrence of right adrenocortical tumor and left adrenal neuroblastoma in an infant with Beckwith-Wiedemann syndrome. Pediatr Blood Cancer 2008;51(5):695–8.
54. Pizzo PA, editor. Principles and practice of pediatric oncology. 5th edition. Philadelphia: Lippincott Williams and Wilkins; 2006.
55. Beckwith JB. Extreme cytomegaly of the adrenal fetal cortex, omphalocele, hyperplasia of kidneys and pancreas, and Leydig cell hyperplasia: another syndrome?. Los Angeles (CA): Western Society for Pediatric Research; 1963.
56. Wiedemann HR. Complexe malformatif famital avec hernie ombilicale et macroglossie; un "syndrome nouveau"? J Genet Hum 1964;13:223–363 [in French].
57. Barlaskar FM, Hammer GD. The molecular genetics of adrenocortical carcinoma. Rev Endocr Metab Disord 2007;8(4):343–8.
58. Malkin HA. Devita, Hellman & Rosenburg's cancer: principles & practice of oncology. section 1: molecular biology of childhood cancers. In: Devita L, Rosenburg, editors. Philadelphia: Lippincott, Williams & Wilkins; 2008. p. 2033–42.
59. Agir H, MacKinnon C, Tan ST. Li-Fraumeni syndrome: a case with 4 separate primary sarcomas and 5 sequential free flaps in the maxillofacial region. J Oral Maxillofac Surg 2008;66(8):1714–9.
60. Bertherat J, Groussin L, Bertagna X. Mechanisms of disease: adrenocortical tumors—molecular advances and clinical perspectives. Nat Clin Pract Endocrinol Metab 2006;2(11):632–41.
61. Gonzalez RJ, et al. Laparoscopic resection of adrenal cortical carcinoma: a cautionary note. Surgery 2005;138(6):1078–85 [discussion: 1085-6].
62. Terzolo M, et al. Adjuvant mitotane treatment for adrenocortical carcinoma. N Engl J Med 2007;356(23):2372–80.
63. Bryant J, et al. Pheochromocytoma: the expanding genetic differential diagnosis. J Natl Cancer Inst 2003;95(16):1196–204.
64. Perren A, et al. Pancreatic endocrine tumors are a rare manifestation of the neurofibromatosis type 1 phenotype: molecular analysis of a malignant insulinoma in a NF-1 patient. Am J Surg Pathol 2006;30(8):1047–51.
65. Korf BR. Statins, bone, and neurofibromatosis type 1. BMC Med 2008;6:22.
66. Bettini R, et al. Ampullary somatostatinomas and jejunal gastrointestinal stromal tumor in a patient with Von Recklinghausen's disease. World J Gastroenterol 2007;13(19):2761–3.
67. Dackiw AP, et al. Adrenal cortical carcinoma. World J Surg 2001;25(7):914–26.
68. Fareau GG, et al. Systemic chemotherapy for adrenocortical carcinoma: comparative responses to conventional first-line therapies. Anticancer Drugs 2008;19(6):637–44.

69. Gonzalez RJ, et al. Response to mitotane predicts outcome in patients with recurrent adrenal cortical carcinoma. Surgery 2007;142(6):867–75 [discussion: 867–75].
70. Davis GB, Berk RN. Intestinal neurofibromas in von Recklinghausen's disease. Am J Gastroenterol 1973;60(4):410–4.
71. Upadhyaya M, et al. Germline and somatic NF1 gene mutations in plexiform neurofibromas. Hum Mutat 2008;29(8):E103–11.
72. Ferner RE, et al. Guidelines for the diagnosis and management of individuals with neurofibromatosis 1. J Med Genet 2007;44(2):81–8.
73. Walther MM, et al. von Recklinghausen's disease and pheochromocytomas. J Urol 1999;162(5):1582–6.
74. House MG, Yeo CJ, Schulick RD. Periampullary pancreatic somatostatinoma. Ann Surg Oncol 2002;9(9):869–74.
75. Fendrich V, et al. Duodenal somatostatinoma associated with Von Recklinghausen's disease. J Hepatobiliary Pancreat Surg 2004;11(6):417–21.
76. Yip L, et al. Surgical management of hereditary pheochromocytoma. J Am Coll Surg 2004;198(4):525–34 [discussion: 534–5].
77. Lee JE, et al. Cortical-sparing adrenalectomy for patients with bilateral pheochromocytoma. Surgery 1996;120(6):1064–70 [discussion: 1070–1].
78. Pacak K. Preoperative management of the pheochromocytoma patient. J Clin Endocrinol Metab 2007;92(11):4069–79.
79. Perrier ND, et al. Posterior retroperitoneoscopic adrenalectomy: preferred technique for removal of benign tumors and isolated metastases. Ann Surg 2008; 248(4):666–74.
80. Woodward ER, Maher ER. Von Hippel-Lindau disease and endocrine tumour susceptibility. Endocr Relat Cancer 2006;13(2):415–25.
81. Hippel EV. Vorstellung eines Patienten mit einem sehr ungewöhnlichen Netzhaut beziehungsweise Aderhautleiden. Heidelberg: Versammlung der Ophthalmologischen Gesellschaft; 1895. [in German].
82. Fulton JF. Harvey Cushing: a biography. Springfield (IL): CC Thomas; 1946. p. 1–755.
83. Delman KA, et al. Abdominal visceral lesions in von Hippel-Lindau disease: incidence and clinical behavior of pancreatic and adrenal lesions at a single center. World J Surg 2006;30(5):665–9.
84. Lewis CE, Yeh MW. Inherited endocrinopathies: an update. Mol Genet Metab 2008;94(3):271–82.
85. Eisenhofer G, et al. Biochemical diagnosis of pheochromocytoma: how to distinguish true- from false-positive test results. J Clin Endocrinol Metab 2003;88(6):2656–66.
86. Toumpanakis CG, Caplin ME. Molecular genetics of gastroenteropancreatic neuroendocrine tumors. Am J Gastroenterol 2008;103(3):729–32.
87. Hammel PR, et al. Pancreatic involvement in von Hippel-Lindau disease. The Groupe Francophone d'Etude de la Maladie de von Hippel-Lindau. Gastroenterology 2000;119(4):1087–95.
88. Hough DM, et al. Pancreatic lesions in von Hippel-Lindau disease: prevalence, clinical significance, and CT findings. AJR Am J Roentgenol 1994;162(5):1091–4.
89. Lubensky IA, et al. Multiple neuroendocrine tumors of the pancreas in von Hippel-Lindau disease patients: histopathological and molecular genetic analysis. Am J Pathol 1998;153(1):223–31.
90. Nadella KS, et al. Targeted deletion of Prkar1a reveals a role for protein kinase A in mesenchymal-to-epithelial transition. Cancer Res 2008;68(8):2671–7.
91. Stratakis CA, Kirschner LS, Carney JA. Clinical and molecular features of the Carney complex: diagnostic criteria and recommendations for patient evaluation. J Clin Endocrinol Metab 2001;86(9):4041–6.

92. Ohara N, et al. Carney's complex with primary pigmented nodular adrenocortical disease and spotty pigmentations. Intern Med 1993;32(1):60–2.
93. Verhoef S, et al. Malignant pancreatic tumour within the spectrum of tuberous sclerosis complex in childhood. Eur J Pediatr 1999;158(4):284–7.
94. Francalanci P, et al. Malignant pancreatic endocrine tumor in a child with tuberous sclerosis. Am J Surg Pathol 2003;27(10):1386–9.
95. Elliott M, et al. Clinical features and natural history of Beckwith-Wiedemann syndrome: presentation of 74 new cases. Clin Genet 1994;46(2):168–74.
96. Hussain K, et al. Hyperinsulinemic hypoglycemia in Beckwith-Wiedemann syndrome due to defects in the function of pancreatic beta-cell adenosine triphosphate-sensitive potassium channels. J Clin Endocrinol Metab 2005; 90(7):4376–82.
97. DeBaun MR, King AA, White N. Hypoglycemia in Beckwith-Wiedemann syndrome. Semin Perinatol 2000;24(2):164–71.
98. Fukuzawa R, et al. Nesidioblastosis and mixed hamartoma of the liver in Beckwith-Wiedemann syndrome: case study including analysis of H19 methylation and insulin-like growth factor 2 genotyping and imprinting. Pediatr Dev Pathol 2001;4(4):381–90.
99. Au KS, Ward CH, Northrup H. Tuberous sclerosis complex: disease modifiers and treatments. Curr Opin Pediatr 2008;20(6):628–33.
100. Jensen RT, et al. Inherited pancreatic endocrine tumor syndromes: advances in molecular pathogenesis, diagnosis, management, and controversies. Cancer 2008;113(suppl 7):1807–43.
101. Libutti SK, et al. Clinical and genetic analysis of patients with pancreatic neuroendocrine tumors associated with von Hippel-Lindau disease. Surgery 2000; 128(6):1022–7 [discussion: 1027–8].
102. Kaelin WG Jr. The von Hippel-Lindau tumour suppressor protein: O_2 sensing and cancer. Nat Rev Cancer 2008;8(11):865–73.

Surgical Management of Zollinger-Ellison Syndrome; State of the Art

Ellen H. Morrow, MD, Jeffrey A. Norton, MD*

KEYWORDS

- Gastrinoma • Surgery • Diagnosis • Localization
- Outcome • MEN-1

Zollinger-Ellison Syndrome (ZES) was originally described in 1955.[1] It is a syndrome of acid hypersecretion caused by a gastrin-producing tumor (gastrinoma). Since the recognition of this disease entity, diagnosis and treatment strategies have changed greatly. The purpose of this review is to describe the current standard in diagnosis and surgical management of ZES and to outline some controversies that have arisen recently.

EPIDEMIOLOGY

The incidence of ZES in the United States is one to three new cases per million per year, making it a rare condition.[2] Eighty percent of gastrinomas occur sporadically, while 20% are associated with Multiple Endocrine Neoplasia Type 1 (MEN-1).[3] ZES causes 0.1% to 1% of peptic ulcer disease.[4] Men are slightly more likely to develop ZES.[5] The mean age at which symptoms begin is 41 years.[6] Patients with MEN-1–associated ZES are likely to present at a younger age; in the third decade of life.[7] ZES occurs in approximately 25% of patients with MEN-1.[8]

PRESENTATION

The presenting signs and symptoms of ZES have also changed with earlier recognition and diagnosis. Initially, it was described as gastric acid hypersecretion, ulcers in unusual locations (jejunum), recurrent ulcers, and nonbeta islet cell tumors of the pancreas.[9] Subsequent studies of large numbers of patients with ZES have demonstrated that common presenting symptoms include abdominal pain, diarrhea, heartburn, nausea, and weight loss.[6] Diarrhea is a common problem as approximately 80% of patients

Division of General Surgery, Department of Surgery, Stanford University School of Medicine, 300 Pasteur Drive, H3591, Stanford, CA 94305-5641, USA
* Corresponding author.
E-mail address: janorton@stanford.edu (J.A. Norton).

Surg Clin N Am 89 (2009) 1091–1103
doi:10.1016/j.suc.2009.06.018
0039-6109/09/$ – see front matter © 2009 Elsevier Inc. All rights reserved.

with ZES have this symptom. Given the nonspecific nature of these symptoms, and the rarity of ZES as compared with more common disorders, such as gastroesophageal reflux disease or routine peptic ulcer disease, there is commonly a significant delay in the diagnosis of ZES. The most common initial diagnosis for patients with ZES is idiopathic peptic ulcer disease.[8] The mean time from onset of symptoms to diagnosis of ZES is 5.9 years.[6] Although the time to diagnosis has remained constant over the past 30 years, there is some evidence that it may prove even more challenging with the widespread use of proton pump inhibitors (PPI).[10] PPI provide very effective acid suppression, which may defer the diagnosis even further.[11,12]

The presentation of ZES in MEN-1 may differ somewhat from patients with sporadic ZES. A recent NIH study demonstrated a higher incidence of severe esophageal disease including Barrett's esophagus in patients with MEN-ZES.[13] Despite the high frequency of ZES in MEN-1, the diagnosis is still usually delayed. Only 5% of patients with MEN-1 are initially diagnosed correctly, compared with 2% of patients with sporadic ZES.[8]

Given the continued delay in diagnosis of ZES, recommendations have been made regarding factors which should increase a clinician's suspicion for the syndrome. Patients who present with the triad of abdominal pain, diarrhea and weight loss, patients who have recurrent or refractory ulcers, patients with prominent gastric rugal folds on endoscopy, or patients with MEN-1 and gastrointestinal symptoms should be tested for ZES.[8] In addition, symptoms of acid hypersecretion associated with diarrhea should indicate the possibility of ZES.[2]

At the time of diagnosis, some patients will have minimal or nonimageable tumor while others may have advanced disease (ie, greater than 40% have lymph node metastases). The duodenum is the most common site of a primary gastrinoma, while the pancreas is the second most common site (**Fig. 1**). Lymph node metastases do not affect survival, while liver metastases do. Hepatic metastases (**Fig. 2**) occur more commonly with pancreatic gastrinomas than duodenal. They may occur in up to 60% of pancreatic cases and less than 10% of duodenal cases.[14]

DIAGNOSIS

Suspicion for the diagnosis of ZES should be aroused when any of the above factors are present. Once the clinician suspects ZES, diagnostic workup should begin with

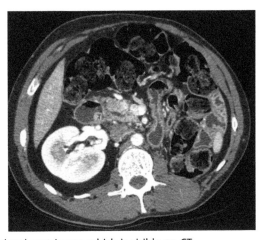

Fig. 1. A large duodenal gastrinoma which is visible on CT.

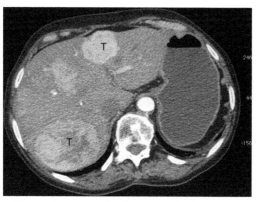

Fig. 2. Arterial phase CT scan demonstrating hypervascular liver metastases.

a fasting serum gastrin level and ascertainment of the presence of gastric acid hyper-secretion. All patients with ZES will have a fasting gastrin greater than 100 pg/mL.[7] A greater than tenfold increase in serum gastrin is more characteristic, and can be diagnostic of ZES with gastric pH less than 2.1.[5] Patients should have PPI held for one week before this test, as acid suppression with PPI will artificially elevate the gastrin level.[2,12,15] H2 blockers should be held for 2 days.[5] **Table 1** outlines other conditions which can cause elevated serum gastrin, including renal failure, short bowel syndrome, antral G cell hyperplasia, atrophic gastritis and retained gastric antrum.[2,3]

Demonstration of acid hypersecretion (in the presence of elevated gastrin) is also critical to make the diagnosis of ZES. Therefore, gastric pH or basal acid output must be measured off medications that inhibit acid secretion, such as PPI, and so forth. Basal acid output greater than 15 mEq/hr is diagnostic as is pH less than 2.[3]

The secretin stimulation test is also confirmatory and can be used to establish the diagnosis in patients with otherwise equivocal results (ie, gastrin between 100 and 500 pg/mL and gastric pH <2.1).[5] However, it is positive in only 85% of patients with ZES.[3] This is a provocative test in which a 2U/kg bolus of secretin is given intravenously (IV), and serum gastrin is subsequently measured at certain time points. A rise in serum gastrin of 200 pg/mL is consistent with ZES. The secretin test can also be used for patients who cannot have their PPI withheld.[8] However, in our experience

Table 1
Differential diagnosis of biochemical abnormalities seen in Zollinger-Ellison syndrome

Hypergastrinemia with Excessive Gastric Acid Production	Hypergastrinemia without Excessive Gastric Acid Production
Zollinger-Ellison syndrome	Pernicious anemia, Atrophic gastritis
Gastric outlet obstruction	Acid reducing medications (H2 antagonists or PPI)
Retained gastric antrum	Renal failure
G-cell hyperplasia	Postvagotomy
	Short gut syndrome

Data from Peterson DA, Dolan JP, Norton JA. Neuroendocrine tumors of the pancreas and gastro-intestinal tract and carcinoid disease. 2nd edition. New York: Springer; 2008.

all patients with ZES can have the PPI held despite grave concerns by referring doctors.

PREOPERATIVE IMAGING

Once the biochemical diagnosis of ZES is established, imaging should be undertaken in an attempt to localize the tumor. **Tables 2** and **3** outline the sensitivities of the various imaging modalities. Somatostatin receptor scintigraphy (SRS) is the study of choice (**Fig. 3**). SRS uses radiolabelled octreotide and single photon emission computed tomography (SPECT) to image the gastrinoma. The sensitivity of SRS has been shown to equal that of all other imaging modalities combined.[16,17] Its sensitivity is estimated between 58% and 78% and it can image tumors in ectopic locations.[16,18,19] The sensitivity of SRS is dependent on tumor size. It detects 96% of tumors larger than 2 cm, but in one study SRS missed 33% of gastrinomas identified at surgery.[16] These tumors were generally small (ie, <1 cm) tumors located within the duodenum. SRS is the best study for localizing primary and metastatic gastrinoma.[17] The use of SRS affects management plans in 19% to 53% of cases.[18,20]

Endoscopic ultrasound (EUS) may be the most sensitive study for pancreatic gastrinomas.[21] However, EUS is not generally helpful for duodenal tumors or liver metastases. EUS may be most useful, therefore, in patients with MEN-1 who are likely to have multiple small pancreatic tumors.

CT provides more anatomic information than SRS, but has lower sensitivity (see **Table 2**). It is critical to exclude large tumors within the pancreas and liver metastases. Gastrinomas are vascular tumors so they are best imaged on the arterial phase of CT (**Fig. 4**). It is an important study, and should be used as one of the two initial imaging modalities. MRI can be used to provide anatomic information if, for some reason, CT is not preferred in a given case.

SURGICAL MANAGEMENT: STANDARD OF CARE

There are two main goals in the treatment of ZES: control of acid production and its sequelae, and treatment of a potentially malignant tumor. Surgical treatment is currently focused on treatment of the tumor, as very effective medical therapy for acid hypersecretion has existed since the development of proton pump inhibitors, such as omeprazole. The typical dose to control acid hypersecretion is 40 mg omeprazole twice a day. Intravenous PPI, such as protonix, are used during surgery and the usual dose in ZES is 80 mg IV every 12 hours. Gastric pH should be measured to be certain acid hypersecretion is controlled. Historically, total gastrectomy was used to treat patients with ZES, but this has not been necessary since the development of PPI, which are much more powerful than H2-receptor antagonists.[22,23]

Table 2	
Results of preoperative imaging studies for primary gastrinoma	
Imaging Modality	**Sensitivity**
SRS	85%
CT	54%–56%
MRI	25%–30%
EUS	67%
Arterial Angiography	28%–59%

Data from Klose KJ, Heverhagen JT. Localisation and staging of gastrin producing umours using cross-sectional imaging modalities. Wien Klin Wochenschr 2007;119(19–20):588–92.

Table 3
Results of imaging studies for metastatic gastrinoma

Imaging Modality	Sensitivity
SRS	92%
CT	42%–56%
MRI	71%–83%
Arterial Angiography	61%–62%

Data from Klose KJ, Heverhagen JT. Localisation and staging of gastrin producing tumours using cross-sectional imaging modalities. Wien Klin Wochenschr 2007;119(19–20):588–92.

Gastrinomas are most frequently located in the duodenum (60%) especially in patients with negative imaging studies. The gastrinoma triangle is an area defined by the junction of the cystic and common bile ducts superiorly, the junction of the second and third portions of the duodenum inferiorly, and the junction of the neck and body of the pancreas medially.[24] Approximately 80% of gastrinomas are found in the gastrinoma triangle, and tumors to the left of the superior mesenteric artery are more malignant than those in the triangle.[19] It is controversial, but there is evidence for the existence of lymph node primary gastrinomas. One study suggests that approximately 15% of patients with ZES may have lymph node-primary gastrinomas. This has been proven by cure of ZES with long-term follow-up following removal of only lymph nodes in the gastrinoma triangle.[25] Others suggest, however, that the primary tumor, probably within the duodenum, was missed and that these patients will recur.

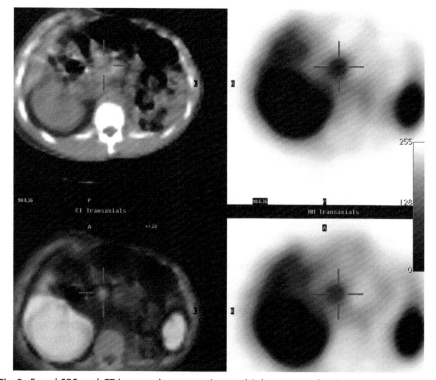

Fig. 3. Fused SRS and CT images demonstrating multiple neuroendocrine tumors.

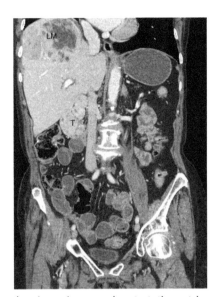

Fig. 4. Coronal CT image showing primary and metastatic gastrinoma.

It is estimated that 60% to 90% of gastrinomas are malignant.[5] Tumor progression and metastases are the chief determinants of survival in patients with ZES whose acid production is controlled medically.[24,26,27] The chief goal of surgery, then, is to cure or control the tumor, and prevent metastases. These goals vary somewhat depending on whether gastrinoma occurs sporadically, or in the setting of MEN-1.

In sporadic ZES, the goal of surgery is to cure the disease. All patients with a biochemical diagnosis of sporadic ZES should undergo surgical exploration. This is recommended because high-cure rates have been demonstrated in patients with sporadic ZES. A series of 123 patients showed an immediate postoperative cure rate of 60%, a 5-year cure rate of 40%, and a 10-year cure rate of 34%.[28] Given that up to 30% of gastrinomas can be missed by preoperative imaging studies, surgical exploration is warranted in all patients with biochemical diagnosis of sporadic ZES regardless of imaging results.

The recommended surgical approach is exploratory laparotomy with extended Kocher maneuver and careful palpation of the pancreas and duodenum for nodules. Intraoperative ultrasound (IOUS) should be used for identification of small pancreatic lesions. IOUS may have higher sensitivity than preoperative imaging methods because it can localize tumors with resolution to 5 mm in the pancreas.[29,30] Enucleation of pancreatic head tumors should be performed, or distal pancreatectomy for tail lesions, and duodenotomy and regional lymphadenectomy.[19] Some also recommend intraoperative gastrin measurements to confirm surgical cure before closure.[31] This is not standard in all centers, however, and may not be necessary since a high-cure rate has been demonstrated with standard surgical procedure including duodenotomy (**Fig. 5**).[32]

Duodenotomy is indicated in all patients undergoing surgery for ZES. Duodenotomy is the most effective method of identifying duodenal gastrinomas, which represent 60% of gastrinomas.[33] Making duodenotomy a standard part of operations for ZES doubled the cure rate from 30% to 60%.[34,35] Lymph node sampling is also an important part of surgery for ZES. In addition to the existence of primary lymph node gastrinomas, there is a high rate of lymph node metastases. Removal of all regional lymph nodes is recommended.[3]

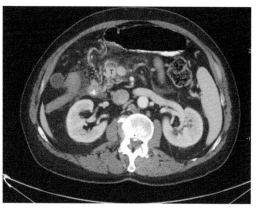

Fig. 5. Gastrinoma in the pancreatic head.

In patients with MEN-1, the management of gastrinomas is somewhat controversial and more complicated. Patients with MEN-1 are unlikely to be cured of ZES with surgery. Some studies have demonstrated cures, but they did not do a full biochemical assessment postoperatively, including negative secretin test and measurement of serial levels of fasting gastrin.[36] A large NIH study demonstrated a 0% cure rate in patients with ZES and MEN-1.[28] This may be secondary to the fact that their tumors tend to be multiple, small, and located in the duodenum.[28,37] There have been cures in patients with MEN-1 treated with Whipple pancreaticoduodenectomy; however, most suggest that the low-grade malignancy rate of duodenal gastrinoma does not warrant this potentially morbid surgery.

Despite the evidence against surgical cure in patients with ZES and MEN-1, there is still significant benefit to surgery in many of these patients. The goal of surgery for patients with ZES and MEN-1 is largely prevention of metastatic disease. The extent of liver metastases is the main determinant of survival.[38] Surgical resection of the primary pancreatic gastrinoma has been shown to prevent the development of liver metastases.[39] The risk of developing liver metastases increases with the size of the primary pancreatic gastrinoma. Patients with gastrinomas less than 1 cm have a 4% rate of liver metastases compared with 28% with gastrinomas that are 1 to 3 cm and a 61% rate of liver metastases with tumors greater than 3 cm.[7,38] For this reason, it is recommended that patients with ZES and MEN-1 undergo surgery to remove any pancreatic gastrinoma greater than 2 cm.[40]

Another aspect of the treatment of patients with ZES in MEN-1 is the sequencing of procedures. The majority of patients with MEN-1 have primary hyperparathyroidism secondary to multigland hyperplasia. Surgical treatment of the parathyroid hyperplasia can reduce the effects of excess gastrin secretion on acid hypersecretion.[41] For this reason, patients with hyperparathyroidism and ZES in the setting of MEN-1 should have their parathyroid surgery first. The recommended procedure is a three and one-half gland parathyroidectomy.

SURGICAL MANAGEMENT; CONTROVERSIES

Although the above guidelines have been established over the past 50 years of research and treatment of ZES, some controversial aspects of treatment remain and some new controversies are arising.

Control of acid hypersecretion is no longer the primary focus of surgical management; however, the question remains as to whether acid-reducing procedures should be performed at the time of laparotomy for tumor resection in ZES. Vagotomy is not a standard part of surgical procedures for ZES at this time, but including parietal cell vagotomy does appear to reduce the long-term need for acid-inhibitory pharmacotherapy in patients who have persistent or recurrent disease.[42] This may be important since there are likely to be some adverse sequelae of long-term acid-inhibition therapy. Achlorhydria occurs frequently in patients using PPI, and may lead to B12 and iron deficiency.[43,44] Further, in patients with MEN-1 and ZES, long-term use of PPI have led to the development of malignant gastric carcinoid tumors. For these reasons, vagotomy may be considered when laparotomy is performed for gastrinoma.

The use of pancreaticoduodenectomy in ZES is also debated. Given the good prognosis of patients with even metastatic gastrinoma, there is hesitation about using a procedure with high morbidity and mortality. Patients with distant metastases still have a 15- year survival of 52% according to some authors.[45] In addition, performing a Whipple makes it more difficult to come back in the future to remove recurrent tumor (**Fig. 6**), or to treat future liver metastases with interventional methods because of the altered anatomy.[40,46,47]

There are studies that have demonstrated the possibility of cure in patients with MEN1 using pancreaticoduodenectomy.[48–51] These small studies did not, however, use a full biochemical assessment serially to rule out recurrent disease. A more recent study demonstrated a cure rate of 77% in patients with MEN1-ZES, but mean follow-up was less than one year.[52] Some also estimate a higher rate of duodenal gastrinomas in patients with MEN, up to 90%, making pancreaticoduodenectomy potentially a more definitive procedure for prevention of recurrence.[53] For these reasons, some authors currently recommend that Whipple be the first line procedure for patients with MEN1-ZES who have their source of gastrin localized to the pancreatic head by selective arterial secretin injection.[9]

Our current recommendation is that Whipple procedure be reserved for young patients with large pancreatic head tumors that are not amenable to enucleation. It is possible that Whipple resection can result in increased cure rates, especially in patients with MEN-1 who are not often cured with more conservative surgical procedures. Further studies need to be done to compare long-term survival and quality of life.[54]

Relative consensus does seem to exist in the surgical management of metastatic disease, although controlled clinical trials do not exist. There is evidence that resection of liver metastases improves survival, although it is difficult to conclude for certain that the demonstrated differences in survival are dependent on surgical treatment, and not

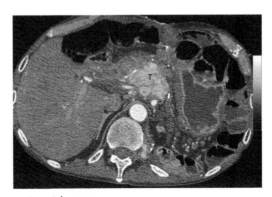

Fig. 6. A large recurrent gastrinoma.

the extent of disease itself.[36,55] A significant percentage of patients with metastatic gastrinoma can undergo liver resections that result in removal of all known disease with 5-year survival up to 85%.[56] In addition to possible survival benefit and surgical cure of metastatic disease, there may be benefit of cytoreductive surgery in ameliorating the functional endocrine tumor syndrome.[57] The current recommendation is to attempt to perform liver resection when at least 90% of the tumor appears to be able to be removed on preoperative imaging studies.

Laparoscopy is increasingly used for complex abdominal procedures, and in particular, the laparoscopic experience with pancreatic resections is growing. There are several reports of laparoscopic resections of pancreatic neuroendocrine tumors especially insulinoma.[58,59] Laparoscopic distal pancreatectomy is a promising procedure with a complication (fistula) rate equal to or less than open procedures.[59] Enucleation also appears to be feasible laparoscopically. Laparoscopic treatment of gastrinoma, however, presents some significant challenges. More than half of gastrinomas occur in the duodenum, or other extra-pancreatic locations. Gastrinomas tend to be larger than other neuroendocrine tumors, and they are more often metastatic. These factors make gastrinomas less amenable to minimally invasive techniques, as evidenced by a higher conversion rate in reported series.[58]

Since many gastrinomas are located in the duodenum, there has been some discussion of the possibility of endoscopic removal. There have been reports using snare polypectomy or band ligation. Some of these cases have reported cure of ZES, but there has also been at least one perforation.[60] Lee and colleagues[61] reported treatment of ZES with endoscopic band ligation. In this case, the patient had refused surgery. The serum gastrin level dropped from 647 to 100 pg/mL, and a postoperative biopsy near the banding site was negative for tumor.

This is an interesting report, but there are several factors that would seem to prevent endoscopic treatment from being equal to surgery in patients who are eligible for surgery. First, gastrinomas occur in a submucosal location, which makes them somewhat less amenable and safe for endoscopic resection. In addition, they are often invasive beyond the submucosa. Secondly, banding does not allow removal of the lesion, but rather causes it to slough. This makes pathologic examination less complete. It is therefore difficult to assess margins. Thirdly, in previous studies endoscopy was inferior to duodenotomy for detection of gastrinomas.[33] It is probable that gastrinomas would be missed if they were detected by endoscopy only. Finally, up to 60% of gastrinomas are associated with lymph node metastases at the time of diagnosis, making endoscopic treatment of the duodenal gastrinoma an incomplete oncologic procedure.[62]

SURVEILLANCE

Gastrin levels and secretin tests are the most sensitive methods for detecting recurrence of gastrinoma.[19,63] SRS should also be used for restaging periodically.

OUTCOMES

Surgery results in cure of ZES for 60% of patients with sporadic disease. The cure rate at 5 years is 40%.[28] Patients with MEN-1 are rarely cured. Surgery also impacts the rate of progression to liver metastases, and the rate of disease-related death. In a large series, 15 year disease-related survival was 98% for operated patients and 74% for unoperated patients.[35] The existence and extent of liver metastases are the main determinants of survival.[45]

SUMMARY

Much has been learned about the diagnosis and treatment of ZES, and certain questions require further investigation. Delay in diagnosis of ZES is still a significant problem, and clinical suspicion should be elevated. The single best imaging modality for localization and staging of ZES is somatostatin receptor scintigraphy. Goals of surgical treatment for ZES differ between sporadic and MEN-1–related cases. All sporadic cases of ZES should be surgically explored, including duodenotomy, even with negative imaging results, because of the high likelihood of finding and removing a tumor for potential cure. Surgery for MEN-1–related cases should be focused on prevention of metastatic disease, with surgery being recommended when pancreatic tumors are greater than 2 cm. The role of Whipple procedure, especially for MEN-1 cases, should be explored further. Laparoscopic and endoscopic treatments are more experimental, but may have a role.

REFERENCES

1. Zollinger RM, Ellison EH. Primary peptic ulcerations of the jejunum associated with islet cell tumors of the pancreas. Ann Surg 1955;142(4):709–23 [discussion, 724–8].
2. Gibril F, Jensen RT. Zollinger-Ellison syndrome revisited: diagnosis, biologic markers, associated inherited disorders, and acid hypersecretion. Curr Gastroenterol Rep 2004;6(6):454–63.
3. Peterson DA, Dolan JP, Norton JA. Neuroendocrine tumors of the pancreas and gastrointestinal tract and carcinoid disease. 2nd edition. New York: Springer; 2008.
4. Isenberg JI, Walsh JH, Grossman MI. Zollinger-Ellison syndrome. Gastroenterology 1973;65(1):140–65.
5. Jensen RT. Gastrinomas: advances in diagnosis and management. Neuroendocrinology 2004;80(Suppl 1):23–7.
6. Roy PK, Venzon DJ, Shojamanesh H, et al. Zollinger-Ellison syndrome. Clinical presentation in 261 patients. Medicine (Baltimore) 2000;79(6):379–411.
7. Norton JA. Gastrinoma: advances in localization and treatment. Surg Oncol Clin N Am 1998;7(4):845–61.
8. Ellison EC, Johnson JA. Current problems in surgery. The Zollinger-Ellison syndrome: a comprehensive review of historical, scientific, and clinical considerations. In brief. Curr Probl Surg 2009;46(1):6–11.
9. Fendrich V, Langer P, Waldmann J, et al. Management of sporadic and multiple endocrine neoplasia type 1 gastrinomas. Br J Surg 2007;94(11):1331–41.
10. Cisco RM, Norton JA. Surgery for gastrinoma. Adv Surg 2007;41:165–76.
11. Corleto VD, Annibale B, Gibril F, et al. Does the widespread use of proton pump inhibitors mask, complicate and/or delay the diagnosis of Zollinger-Ellison syndrome? Aliment Pharmacol Ther 2001;15(10):1555–61.
12. Jensen RT, Fraker DL. Zollinger-Ellison syndrome. Advances in treatment of gastric hypersecretion and the gastrinoma. JAMA 1994;271(18):1429–35.
13. Hoffmann KM, Gibril F, Entsuah LK, et al. Patients with multiple endocrine neoplasia type 1 with gastrinomas have an increased risk of severe esophageal disease including stricture and the premalignant condition, Barrett's esophagus. J Clin Endocrinol Metab 2006;91(1):204–12.
14. Imamura M, Komoto I, Ota S. Changing treatment strategy for gastrinoma in patients with Zollinger-Ellison syndrome. World J Surg 2006;30(1):1–11.

15. Frucht H, Howard JM, Slaff JI, et al. Secretin and calcium provocative tests in the Zollinger-Ellison syndrome. A prospective study. Ann Intern Med 1989;111(9): 713–22.
16. Alexander HR, Fraker DL, Norton JA, et al. Prospective study of somatostatin receptor scintigraphy and its effect on operative outcome in patients with Zollinger-Ellison syndrome. Ann Surg 1998;228(2):228–38.
17. Gibril F, Reynolds JC, Doppman JL, et al. Somatostatin receptor scintigraphy: its sensitivity compared with that of other imaging methods in detecting primary and metastatic gastrinomas. A prospective study. Ann Intern Med 1996;125(1):26–34.
18. Gibril F, Jensen RT. Diagnostic uses of radiolabelled somatostatin receptor analogues in gastroenteropancreatic endocrine tumours. Dig Liver Dis 2004; 36(Suppl 1):S106–20.
19. Gibril F, Jensen RT. Advances in evaluation and management of gastrinoma in patients with Zollinger-Ellison syndrome. Curr Gastroenterol Rep 2005;7(2): 114–21.
20. Termanini B, Gibril F, Reynolds JC, et al. Value of somatostatin receptor scintigraphy: a prospective study in gastrinoma of its effect on clinical management. Gastroenterology 1997;112(2):335–47.
21. Klose KJ, Heverhagen JT. Localisation and staging of gastrin producing tumours using cross-sectional imaging modalities. Wien Klin Wochenschr 2007; 119(19–20):588–92.
22. Fox PS, Hofmann JW, Decosse JJ, et al. The influence of total gastrectomy on survival in malignant Zollinger-Ellison tumors. Ann Surg 1974;180(4):558–66.
23. McCarthy DM. Report on the United States experience with cimetidine in Zollinger-Ellison syndrome and other hypersecretory states. Gastroenterology 1978; 74(2 Pt 2):453–8.
24. Stabile BE, Morrow DJ, Passaro E Jr. The gastrinoma triangle: operative implications. Am J Surg 1984;147(1):25–31.
25. Norton JA, Alexander HR, Fraker DL, et al. Possible primary lymph node gastrinoma: occurrence, natural history, and predictive factors: a prospective study. Ann Surg 2003;237(5):650–7 [discussion: 657–9].
26. Norton JA, Doppman JL, Jensen RT. Curative resection in Zollinger-Ellison syndrome. Results of a 10-year prospective study. Ann Surg 1992;215(1):8–18.
27. Sutliff VE, Doppman JL, Gibril F, et al. Growth of newly diagnosed, untreated metastatic gastrinomas and predictors of growth patterns. J Clin Oncol 1997; 15(6):2420–31.
28. Norton JA, Fraker DL, Alexander HR, et al. Surgery to cure the Zollinger-Ellison syndrome. N Engl J Med 1999;341(9):635–44.
29. Doppman JL. Pancreatic endocrine tumors–the search goes on. N Engl J Med 1992;326(26):1770–2.
30. Norton JA, Cromack DT, Shawker TH, et al. Intraoperative ultrasonographic localization of islet cell tumors. A prospective comparison to palpation. Ann Surg 1988;207(2):160–8.
31. Proye C, Pattou F, Carnaille B, et al. Intraoperative gastrin measurements during surgical management of patients with gastrinomas: experience with 20 cases. World J Surg 1998;22(7):643–9 [discussion: 649–50].
32. Norton JA, Alexander HR, Fraker DL, et al. Does the use of routine duodenotomy (DUODX) affect rate of cure, development of liver metastases, or survival in patients with Zollinger-Ellison syndrome? Ann Surg 2004;239(5):617–25 [discussion 626].
33. Norton JA. Intraoperative methods to stage and localize pancreatic and duodenal tumors. Ann Oncol 1999;10(Suppl 4):182–4.

34. Doherty GM, Thompson NW. Multiple endocrine neoplasia type 1: duodeno-pancreatic tumours. J Intern Med 2003;253(6):590–8.

35. Norton JA, Fraker DL, Alexander HR, et al. Surgery increases survival in patients with gastrinoma. Ann Surg 2006;244(3):410–9.

36. Norton JA, Jensen RT. Resolved and unresolved controversies in the surgical management of patients with Zollinger-Ellison syndrome. Ann Surg 2004; 240(5):757–73.

37. Thompson NW. Surgical treatment of the endocrine pancreas and Zollinger-Ellison syndrome in the MEN 1 syndrome. Henry Ford Hosp Med J 1992;40(3–4):195–8.

38. Weber HC, Orbuch M, Jensen RT. Diagnosis and management of Zollinger-Ellison syndrome. Semin Gastrointest Dis 1995;6(2):79–89.

39. Fraker DL, Norton JA, Alexander HR, et al. Surgery in Zollinger-Ellison syndrome alters the natural history of gastrinoma. Ann Surg 1994;220(3):320–8 [discussion: 328–30].

40. Norton JA, Fang TD, Jensen RT. Surgery for gastrinoma and insulinoma in multiple endocrine neoplasia type 1. J Natl Compr Canc Netw 2006;4(2):148–53.

41. Norton JA, Cornelius MJ, Doppman JL, et al. Effect of parathyroidectomy in patients with hyperparathyroidism, Zollinger-Ellison syndrome, and multiple endocrine neoplasia type I: a prospective study. Surgery 1987;102(6):958–66.

42. McArthur KE, Richardson CT, Barnett CC, et al. Laparotomy and proximal gastric vagotomy in Zollinger-Ellison syndrome: results of a 16-year prospective study. Am J Gastroenterol 1996;91(6):1104–11.

43. Koop H, Bachem MG. Serum iron, ferritin, and vitamin B12 during prolonged omeprazole therapy. J Clin Gastroenterol 1992;14(4):288–92.

44. Termanini B, Gibril F, Sutliff VE, et al. Effect of long-term gastric acid suppressive therapy on serum vitamin B12 levels in patients with Zollinger-Ellison syndrome. Am J Med 1998;104(5):422–30.

45. Weber HC, Venzon DJ, Lin JT, et al. Determinants of metastatic rate and survival in patients with Zollinger-Ellison syndrome: a prospective long-term study. Gastroenterology 1995;108(6):1637–49.

46. Ruszniewski P, Malka D. Hepatic arterial chemoembolization in the management of advanced digestive endocrine tumors. Digestion 2000;62(Suppl 1):79–83.

47. Ruszniewski P, Rougier P, Roche A, et al. Hepatic arterial chemoembolization in patients with liver metastases of endocrine tumors. A prospective phase II study in 24 patients. Cancer 1993;71(8):2624–30.

48. Delcore R, Friesen SR. Role of pancreatoduodenectomy in the management of primary duodenal wall gastrinomas in patients with Zollinger-Ellison syndrome. Surgery 1992;112(6):1016–22 [discussion: 1022–33].

49. Imamura M, Kanda M, Takahashi K, et al. Clinicopathological characteristics of duodenal microgastrinomas. World J Surg 1992;16(4):703–9 [discussion: 709–10].

50. Stabile BE, Passaro E Jr. Benign and malignant gastrinoma. Am J Surg 1985; 149(1):144–50.

51. Stadil F. Treatment of gastrinomas with pancreaticoduodenectomy. In: Mignon M, Jensen RT, editors. Frontiers in gastrointestinal research. Basel, Switzerland: S. Karger; 1995.

52. Tonelli F, Fratini G, Nesi G, et al. Pancreatectomy in multiple endocrine neoplasia type 1-related gastrinomas and pancreatic endocrine neoplasias. Ann Surg 2006;244(1):61–70.

53. Pipeleers-Marichal M, Somers G, Willems G, et al. Gastrinomas in the duodenums of patients with multiple endocrine neoplasia type 1 and the Zollinger-Ellison syndrome. N Engl J Med 1990;322(11):723–7.

54. Norton JA. Surgical treatment and prognosis of gastrinoma. Best Pract Res Clin Gastroenterol 2005;19(5):799–805.
55. Chen H, Hardacre JM, Uzar A, et al. Isolated liver metastases from neuroendocrine tumors: does resection prolong survival? J Am Coll Surg 1998;187(1): 88–92 [discussion: 92–3].
56. Norton JA, Doherty GM, Fraker DL, et al. Surgical treatment of localized gastrinoma within the liver: a prospective study. Surgery 1998;124(6):1145–52.
57. Sarmiento JM, Que FG. Hepatic surgery for metastases from neuroendocrine tumors. Surg Oncol Clin N Am 2003;12(1):231–42.
58. Assalia A, Gagner M. Laparoscopic pancreatic surgery for islet cell tumors of the pancreas. World J Surg 2004;28(12):1239–47.
59. Pierce RA, Spitler JA, Hawkins WG, et al. Outcomes analysis of laparoscopic resection of pancreatic neoplasms. Surg Endosc 2007;21(4):579–86.
60. Straus E, Raufman JP, Samuel S, et al. Endoscopic cure of the Zollinger-Ellison syndrome. Gastrointest Endosc 1992;38(6):709–11.
61. Lee SH, Hong YS, Lee JM, et al. Duodenal gastrinoma treated with endoscopic band ligation. Gastrointest Endosc 2009;69(4):964–7.
62. Thom AK, Norton JA, Axiotis CA, et al. Location, incidence, and malignant potential of duodenal gastrinomas. Surgery 1991;110(6):1086–91 [discussion: 1091–3].
63. Gibril F, Jensen RT. Comparative analysis of diagnostic techniques for localization of gastrointestinal neuroendocrine tumors. Yale J Biol Med 1997;70(5–6):509–22.

Insulinoma

Aarti Mathur, MD[a], Philip Gorden, MD[b], Steven K. Libutti, MD, FACS[c,d,e],*

KEYWORDS

- Insulinoma • Pancreatic neuroendocrine tumor
- Metastatic insulinoma • Management • Surgery

Insulinoma is a rare neuroendocrine tumor with an incidence of 4 per 1 million persons per year.[1] Insulinoma may occur as a unifocal sporadic event in patients without an inherited syndrome or as a part of multiple endocrine neoplasia type 1. Key neuroglycopenic and hypoglycemic symptoms in conjunction with biochemical proof establish the diagnosis. Once the diagnosis is established, the insulinoma is preoperatively localized within the pancreas with the goal of surgical excision for cure. This review discusses the historical background, diagnosis, and management of sporadic insulinoma.

HISTORICAL BACKGROUND

Paul Langerhans, while a medical student, first described pancreatic islet cells in 1869.[2] Several decades later, in 1922, Banting and Best isolated insulin, or "isletin," as they called it, from a solution extract of a dog's pancreas. One year later, in 1923, Harris suggested a clinical possibility of hyperinsulinism and contrasted it with the hypoinsulinism of diabetes.[2] His suspicion was confirmed the following year, when several case reports of patients with symptomatic hyperinsulinism were published.[2]

However, it was not until 3 years later that the association between hyperinsulinism and a functional islet cell tumor was first established by Wilder and colleagues[3] after he performed an operation in a patient with hypoglycemia and found an islet cell carcinoma with hepatic metastases. The first surgical cure of an islet cell tumor was achieved by Graham in 1929.[2] Several years later, Whipple observed that symptoms of hypoglycemia provoked by fasting, a circulating glucose level of less than 50 mg/100 mL when these symptoms presented, and relief of these symptoms with

[a] Surgery Branch, National Cancer Institute, National Institutes of Health, 10 Center Drive, Building 10, Bethesda, MD 20892, USA
[b] Clinical Endocrinology Branch-NIDDK, National Institutes of Health, NIDDK, MSC 1612, 10 Center Drive, Bethesda, MD 20892, USA
[c] Montefiore-Einstein Center for Cancer Care, 3400 Bainbridge Avenue, Bronx, NY 10467, USA
[d] Albert Einstein Cancer Center, 3400 Bainbridge Avenue, Bronx, NY 10467, USA
[e] Department of Surgery, Montefiore Medical Center/Albert Einstein College of Medicine, Greene Medical Arts Pavilion, 4th Floor, 3400 Bainbridge Avenue, Bronx, NY 10467, USA
* Corresponding author.
E-mail address: slibutti@montefiore.org (S.K. Libutti).

Surg Clin N Am 89 (2009) 1105–1121
doi:10.1016/j.suc.2009.06.009
0039-6109/09/$ – see front matter © 2009 Published by Elsevier Inc.
surgical.theclinics.com

administration of glucose was the basis for the diagnosis of an insulinoma, thus establishing the "Whipple triad" that we now use today.[2]

SPORADIC VERSUS MULTIPLE ENDOCRINE NEOPLASIA TYPE 1

Insulinoma can occur sporadically, or it can be associated with multiple endocrine neoplasia type 1 (MEN-1). MEN-1 syndrome is an autosomal dominant condition that occurs as a result of inactivating mutations of the MEN1 gene located on chromosome 11.[4] This syndrome is characterized by primary hyperparathyroidism, anterior pituitary adenomas, and tumors of the endocrine pancreas and duodenum. The most common functioning islet cell tumors in MEN-1 are gastrinomas and insulinomas.[4]

Insulinoma affects approximately 10% of MEN-1 patients.[4] In contrast to sporadic insulinomas, which typically present as solitary, benign, encapsulated lesions, MEN-1 associated insulinomas develop earlier and tend to be multifocal, occurring throughout the pancreas.[5,6] This review focuses on the diagnosis, localization, and management of sporadic insulinomas.

DIAGNOSIS

As described by "Whipple's triad," hypoglycemia and neuroglycopenic symptoms that are corrected by the administration of carbohydrate are the hallmarks of the diagnosis of insulinoma. Inappropriately elevated insulin levels cause hypoglycemic episodes characterized by neuroglycopenic symptoms and sympathetic overdrive (**Table 1**). These symptoms are typically precipitated by fasting or exercise, but can also occur postprandially, or have no relationship to eating.[7]

Neuroglycopenic symptoms vary in spectrum and include difficulty awakening, visual disturbances, confusion, lethargy, weakness, abnormal behavior, seizures, loss of consciousness, or coma.[7,8] In addition, hypoglycemia also results in catecholamine release with adrenergic sympathetic nervous system activation resulting in sweating, anxiety, and palpitations.[7,8] Erroneous psychiatric or neurologic diagnoses are common in this situation, resulting in a delayed diagnosis.

The diagnosis of insulinoma can only be established by documenting symptomatic hypoglycemia with inappropriately elevated insulin levels during a 48-hour monitored fast (**Fig. 1**).[9] Hypoglycemia is defined as a blood sugar level less than 50 mg/dL in the

Table 1 Symptoms and frequency of clinical symptoms[7,8]	
Neuroglycopenic Symptoms	
Visual disturbances	59%
Altered mental state ± confusion	75%–80%
Coma or amnesia	47%
Abnormal behavior	36%
Weakness	24%–32%
Seizures	17%–23%
Sympathetic Adrenergic Symptoms	
Palpitations	10%–12%
Sweating	12%–69%
Tremors	17%–24%
Hyperphagia/obesity	25%–50%

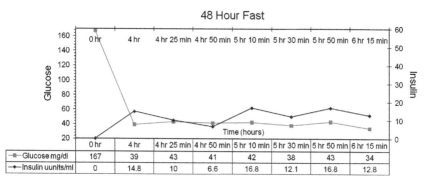

Fig. 1. Forty-eight hour fast. This patient has elevated serum insulin levels (>10 μU/mL) despite hypoglycemia indicating an insulinoma. (*Courtesy of* National Institutes of Health, Bethesda, MD).

fasting state. In healthy individuals, the blood glucose level does not fall below 70 mg/dL after an overnight fast.[10] For many years, well before tests for determination of insulin and proinsulin were readily available, the 72-hour monitored fast was the cornerstone for diagnosis. However, in more than 97% of individuals, a supervised fast of 48 hours in conjunction with biochemical testing, including plasma insulin and proinsulin measurements every 6 hours, is sufficient to diagnose insulinoma.[11] In addition, patients with this diagnosis typically have serum insulin levels higher than 5 to 10 μU/mL and an insulin to glucose ratio greater than 0.3.[9] In obese patients with peripheral insulin resistance, these values may be elevated and mimic the pattern of an insulinoma.[9]

Other conditions may cause fasting hypoglycemia with elevated insulin levels.[10] These conditions include pancreatic islet disease other than insulinoma, and factitious use of excessive insulin or hypoglycemic agents. To differentiate from these conditions, tests such as a plasma proinsulin, C peptide, sulfonylurea must be used. Endogenous insulin is synthesized as a precursor, proinsulin, which can be quantified. Proinsulin values are poorly suppressible in these patients in contrast to noninsulinoma patients.[12] Eighty-seven percent of patients with insulinoma have a plasma proinsulin component equal to or greater than 25% of the total immunoreactive insulin or specific proinsulin concentration of 22 pmol or more. In patients with surreptitious use of insulin or an oral hypoglycemic agent, the proinsulin level is either normal or decreased.

During the body's production of insulin C-peptide is cleaved from proinsulin, making it another useful indicator of surreptitious insulin use. Commercial insulin preparations do not contain it. Therefore, an elevated C-peptide indicates endogenous hyperinsulinism.

In summary, key neuroglycopenic and sympathetic symptoms together with biochemical proof establish a diagnosis of insulinoma. To diagnose an insulinoma, in addition to documenting blood glucose levels below 50 mg/dL during monitored symptomatic episodes that improve with oral intake, the patient should have elevated C-peptide levels (>200 pmol/L) and absence of plasma sulfonylurea. **Box 1** shows the common diagnostic criteria for insulinoma.

LOCALIZATION

After establishing a diagnosis of insulinoma, a variety of imaging modalities with different sensitivities can localize the tumor. The role of preoperative imaging is 2-fold. First, imaging is used to evaluate for evidence of metastatic disease; second,

---

Box 1
Common diagnostic criteria for insulinoma

Documentation of blood glucose of <50 mg/dL with hypoglycemic symptoms

Relief of symptoms after eating

Elevated C-peptide (>200 pmol/L)

Absence of plasma sulfonylurea

Increased serum insulin level (>5–10 μU/mL)

Increased proinsulin level (≥25% or ≥22 pmol)

---

localization can better facilitate discussions with the patient with regard to extent and type of operation. Because virtually all sporadic insulinomas are small and intrapancreatic, preoperative localization fails 10% to 27% of the time.[13] The extent of imaging necessary to ensure an operative cure has not been clearly defined and varies between institutions. In fact, some suggest that preoperative localization within the pancreas is not even necessary because the insulinoma can be localized successfully intraoperatively.[14]

Results of noninvasive localization studies, including transabdominal ultrasound, multiphase helical computed tomography (CT), magnetic resonance imaging (MRI), and somatostatin receptor scintigraphy (SRS) are disappointing. The success rate of transabdominal ultrasound for localization varies widely across institutions, from 9% to 66%.[7,13,15–17] Multiphase helical CT localizes 50% to 80% (**Fig. 2**), MRI 40% to 70%, and SRS 17% of all insulinomas.[7,13,15–19] All of the these imaging studies combined can localize around 80% of tumors.[13,16,17] CT and MRI are useful to evaluate for metastatic disease, although MRI may be more sensitive than CT in identifying liver metastases.[9]

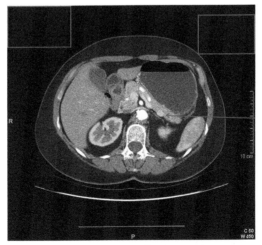

Fig. 2. Lesion successfully localized by computed tomography scan. A round, well-circumscribed, hyperenhancing lesion can be seen at the tail of the pancreas (*arrow*). (*Courtesy of* National Institutes of Health, Bethesda, MD.)

When preoperative noninvasive studies fail to localize tumors, invasive studies may aid in regional localization. Pancreatic arteriography was historically considered the gold standard, with early reports quoting success rates of 90%.[13] However, more recent studies show a much lower rate of localization in the range of 25% to 50%.[7,13,15–17]

Transhepatic portal venous sampling (THPVS) involves percutaneous and transhepatic catheterization of a branch of the portal vein followed by advancement into the small draining veins of the pancreas, including the superior mesenteric, portal, and splenic veins, to sample blood for insulin.[13,20] A step-up in the insulin level reflects the region of the pancreas where the insulinoma resides. This technique has shown a 77% to 100% success in localization.[17,20,21] However, THPVS requires special skills and experience and is associated with slight, but significant morbidity; it has therefore been abandoned.

THPVS has been replaced by intra-arterial calcium stimulation (IAC), which relies on calcium as a secretagogue for insulin secretion from the tumor.[15,16] IAC involves catheterization of the gastroduodenal, superior mesenteric, and proximal and distal splenic arteries, which are then subsequently injected with calcium.[15,16] Blood is sampled for insulin from a second catheter, which is placed first in the right hepatic vein and then the left hepatic vein for corroboration. A step-up in the insulin concentration localizes the insulinoma to a particular region of the pancreas (**Figs. 3** and **4**). IAC has a reported sensitivity from 80% to 94% in localizing insulinomas to a particular region of the pancreas.[15,16]

The use of endoscopic ultrasound for tumor localization has steadily increased over the past several years. Reported sensitivities range from 40% to as high as 93%.[21,22] The sensitivity has shown to vary by tumor location, and is also operator dependent. The authors' experience with endoscopic ultrasound is limited, as this modality is not employed at our institution.

The use of intraoperative ultrasound (IOUS), introduced in 1981, is useful to localize intrapancreatic, nonpalpable lesions, and to determine the proximity of those lesions to the pancreatic or biliary duct. IOUS performed during an open or laparoscopic exploration can localize an insulinoma in 86% of cases.[16,21]

The practice at the authors' institution once the diagnosis of insulinoma has been made is to obtain a CT scan to evaluate for metastatic disease and to assist with localization of the lesion. If the CT scan successfully localizes the lesion, the patient is taken to the operating room for either an open or laparoscopic exploration with IOUS. If the CT scan does not show a lesion, the patient undergoes intra-arterial calcium stimulation to regionalize the tumor, then is taken to the operating room.

MANAGEMENT
Medical Management

For patients who are not surgical candidates or those who are waiting for an operation, several measures can be taken to manage the symptoms, including dietary modification and pharmacologic agents. Dietary modification includes consumption of frequent, small meals throughout the day and middle of the night to avoid symptomatic hypoglycemia. The initial drug of choice, and the most well studied, is diazoxide, a benzothiadiazide. Diazoxide directly inhibits insulin release from β cells via stimulation of α-adrenergic receptors. Diazoxide also inhibits cyclic adenosine monophosphate phosphodiesterase (cAMP), which enhances glycogenolysis and has a hyperglycemic effect. Initiation doses of 150 to 200 mg given in 2 to 3 divided doses per day should be titrated to maximum dose of 400 mg daily. Diazoxide offers

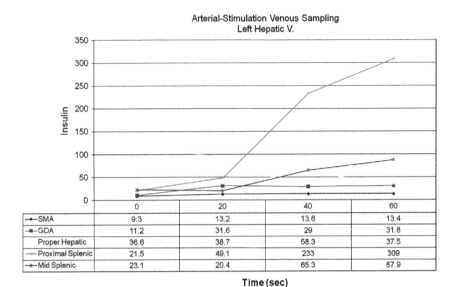

	0	20	40	60
SMA	9.3	13.2	13.6	13.4
GDA	11.2	31.6	29	31.8
Proper Hepatic	36.6	38.7	58.3	37.5
Proximal Splenic	21.5	49.1	233	309
Mid Splenic	23.1	20.4	65.3	87.9

Time (sec)

Fig. 3. Left hepatic vein insulin concentrations after intra-arterial calcium injection. Injections of the superior mesenteric artery (SMA), gastroduodenal artery (GDA), and proper hepatic artery do not show any suspicious areas. However, the increase in insulin concentration after injection into the proximal and mid splenic arteries help localize this lesion to the tail of the pancreas. (*Courtesy of* National Institutes of Health, Bethesda, MD.)

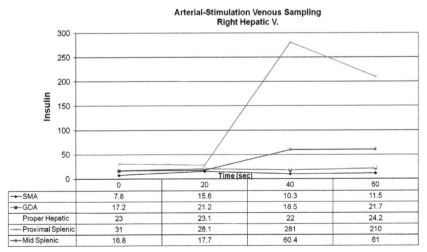

	0	20	40	60
SMA	7.8	15.6	10.3	11.5
GDA	17.2	21.2	18.5	21.7
Proper Hepatic	23	23.1	22	24.2
Proximal Splenic	31	28.1	281	210
Mid Splenic	16.8	17.7	60.4	61

Fig. 4. Right hepatic vein insulin concentration after intra-arterial calcium injection. Injections of the SMA, GDA, and proper hepatic artery do not show any suspicious areas. However, the increase in insulin concentration after injection into the proximal and mid splenic arteries helps to localize and confirm that this lesion is in the tail of the pancreas. (*Courtesy of* National Institutes of Health, Bethesda, MD.)

symptom control in about 50% to 60% of patients.[7] Sodium retention and edema, which occur in about 50% and may require addition of a diuretic, complicate the use of diazoxide. Gastrointestinal symptoms such as nausea, and occasional hirsutism, can also occur.

The somatostatin analogues octreotide and lantreotide bind with high affinity to the second of the 5 subtypes of the somatostatin receptor, sst2.[23,24] This receptor is present in varying degrees on insulinomas, accounting for the variability of response. However, this class of agents can decrease plasma insulin levels and alleviate symptoms in 40% to 60% of patients.[23,24] Initiation doses of 50 µg subcutaneously 2 or 3 times daily may be increased to 1500 µg daily. Major side effects include gastrointestinal bloating, abdominal cramping, malabsorption, and cholelithiasis.[23,24] Octreotide can also decrease glucagon and growth hormone levels, resulting in a worsening hypoglycemia in some patients. The mean duration of octreotide treatment in studies is 1 year and frequently tachyphylaxis develops.[8]

Phenytoin (Dilantin), at a maintenance dose of 300 to 600 mg daily, inhibits the release of insulin from β cells and has been used to treat a small number of patients with insulinoma.[8,9] Only in about one third of the patients does a clinically significant hyperglycemic effect occur. Verapamil, a calcium channel blocker, and propranolol, a β-blocker, have been used in a few patients either alone or in combination with other drugs to help control symptoms.[8,9] Glucocorticoids and glucagon have also been given alone or in conjunction with diazoxide to a few patients, with some palliation achieved.[9]

Surgical Management

Most sporadic insulinomas are benign, solitary lesions that are amenable to complete surgical excision for cure. At surgical exploration, the entire abdomen is inspected for evidence of metastatic disease or extrapancreatic tumors that secrete insulinoma-related growth factors.[9] Next, the entire pancreas is exposed to palpate any tumors.

Palpation of the pancreas effectively localizes the insulinoma 70% of the time. Next, intraoperative ultrasound, which has an 86% rate of detection, is performed. Intraoperative detection of an insulinoma with the combination of palpation and ultrasound ranges from 83% to 98%.[17,25] In addition, IOUS also allows identification of the pancreatic duct and vessels and determination of the proximity of the tumor to these structures.

Because most insulinomas are benign, tumor enucleation is the procedure of choice, when possible.[26,27] Insulinomas tend to be compact and encapsulated, presenting a clear dissection plane between the tumor and the surrounding pancreas (**Fig. 5**). It is important to remove the tumor with the capsule completely to prevent a local recurrence. A segmental resection of the pancreas, distal pancreatectomy, or rarely a pancreaticoduodenectomy, may be required for lesions in close proximity to the pancreatic duct or involving a large portion of the pancreatic substance. Tumors that are hard, infiltrating, create puckering of surrounding tissue, or cause pancreatic duct dilation should raise a suspicion of malignancy, and therefore also be removed by formal resection.

Historically, if the tumor could not be localized intraoperatively, blind distal pancreatectomy would be performed. However, because insulinomas may occur throughout the pancreas with relatively equal frequency, a blind distal pancreatectomy for an occult tumor is an inadvisable procedure.[28] In addition, with the current status of localization studies this practice is largely unnecessary.

With the recent advances in laparoscopic technique and instrumentation, the surgical management of an insulinoma has moved toward a minimally invasive

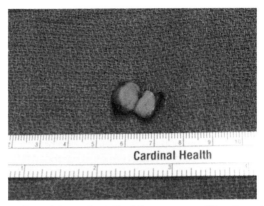

Fig. 5. Insulinoma enucleated from the tail of the pancreas. (*Courtesy of* Steven K. Libutti, MD, Bethesda, MD.)

approach. Laparoscopic ultrasound detects 86% of insulinomas.[21] Some institutions also favor placing a handport for palpation to aid in detection.[29] Laparoscopic resection is successful in 70% to 100% of cases.[29,30] However, it is still performed in only a minority of cases.

Complications related to the actual pancreatic procedure are similar for both the open and laparoscopic approach, and are as high as 45%.[29–31] Pancreatic duct leak causing pseudocyst, abscess, or fistula formation comprise the main source of this morbidity. Rates of pancreatic fistula are reported to be 15% to 43%.[26,29,31] Fernandez-Cruz and colleagues[29] noted a higher incidence of pancreatic fistula after enucleation than with distal pancreatectomy and splenectomy (38% vs 12.5%). Most these fistulas can be managed conservatively with drainage, parenteral nutrition, and somatostatin analogues to decrease the output. Some may require placement of a stent in the pancreatic duct or rarely, reoperation. Intra-abdominal abscess requiring percutaneous drainage occurs at a rate of 4% to 6% postoperatively, and 4% to 8% patients develop temporary delayed gastric emptying, which can be managed with pharmacologic agents.[17,29,32]

METASTATIC DISEASE

The documentation of metastatic disease, either at the time of surgery or by imaging studies, is the only accurate means of diagnosing a malignant insulinoma. Metastases predominantly present in the liver or lymph nodes but can also be found in the bone and peritoneal tissue, resulting in uncontrolled insulin secretion.[33,34] Life-threatening and debilitating hypoglycemia can occur from these hormone active lesions.[33,35,36] Achievement of glycemic control becomes critical and pharmacologic palliation with diazoxide, octreotide, or glucagon must be used.[36]

In a retrospective review, Danforth and colleagues[37] found that primary malignant tumors were usually single, with a mean diameter of 6 cm. These investigators reported median disease-free survival of 5 years with recurrence rate of 63% at a median of 2.8 years after curative resection.[37] However, the clinical course of patients with metastatic disease is variable. Some patients with indolent tumors may remain symptom-free for years without treatment, whereas others have symptomatic disease progression from hypersecretion of insulin or tumor bulk.[36] Long-term survival is not unusual, and 25% to 35% of patients may survive longer than 5 years.[33,36] After initial tumor resection, the biology of the tumor rather than any treatment modality most likely determines long-term survival.[33]

Because malignant insulinomas are rare, occurring in only 5% to 15% of all reported cases, controlled studies that address a specific therapeutic approach to treatment have not been performed and are probably not feasible.[33,34,38] Affected patients usually are included with other neuroendocrine tumor patients on various protocols intended to evaluate the effectiveness of a particular therapy. Despite the various therapies including surgery, chemotherapy, biotherapy, hepatic embolization, hepatic perfusion, radiofrequency ablation, and peptide-receptor radionuclide therapy, prognosis remains poor with a median survival of approximately 2 years.[25]

Surgery

The goals of surgery are to maximize local control and minimize hypoglycemic symptoms to improve quality and duration of patient survival. Cytoreductive surgery can alleviate symptoms in metastatic insulinoma in a select group of patients. Patients with a reasonable performance status, with minimal extrahepatic disease, and whose primary tumor has been or can be removed, are candidates for cytoreductive surgery. The current mortality rate of less than 2% and major morbidity rate of less than 20% represent the success of the operative approach and justify this intervention.[38–41] Unfortunately, however, curative cytoreduction is possible in less than 10% of all patients with metastatic insulinoma.[36,42,43]

A large retrospective study of 170 patients with neuroendocrine tumors, consisting of 108 patients with hormonally active tumors and 18 patients with functional islet cell tumors, reported a 95% biochemical response that lasted for a median of 45 months.[39] Overall survival for 170 patients was 61% and 35% at 5 and 10 years, respectively.[39] However, disease recurrence was 85% at 5 years.[39] Recently, Osborne and colleagues[44] reported the first series of 120 patients comparing embolization to curative or palliative resection. In patients who underwent cytoreduction, complete and partial symptomatic relief was achieved in 69% and 23%, respectively, compared with 59% and 32% in the embolization group.[44] The cytoreduction group had a statistically significantly longer mean duration of symptom relief (35 ± 22 months vs 22 ± 13.6 months), and increased mean survival (43 ± 26 months vs 24 ± 16 months).[44] The curative cytoreduction group had an increased survival compared with the palliative cytoreductive group (50 ± 27.6 months vs 32 ± 18.9 months).[44] Several other single-institution studies have reported 5-year survival benefit from 60% to 70% after curative resection; however, this benefit has yet to be proven in randomized clinical trials.[34,36,38–40]

Hepatic transplantation

For clearly unresectable liver metastases, there has been some limited experience with hepatic transplantation. An early report on liver transplantation for 30 patients with metastatic gastroenteropancreatic neuroendocrine tumors showed a 1-year survival of only 52%.[45] However, a later review of 103 patients reported a 2-year and a 5-year survival rate of 60% and 47%, respectively.[46] In 2002, the largest, single-center study of liver transplantation for gastroenteropancreatic neuroendocrine tumors consisting of 19 patients reported a 5-year survival of 80%.[45] Patients younger than 50 years old, who have had their primary pancreatic tumor completely resected and have no extrahepatic disease, tend to have a more favorable prognosis.[45] Various other studies report 5-year survival after liver transplant for neuroendocrine tumors in the range of 36% to 80%.[47,48] In addition, the aforementioned studies included carcinoid tumors, which also portend a better prognosis with transplantation. Given the morbidity of this procedure and the questionable survival benefit, hepatic transplantation may be considered in highly selected patients and should still be considered investigational.

Biotherapy with Octreotide/Interferon

Biotherapy with somatostatin analogues is frequently instituted in patients with enlarging tumor burdens, especially in slow-growing neuroendocrine tumors without extensive liver involvement. Proposed mechanisms include inhibition of endocrine growth factors, such as insulin-like growth factor-1, direct binding of somatostatin receptors, and antiangiogenic properties.[9,36,49] Octreotide can also inhibit endothelial cell proliferation through somatostatin receptors present on endothelial cells.[9] Studies suggest that this drug is well tolerated and has mostly a tumoristatic effect, causing a decrease or cessation of growth in 30% to 80% of patients with neuroendocrine tumors.[8] Objective tumor responses are typically less than 10% with a median duration of 7 months.[50] The presumption that a tumoristatic effect will result in improved progression free or overall survival has yet to be clearly demonstrated. Somatostatin analogues must be used with caution in patients with metastatic insulinoma, as these tumors frequently do not express the sst2 receptor to which this drug binds.[24,30,33,50] In addition, inhibition of glucagon may worsen hypoglycemia.

Interferon has been extensively studied in low-grade neuroendocrine tumors and a small proportion of pancreatic neuroendocrine tumors (PNETs).[8,13,36,51] The exact mechanism of action is unclear at this time, but similar to octreotide, its major effect is tumor growth stabilization rather than inducing regression.[34] Interferon-a at doses of 5 to 6 million units given 3 to 5 times weekly has shown a radiological response in less than 20% patients with PNETs.[8,36] Unfortunately, interferon causes a multitude of side effects including flulike symptoms, fatigue, weight loss, lipid, thyroid, and liver function abnormalities, and overall is not well tolerated by most patients.[8,13,36,51] Combination treatments with interferon with somatostatin remain investigational.[52]

Chemotherapy

Systemic chemotherapy for advanced or metastatic pancreatic endocrine tumors has been studied with various single as well as combinations of agents over the past 3 decades. In general, responses range from 6% to 69%, with median overall survival ranging from 17 to 38 months with chemotherapy.[36,41,53–55]

Streptozocin was approved by the Food and Drug Administration (FDA) in 1976 for use in PNETs after a 50% response rate was observed among 52 patients who were treated.[13] Subsequent studies have shown response rates of 36% to 50% with limited duration. In addition, patients suffer significant nausea, vomiting, and renal and hematological toxicity.[8] Doxorubicin has also demonstrated single-agent activity with a response rate of 33% in a phase II trial that included 42 patients.[8,9,36]

Combination chemotherapy consists of various streptozocin-based regimens allowing for the use of smaller doses of streptozocin to reduce toxicity. The Eastern Cooperative Oncology group compared 5-fluorouracil (5-FU) with streptozocin to streptozocin with doxorubicin to chlorozotocin monotherapy, and found response rates of 45%, 69%, and 30%, respectively.[53] In addition, compared with the streptozocin with 5-FU, the streptozocin with doxorubicin showed an increased median time to progression (20 months vs 7 months), increase median overall survival (2.2 years vs 1.4 years), and a mean duration of response of 18 months.[53]

Because response criteria used in older studies was not standardized, the reported response rates may be exaggerated. Two more recent retrospective studies show response rates of 6% after combination of streptozocin and doxorubicin.[41,55] In the largest series of 84 patients treated with combination streptozocin, doxorubicin, and 5-FU, the response rate was 39%, median progression free survival 18 months, and median overall survival 37 months.[54] That study showed a median time to response of 4 months, indicating that patients who do not have disease progression should be continued on this regimen for at least 4 months.[54]

Temozolamide, an oral alkylating agent, has been studied in combination with several other agents. In a phase II trial, temozolamide plus thalidomide showed a response rate of 45%.[56] Temozolamide with bevacizumab, a vascular endothelial growth factor inhibitor, showed a response rate of 24% among 17 PNETs treated.[9] Temozolamide in combination with capecitabine showed a response rate of 59% among 17 patients with metastatic neuroendocrine tumors of the pancreas.[9]

Several novel therapies are now available that are directed at multiple various growth factors produced by these tumors. These treatments include the tyrosine kinase inhibitors, sutinib and imatinib, with response rates of 17%, as well as agents targeting downstream targets of tyrosine kinase receptor activation, such as mammalian target of rapamycin, a threonine kinase involved in regulating cell cycle progression.[8] Despite the multitude of publications, the role of cytotoxic chemotherapy continues to be debated. At this time, due to lack of randomized controlled trials, which are difficult to perform because of the rarity of these tumors, it is unclear which chemotherapy regimen is best.

Liver-Directed Therapy

Hepatic artery embolization, chemoembolization, and infusion

Hepatic artery embolization (HAE) takes advantage of the liver's dual blood supply. The normal liver derives most of its blood supply from the portal circulation, whereas metastatic lesions derive most of their blood supply from the hepatic artery. Therefore, interruption of the hepatic artery preferentially causes ischemic necrosis of hepatic metastases while preserving normal liver. The generally accepted indications for embolization in patients with neuroendocrine tumors metastatic to the liver include unresectable disease producing symptoms related to either hormonal excess or tumor bulk, or rapid disease progression.

At present a variety of small particles are available to occlude the hepatic artery including lipiodol or ethiodized oil, a cottonseed oil-based contrast material, small plastic particles, and gelatin foam particles.[8] Comparative studies among these agents are lacking. Hepatic arterial vascular occlusion for islet cell carcinomas has produced objective tumor responses in 17% to 82%.[42]

Addition of chemotherapy to the embolic material, or hepatic artery chemoembolization (HACE) has several theoretical advantages. Regional delivery of chemotherapy can offer pharmacokinetic advantages and may increase intratumoral drug concentration as well as time of exposure. In addition, certain chemotherapeutic agents such as doxorubicin, mitomycin C, and streptozocin are more active in hypoxic tumor cells.[42,49] Small series have reported biochemical response rates 47% to 91% and tumor response rates that vary across the board from 0% to 100%.[42,44,49] Median survival ranges from 9 to 20 months for islet cell carcinomas in various studies.[42] Although several studies have established beneficial therapeutic effects of HAE and HACE, it is unclear whether chemoembolization confers therapeutic advantage over bland embolization.

Hepatic artery infusion (HAI) involves administration of high-dose chemotherapy with streptozocin or 5-FU via the left, right, or main hepatic artery.[34,57] This procedure is usually followed up by HACE. In a small series of patients treated with 4 monthly cycles of 5-FU, median response rate for patients with functional PNETs was 91%

with median survival of 46 months. Response rates for HAI range from 0% to 100% for islet cell neoplasms in various studies.[34,49,57]

Isolated hepatic perfusion (IHP) is a regional treatment strategy that requires a laparotomy to completely isolate the vascular supply of the liver, permitting hepatic perfusion with high-dose chemotherapy using an extracorporeal perfusion circuit (see **Fig. 1**).[58–60] The perfusion circuit provides inflow with chemotherapeutic agents via the gastroduodenal artery and receives outflow from the suprarenal and retrohepatic inferior vena cava (IVC). Systemic blood flow is maintained by venovenous bypass from the infrarenal IVC, cannulated via a saphenous vein cut down to the left axillary vein.[58–60] Separation of the hepatic and systemic circulation permits usage of higher doses of chemotherapy, administration of agents such as tumor necrosis factor (TNF), and allows for manipulation of various conditions such as hyperthermia or hypoxia. IHP with melphalan or melphalan and TNF in patients with progressive liver metastases from pancreatic and gastric neuroendocrine tumors has shown a response rate of 50%, with a mean duration of 15 months.[60] The major disadvantage of this approach is that only a single treatment can be applied and it requires an open surgical procedure with associated morbidity.[61]

Percutaneous hepatic perfusion evolved from IHP as a minimally invasive approach allowing multiple treatments with the same principles as an open hepatic perfusion.[61] The procedure requires cannulation of bilateral internal jugular veins and the common femoral artery while the patient is under general anesthesia. Complete vascular isolation is accomplished using a double balloon IVC catheter system (Delcath Systems, New York, NY), placed percutaneously.[61] Melphalan is infused directly into the hepatic artery. Hepatic venous outflow is collected via the double balloon catheter, which sits in the retrohepatic IVC, and is run through a pair of activated charcoal filters before returning to the systemic circulation by a catheter in the internal jugular vein. In a phase I study of hepatic arterial melphalan infusion with hepatic venous hemofiltration, a 30% response rate was observed.[61] A phase II trial is currently under way.

Ablative techniques

Patients may occasionally have too many small lesions to be considered resectable; however, they may be candidates for an ablative approach. Radiofrequency ablation (RFA) destroys tumors by heat. A probe is inserted directly into the tumor during laparoscopy or laparotomy, or percutaneously with image guidance. This probe emits high-frequency radio waves that generate frictional heat from ionic vibration of tissue particles. This thermal energy produces temperatures higher than 60°C, resulting in coagulation necrosis of the tumor.[62] The symptomatic response rate to RFA ranges from 71% to 95% that lasts for a mean duration of 8 to 10 months.[62] In one of the largest series, new liver lesions developed in 28% of patients at a mean of 1.6 years and local liver recurrence was reported to be 13%.[63]

Cryoablation is similar to RFA, with the exception that it relies on freezing as the method of tumor destruction. A probe inserted into the tumor passes liquid nitrogen into the tumor, subjecting it to multiple freeze and thaw cycles. Although RFA is used more commonly today, there are small series in the literature that report cryoablation as an effective approach.[8]

Percutaneous ethanol injection (PEI) can be incorporated for treatment of liver metastases from neuroendocrine tumors. In one study, complete responses were observed in all 4 neuroendocrine hepatic metastases.[64] Others have performed PEI of metastases located adjacent to vital structures such as the hepatic flexure of the colon, metastases adjacent to large vessels vulnerable to the heat-sink effect, and metastases adjacent to central bile ducts, where subsequent biliary stricture may occur.[65] Various studies have shown that complete necrosis of liver metastases can be obtained. This technique is usually employed for hepatocellular carcinoma and is not effective for metastatic PNETs. PEI has largely been replaced by radiofrequency thermal ablation and cryoablation.[66]

Peptide Receptor Radionuclide Therapy

Peptide receptor radionuclide therapy (PRRT) is an emerging treatment modality for patients with unresectable, somatostatin-receptor positive neuroendocrine tumors. This treatment relies on the fact that some insulinomas express somatostatin receptors and internalize radiolabeled analogues, facilitating delivery of cytotoxic doses of localized radiation to the tumor. With this approach roughly 25% patients had an objective tumor response, with greater than 50% shrinkage.[67,68] Over the past decade, the most frequently used somatostatin analogues intravenously injected include indium-111 (^{111}In), yttrium-90 (^{90}Y), and lutetium-177 (^{177}Lu).[67] Whereas complete responses are rare, partial response rates vary from 0% to as high as 40% with a median duration ranging from 12 to 37 months. Side effects include hematologic toxicity and renal toxicity, which can be reduced by coadministration of amino acids. This form of therapy is currently under evaluation at several centers to further define its utility.

Selective Internal Radiation Therapy

There has been considerable interest in 2 radioactive microsphere devices recently approved by the FDA for liver-directed therapy. TheraSphere (MDS Nordion, Ottawa, Canada), which consists of nonbiodegradable glass microspheres, is FDA approved for unresectable hepatocellular carcinoma. SIR-Spheres (Sirtex, Wilmington, MA) consists of resin microspheres and is approved for metastatic colon cancer to the liver. Both devices contain ^{90}Y. The principle underlying this technology is the preferential distribution of microspheres via direct hepatic transarterial injection into the peritumoral vasculature, allowing delivery of high doses of radiation into the tumor and sparing normal liver. Selective internal radiation therapy with ^{90}Y microspheres has been used to treat hepatic metastases from neuroendocrine tumors in a limited number of patients. A recent study of 84 patients who received a tumor dose of 1000 Gy reported stable disease in 67% of patients for 12 months, symptomatic palliation in 80%, and few responses.[62,69] King and colleagues[69] reported a symptomatic response rate of 50% at 6 months with 18% complete tumor responses, 32% partial responses, and mean overall survival of 29.4 ± 3.4 months. Further investigation of the agents will help delineate its role in metastatic neuroendocrine tumors.

SUMMARY

Insulinoma is a rare, usually benign, pancreatic islet cell tumor. A patient with a suspected insulinoma should undergo a monitored 48-hour fast with appropriate confirmatory laboratory values to establish the diagnosis. Next, a CT scan is carried out evaluate for metastatic disease as well as to localize the lesion within the pancreas. If CT is unable to localize the lesion, intra-arterial calcium stimulation to regionalize the tumor is recommended.

The patient is then taken to the operating room for either an open or laparoscopic exploration with intraoperative ultrasound. Because most insulinomas are solitary and benign, enucleation, if feasible, is the procedure of choice. However, a tumor in close proximity to the pancreatic duct, a large or hard tumor creating puckering of the surrounding tissue requires a formal resection. Medical management, including diazoxide, should be initiated while awaiting surgical excision to temporize symptoms.

On rare occasions patients present with metastatic disease, most commonly to the liver and lymph nodes. In patients with metastatic disease surgical debulking, if possible, provides long-term survival. However, if surgical resection is not possible then other options exist. For hepatic predominant disease, treatments such as RFA, HAE, chemoembolization, and hepatic perfusion may be used. Other potential treatment options for metastatic disease include cytotoxic chemotherapy, molecularly targeted therapy, or targeted radiotherapy. Because of the infrequent occurrence of metastatic insulinoma, prospective randomized trials have not been conducted to evaluate the superiority of these therapies.

REFERENCES

1. Available at: www.Seer.cancer.gov. Accessed 2008.
2. Whipple AO, Frautz VK. Adenomas of islet cells with hyperinsulinism: a review. Ann Surg 1935;101:1299–335.
3. Wilder RM, Allan FN, Power MH, et al. Carcinoma of the islets of the pancreas: hyperinsulinism and hypoglycemia. J Am Med Assoc 1927;89:348–55.
4. Rich TA, Perrier ND. Multiple endocrine neoplasia syndromes. Surg Clin North Am 2008;88(4):863–95.
5. Demeure MJ, Klonoff DC, Karam JH, et al. Insulinomas associated with multiple endocrine neoplasia type I: the need for a different surgical approach. Surgery 1991;110:998–1005.
6. O'Riordain DS, Brien T, van Heerden JA, et al. Surgical management of insulinoma associated with multiple endocrine neoplasia type I. World J Surg 1994;18: 488–94.
7. Boukhman MP, Karam JH, Shaver J, et al. Insulinoma—experience from 1950 to 1995. West J Med 1998;169:98–104.
8. Metz DC, Jensen RT. Gastrointestinal neuroendocrine tumors: pancreatic endocrine tumors. Gastroenterology 2008;135:1469–92.
9. Yao JC, Rindi G, Evans DB. Pancreatic endocrine tumors. In: Devita Jr. VT, Hellman S, Rosenberg SA, editors. Cancer principles and practice of oncology. 8th edition. Philadelphia: Lippincott Williams & Wilkins; 2007. p. 1702–16.
10. Service FJ. Diagnostic approach to adults with hypoglycemic disorders. Endocrinol Metab Clin North Am 1999;28(3):519–32, vi.
11. Hirshberg B, Andrea L, Bartlett DL, et al. Forty-eight-hour fast: the diagnostic test for insulinoma. J Clin Endocrinol Metab 2000;85:3222–6.
12. Gorden P, Skarulis MC, Roach P, et al. Plasma proinsulin-like component in insulinoma: a 25-year experience. J Clin Endocrinol Metab 1995;80:2884–7.
13. Grant CS. Insulinoma. Best Pract Res Clin Gastroenterol 2005;19:783–98.
14. Hashimoto LA, Walsh RM. Preoperative localization of insulinomas is not necessary. J Am Coll Surg 1999;189:368–73.
15. Guettier JM, Kam A, Chang R, et al. Localization of insulinomas to regions of the pancreas by intraarterial calcium stimulation: the NIH experience. J Clin Endocrinol Metab 2009;94:1074–80.
16. Brown CK, Bartlett DL, Doppman JL, et al. Intraarterial calcium stimulation and intraoperative ultrasonography in the localization and resection of insulinomas. Surgery 1997;122:1189–94.
17. Nikfarjam M, Warshaw AL, Axelrod L, et al. Improved contemporary surgical management of insulinomas. A 25-year experience at the Massachusetts General Hospital. Ann Surg 2008;247:165–72.

18. Fidler JL, Fletcher JG, Reading CC, et al. Preoperative detection of pancreatic insulinomas on multiphasic helical CT. AJR Am J Roentgenol 2003;181:775–80.
19. Gibril F, Jensen RT. Diagnostic uses of radiolabelled somatostatin receptor analogues in gastroenteropancreatic endocrine tumors. Dig Liver Dis 2004;36: S106–20.
20. Doherty GM, Doppman JL, Shawker TH, et al. Results of a prospective strategy to diagnose, localize, and resect insulinomas. Surgery 1991;110:989–96.
21. Grover AC, Skarulis M, Alexander R, et al. A prospective evaluation of laparoscopic exploration with intraoperative ultrasound as a technique for localizing sporadic insulinomas. Surgery 2005;138:1003–8.
22. Anderson MA, Carpenter S, Thompson NW. Endoscopic ultrasound is highly accurate and directs management in patients with neuroendocrine tumors of the pancreas. Am J Gastroenterol 2000;95:2271–7.
23. Gorden P, Comi RJ, Maton PN, et al. NIH conference. Somatostatin and somatostatin analogue (SMS 201–995) in treatment of hormone-secreting tumors of the pituitary and gastrointestinal tract and non-neoplastic diseases of the gut. Ann Intern Med 1989;110:35–50.
24. Arnold R, Wied M, Behr TH. Somatostatin analogues in the treatment of endocrine tumours of the gastrointestinal tract. Expert Opin Pharmacother 2002;3(6): 643–56.
25. Norton JA, Cromack DT, Shawker TH, et al. Intraoperative ultrasonographic localization of islet cell tumors. A prospective comparison to palpation. Ann Surg 1988;207:160–8.
26. Park BJ, Alexander HR, Libutti SK, et al. Operative management of islet-cell tumors arising in the head of the pancreas. Surgery 1998;124:1056–61.
27. Sweet MP, Izumisato Y, Way LW, et al. Laparoscopic enucleation of insulinomas. Arch Surg 2007;142:1202–4.
28. Hirshberg B, Libutti SK, Alexander HR, et al. Blind distal pancreatectomy for occult insulinoma, an inadvisable procedure. J Am Coll Surg 2002;194:761–4.
29. Fernández-Cruz Laureano, Blanco Laia, Cosa Rebeca, et al. Is laparoscopic resection adequate in patients with pancreatic neuroendocrine tumors? World J Surg 2008;32(5):904–17.
30. Finlayson E, Clark OH. Surgical treatment of insulinomas. Surg Clin North Am 2004;84:775–85.
31. Menegaux F, Schmitt G, Mercadier M, et al. Pancreatic insulinomas. Am J Surg 1992;165:243–8.
32. Phan Giao Q, Yeo Charles J, Hruban Ralph H, et al. Surgical experience with pancreatic and peripancreatic neuroendocrine tumors: review of 125 patients. J Gastrointest Surg 1998;2:399–492.
33. Hirshberg B, Cochran C, Skarulis MC, et al. Malignant insulinoma: spectrum of unusual clinical features. Cancer 2005;104:264–72.
34. Starke A, Saddig C, Mansfeld L, et al. Malignant metastatic insulinoma—postoperative treatment and follow-up. World J Surg 2005;29:789–93.
35. Arioglu E, Gottlieb NA, Koch CA, et al. Natural history of a proinsulin-secreting insulinoma: from symptomatic hypoglycemia to clinical diabetes. J Clin Endocrinol Metab 2000;85:3628–30.
36. Phan AT, Yao JC, Evans DB. Treatment options for metastatic neuroendocrine tumors. Surgery 2008;144(6):895–8.
37. Danforth DN, Gorden P, Brennan MF. Metastatic insulin-secreting carcinoma of the pancreas: clinical course and the role of surgery. Surgery 1984;96: 1027–37.

38. Norton JA, Warren RS, Kelly MG, et al. Aggressive surgery for metastatic neuro-endocrine liver tumors. Surgery 2003;134:1057–63.
39. Sarmiento JM, Que FG. Hepatic surgery for metastases from neuroendocrine tumors. Surg Oncol Clin N Am 2003;12(1):231–42.
40. Sarmiento JM, Que FG, Grant CS, et al. Concurrent resections of pancreatic islet cell cancers with synchronous hepatic metastases: outcomes of an aggressive approach. Surgery 2002;132:976–82.
41. McCollum AD, Kilke MH, Ryan DP, et al. Lack of efficacy of streptozocin and doxorubicin in patients with advanced pancreatic endocrine tumors. Am J Clin Oncol 2004;27:485–8.
42. Madoff DC, Gupta S, Ahrar K, et al. Update on management of neuroendocrine hepatic metastases. J Vasc Interv Radiol 2006;17(8):1235–49.
43. Sarmiento JM, Heywood G, Rubin J, et al. Surgical treatment of neuroendocrine metastases to the liver: a plea for resection to increase survival. J Am Coll Surg 2003;197:29–37.
44. Osborne DA, Zervos EE, Strosberg J, et al. Improved outcome with cytoreduction versus embolization for symptomatic hepatic metastases of carcinoid and neuro-endocrine tumors. Ann Surg Oncol 2006;13:572–81.
45. Van Vilsteren FG, Baskin-Bey ES, Nagorney DM, et al. Liver transplantation for gastroenteropancreatic neuroendocrine cancers: defining selection criteria to improve survival. Liver Transpl 2006;12:448–56.
46. Lenhert T. Liver transplantation for metastatic neuroendocrine carcinoma. An analysis of 103 patients. Transplantation 1998;27:1307–12.
47. Florman S, Toure B, Kim L, et al. Liver transplantation for neuroendocrine tumors. J Gastrointest Surg 2004;8:208–12.
48. Castaldo ET, Pinson WC. Liver transplant for non-hepatocellular carcinoma malignancy. HPB (Oxford) 2007;9(2):98–103.
49. Gupta S, Johnson MM, Murthy R, et al. Hepatic arterial embolization and chemoembolization for the treatment of patients with metastatic neuroendocrine tumors: variables affecting response rates and survival. Cancer 2005;104:590–602.
50. Arnold R, Trautmann ME, Creutzfeldt W, et al. Somatostatin analogue octreotide and inhibition of tumor growth in metastatic neuroendocrine gastroenteropancreatic tumors. Gut 1996;38:430–8.
51. Kulke MH. Gastrointestinal neuroendocrine tumors: a role for targeted therapies? Endocr Relat Cancer 2007;14:207–19.
52. Wang HS, Oh DS, Ohning GV, et al. Cyto-reduction of neuroendocrine tumours using sandostatin LAR in combination with Infergen: results of a case series. J Pharm Pharmacol 2006;58:1623–8.
53. Moertel CG, Lefkopoulo M, Lipsitz S, et al. Streptozocin-doxorubicin, streptozocin-fluorouracil or chlorozotocin in the treatment of advanced islet-cell carcinoma. N Engl J Med 1992;326:519–23.
54. Kouvaraki MA, Ajani JA, Hoff P, et al. Fluorouracil, doxorubicin, and streptozocin in the treatment of patients with locally advanced and metastatic pancreatic endocrine carcinoma. J Clin Oncol 2004;22:4762–71.
55. Cheng PN, Saltz LB. Failure to confirm major objective antitumor activity for streptozocin and doxorubicin in the treatment of patients with advanced islet cell carcinoma. Cancer 1999;86:944–8.
56. Kulke MH, Stuart K, Enzinger PC, et al. Phase II study of temozolamide and thalidomide in patients with metastatic neuroendocrine tumors. J Clin Oncol 2006;24:401–6.

57. Christante D, Pommiers J, Givi B, et al. Hepatic artery chemoinfusion with chemo-embolization for neuroendocrine cancer with progressive hepatic metastases despite octreotide treatment. Surgery 2008;144:885–94.
58. Alexander HR, Libutti SK, Bartlett DL, et al. A phase I-II study of isolated hepatic perfusion using melphalan with or without tumor necrosis factor for patients with ocular melanoma metastatic to the liver. Clin Cancer Res 2000;6:3062–5.
59. Jones A, Alexander HR. Development of isolated hepatic perfusion for patients who have unresectable hepatic malignancies. Surg Oncol Clin N Am 2008;17: 857–76.
60. Grover AC, Libutti SK, Pingpank JF, et al. Isolated hepatic perfusion for the treatment of patients with advanced liver metastases from pancreatic and gastrointestinal neuroendocrine neoplasms. Surgery 2004;136:1176–82.
61. Pingpank JF, Libutti SK, Chang R, et al. Phase I study of hepatic arterial melphalan infusion and hepatic venous hemofiltration using percutaneously placed catheters in patients with unresectable hepatic malignancies. J Clin Oncol 2005;23:3465–74.
62. Vogl TJ, Naguib NN, Zangos S, et al. Liver metastases of neuroendocrine carcinomas: interventional treatment via transarterial embolization, chemoembolization, and thermal ablation. Eur J Radiol, 2008, Doi:10.1016/j.ejrad.2008.08.008.
63. Berber E, Flesher N, Siperstein AE. Laparoscopic RFA of neuroendocrine liver metastases. World J Surg 2002;26:985–90.
64. Livraghi T, Vettori C, Lazzaroni S. Liver metastases: results of percutaneous ethanol injection in 14 patients. Radiology 1991;179:709–12.
65. Atwell TD, Charboneau JW, Que FG, et al. Treatment of neuroendocrine cancer metastatic to the liver: the role of ablative techniques. Cardiovasc Intervent Radiol 2005;28:409–21.
66. Giovanni M. Percutaneous alcohol ablation for liver metastasis. Semin Oncol 2002;29:192–5.
67. Forrer F, Valkerma R, Kwekkeboom DJ, et al. Peptide receptor radionuclide therapy. Best Pract Res Clin Endocrinol Metab 2007;21:111–29.
68. Kwekkeboom DJ, Teunissen JJ, Bakker WH, et al. Radiolabeled somatostatin analogue [^{177}Lu-DOTA^0, Tyr^3]octreotate in patients with endocrine gastropancreatic tumors. J Clin Oncol 2005;23:2754–62.
69. King J, Quinn R, Glenn DM, et al. Radioembolization with selective internal radiation microspheres for neuroendocrine liver metastases. Cancer 2008;113(5): 921–9.

Carcinoid Tumors

Janice L. Pasieka, MD, FRCSC, FACS*

KEYWORDS

- Carcinoid • Neuroendocrine tumors • Treatment of prognosis
- Review

TERMINOLOGY

Carcinoid tumors, now referred to as neuroendocrine tumors (NETs), encompass a wide range of neoplasms and clinical behaviors depending on their site of origin, hormonal production, and differentiation. First described in 1888 by Lubarsch, the term Karznoid, or carcinoma-like, was introduced by Oberndorfer in 1907 when he described a distinct intestinal tumor that was biologically less aggressive than intestinal adenocarcinoma.[1] With time Oberndorfer recognized the potential malignant nature of many of these tumors and modified his early stance in regard to their "benign" behavior. It was however years earlier, in 1890, that Ransom reported similar tumors from the ileum that were associated with diarrhea and wheezing.[2] The secretion of hormones and peptides from these tumors was not appreciated at that time. In 1914, Gosset and Mason suggested that carcinoid tumors arose from the enterochromaffin cells of the gastrointestinal (GI) tract.[3] This recognition that carcinoid tumors were endocrine related was not widely appreciated until Erspamer succeeded in demonstrating serotonin (5-HT) in the enterochromaffin cells and in 1953 Lembeck was able to extract 5-HT from a carcinoid tumor.[4,5]

In 1968, Williams and Sandler proposed an embryologic classification of these tumors: foregut (bronchial, thymus, stomach, duodenum, pancreas), midgut (small bowel, appendix, right colon), hindgut (transverse and descending colon, rectum). These investigators demonstrated that tumors arising from different segments of the embryologic gut varied in their histologic, immunohistochemical, and bioactive amine production. Foregut carcinoids are generally argentaffin-negative and lack the decarboxylation enzyme that converts 5-hydroxytryptophan (5-HTP) to 5-HT. Therefore, these tumors have low serotonin levels and often secrete 5-HTP and histamine. Midgut carcinoids are argentaffin-positive and have high 5-HT content. Midgut carcinoids have been shown to also secrete tachykinins, prostaglandins, and bradykinins into the circulation.[6] Hindgut carcinoids are argentaffin-negative and rarely contain 5-HT or secrete 5-HTP. Although this classification emphasized

Division of Surgical Oncology and General Surgery, Department of Surgery, University of Calgary, 1403 29th Street NW, Calgary, AB T2N 2T0, Canada
* Corresponding author.
E-mail address: Janice.pasieka@albertahealthservices.ca

Surg Clin N Am 89 (2009) 1123–1137
doi:10.1016/j.suc.2009.06.008
0039-6109/09/$ – see front matter © 2009 Elsevier Inc. All rights reserved.

surgical.theclinics.com

clinicopathologic differences between the various gastrointestinal neuroendocrine tumors (GI-NETs), it proved to be too imprecise in predicting the biologic behavior of each tumor.[7] It became particularly apparent in foregut tumors that varied greatly in function and prognosis, and morphologically that a single group classification was not clinically useful. In 2000 a newer classification was developed by the World Health Organization, which included not only the site of origin but also histologic variations that were more predictive of biologic behavior.[4,6,8] Using this system, tumors are classified into well-differentiated NET tumors and well-differentiated and poorly differentiated NET carcinomas (**Box 1**). Today the term carcinoid is preferably used for tumors that arise in the GI tract that can produce serotonin or cause carcinoid syndrome. This term refers to primarily midgut small bowel carcinoids, whereas the remaining "carcinoid" tumors should be termed NETs, followed by their site of origin and the endocrinopathy if present.

Neuroendocrine cells occur throughout the length of the GI tract and are the largest group of hormone-producing cells in the body.[7,9] Neuroendocrine cells are derived from multipotent stem cells and not, as originally thought, from the migration of neural crest cells. There are at least 13 gut neuroendocrine cells, which produce various bioactive peptides and amines including serotonin, gastrin, and histamine. The secretory products are stored in vesicles within the cells. Chromogranin A (CgA) and synaptophysin are some of the proteins that make up these vesicles, and therefore have become useful tumor markers. CgA has been shown to have a high sensitivity and variable specificity for NETs. CgA is elevated in 80% of patients with NETs from all sites and seems to correlate with tumor load.[6,10,11]

The density of these various neuroendocrine cells in a given anatomic segment of the gut is dictated by the physiologic needs of that site. For example, histamine-producing enterochromaffin-like (ECL) cells play a pivotal role in gastric acid secretion and are therefore located predominantly in the fundus of the stomach.[4] It is postulated that GI-NETs arise as a result of one or more genetic mutations in "neuroendocrine-committed cells." The resulting tumor adopts the phenotype of the parent cell that is normally present in that part of the gut.[4] Thus, NETs most often originate in the midgut serotonin-producing neuroendocrine cells, whereas ECL

Box 1
Classification of neuroendocrine tumors

Well-differentiated neuroendocrine tumors

    Solid trabecular or glandular structure, *Ki67* <2%, absent cytological atypia, absence of angioinvasion

Well-differentiated neuroendocrine carcinomas

    Well-differentiated, >2 cm, absent or low cytological atypia, evidence of lymphovascular invasion, *Ki67* <2%, presence of metastases

Poorly differentiated neuroendocrine carcinomas

    Predominate solid structure with necrosis and cellular atypia, *Ki67* >15%

Mixed exocrine/endocrine carcinoma

    Previously termed adenocarcinoid

Tumor-like lesions

tumors are found in the normal distribution of the histamine-producing ECL cells of the stomach.

EPIDEMIOLOGY

Overall the incidence of GI-NETs is 2.5 to 5 per 100,000.[9,12,13] Using the SEER (Surveillance Epidemiology and End Results) database, the incidence and prevalence of these tumors has increased significantly over the last few decades.[12–14] In an analysis of 13,715 NETs, 68% arose from the GI tract and 25% from the bronchopulmonary tract.[13] Within the GI tract, small bowel carcinoids accounted for 42%, rectal 27%, and stomach 9%. The age-adjusted incidence of small bowel carcinoids has increased by 460% over 30 years. Furthermore, the prevalence over this period increased by 274% in whites and 500% in blacks. The cause for this increase is not clearly understood and may partly reflect an increase in reporting and enhanced detection with radiographic and endoscopic advances.

GASTRIC CARCINOIDS

Gastric carcinoids constitute 4% of all GI-NETs and 1% of gastric neoplasms,[9,12,15,16] and can be divided into 4 types. The first 3 originate from the ECL cells in the gastric mucosa and types 1 and 2 are gastrin-dependent. The percentage of gastric carcinoids among NETs has been shown to be increasing. Early data in the 1970s demonstrated an incidence of 2.5% whereas late SEER data found an incidence approaching 6%.[13] It has also been shown that the percentage of gastric carcinoids in relation to all gastric neoplasms has also increased from 0.4% to 1.8%. Whether this represents a true biologic increase or reflects a change in awareness and improved diagnosis, or increase in reporting, remains unclear.[13] The true incidence of gastric carcinoids was not really appreciated prior to the increased application of upper endoscopy.[17]

Type 1 Gastric Carcinoids

Type 1 gastric carcinoids account for 70% to 80% of gastric carcinoids and develop as a result of the trophic effect of gastrin on the ECL cells.[15,17,18] These tumors are associated with autoimmune chronic atrophic gastritis. The loss of hydrochloric acid-producing parietal cells leads to achlorhydria, which in turn stimulates the G cells of the antrum to produce gastrin. It is thought that the hypergastrinemia promotes the growth of the ECL cells, first resulting in hyperplasia out of which multiple ECL tumors arise.[17,19] These tumors are typically multiple, usually small (<2 cm) and, because of their association with autoimmune atrophic gastritis, occur more frequently in women aged 50 years or older, commonly associated with B12 malabsorption and pernicious anemia.[15,18] The diagnosis is commonly made incidentally on upper endoscopy as these patients are usually asymptomatic. Most of these tumors are benign, but metastases have been reported in 3% to 5% of patients.[16] Histologically these tumors fall into the classification of well-differentiated NETs, demonstrating little evidence of invasion and having a low proliferation index. Small tumors can be removed endoscopically, whereas larger tumors or those demonstrating invasion require surgical excision. Ongoing endoscopic surveillance is required every 6 months because recurrence remains high. The role of concomitant antrectomy aimed at reducing the hypergastrinemia should be considered when surgical excision is required for removal, although it must be individualized to each patient.[15,20] Somatostatin analogues have been used to reduce the gastrin levels and have been shown to reduce recurrences, although current guidelines do not advocate their routine use.[18,20,21] Five-year survival rates, approaching 98%, illustrate the benign nature of this type of tumor.[20]

Type 2 Gastric Carcinoids

These tumors, like Type 1 gastric carcinoids, are gastrin-dependent and often multi-focal. Type 2 gastric carcinoids develop secondarily in the context of hypergastrine-mia due to Zollinger-Ellison syndrome (ZES) associated with multiple endocrine neoplasia type 1 (MEN-1). ECL cell hyperplasia is common in MEN-1/ZES patients, and it is possible that 15% to 30% of these patients will develop carcinoids in the body and fundus of the stomach.[15] In contrast to type 1 patients, these patients have elevated gastric acid and present with the clinical manifestations of ZES. Type 2 gastric tumors represent 5% of gastric carcinoids and are equally distributed between males and females.[17] Histologically they appear similar to Type 1 tumors, but their malignant potential is greater.[15] Regional lymph nodes have been reported in up to 30% of cases and liver metastases in 10%.[15,18] Therefore Type 2 gastric carci-noids commonly are classified as well-differentiated neuroendocrine carcinomas when invasion or metastases are present.

Treatment of these tumors is focused on removal of the source of gastrin (typi-cally a duodenal gastrinoma), together with resection of the gastric carcinoid. This result can be achieved endoscopically for small tumors (<2 cm) or with surgical resection for large lesions and those with invasion ECL lymph node involvement.[20] The 5-year survival is approximately 90% for type 2 gastric carcinoids.

Type 3 Gastric Carcinoids

Type 3, or sporadic tumors, account for 20% of gastric carcinoids. Unlike types 1 and 2, these tumors are not associated with elevated gastrin levels. Type 3 tumors are usually solitary, large (>2 cm), and occur most frequently in men older than 50 years.[17,18,20] Histologically they can be well-differentiated NET carcinomas; however, large lesions tend to have atypical histology with pleomorphism, high mitoses, and often a high Ki67 index. Therefore many of these tumors are classified as poorly differentiated neuro-endocrine carcinomas.[15,16,18] Regional lymph node involvement is found in up to 50% of cases, and liver metastases develop in over two-thirds of the patients.[15–18,20]

An "atypical" carcinoid syndrome can develop in 5% to 10% in patients with type 3 carcinoids. The syndrome is a result of histamine release and is characterized by a patchy bright red flush, cutaneous edema, salivary gland swelling, and increased lacrimation.[15,22] Urinary measurements of histamine levels and serum CgA serve as tumor markers and can be useful in following response to therapy. Sporadic gastric carcinoid should be treated similar to adenocarcinoma of the stomach, with an en bloc resection and an appropriate D1 and D2 lymph node clearance. Unfortunately, unlike type 1 and 2 carcinoid, type 3 has a 5-year survival of only 50% overall and 10% in those patients with distant metastases.[15,16,23]

Type 4 Gastric Carcinoids

These tumors consist of poorly differentiated endocrine carcinomas and mixed exocrine-endocrine carcinomas. Atrophic gastritis has been seen in up to 50% of these patients. The tumors are usually larger than 5 cm, often ulcerating and surgically unresectable. The prognosis is poor, with a median survival of only 8 months reported in the literature.[15,16,24] Platinum-based chemotherapy has been attempted in a limited number of patients.

MIDGUT CARCINOIDS

Midgut carcinoids are the most common carcinoid tumor, accounting for 25% of all abdominal-NETs. Midgut carcinoids originate most frequently in the terminal ileum, followed by the appendix and right colon.[15] Although these tumors share the same embryologic development, they appear to be biologically different. Appendiceal carcinoids differ from the small bowel tumors in that they are usually small, rarely metastasize, and rarely are a cause of carcinoid syndrome. On the other hand, carcinoid syndrome occurs in a third of the patients with small bowel tumors, and regional and distant spread is common. Most small bowel carcinoids are well-differentiated neuroendocrine carcinomas, whereas right colon carcinoids are more likely to be poorly differentiated.[15]

Small Bowel Carcinoids

Small bowel carcinoids most frequently arise in the submucosa of the terminal ileum. Unlike appendiceal carcinoids, the size of these tumors is an unreliable predictor of metastatic potential.[9] Metastatic spread is common, with regional nodal disease occurring in 70% of patients and liver metastases in more than 50%. Multiple tumors may be found in a third of the patients. Fibrosis induced around the mesenteric nodal metastases causes contraction of the mesentery and kinking of the bowel (**Fig. 1**). The mesenteric vessels become occluded from this desmoplastic reaction, leading to chronic ischemic changes of the antimesenteric border of the bowel (**Fig. 2**). As a result, patients often present with nonspecific abdominal pain and a history consistent with intermittent ischemia. Due to the indolent behavior of these tumors, patients usually have symptoms for a mean of 5 years before the diagnosis is made.[25] Forty percent of patients are discovered during emergency surgery for small bowel obstruction. In other patients, the diagnosis is made "incidentally" on imaging studies that identify the small bowel mesenteric nodal disease or liver metastases (**Figs. 3** and **4**).

Carcinoid syndrome occurs in 20% to 30% of patients with small bowel carcinoids. This syndrome is a constellation of symptoms resulting from excess biogenic amines, peptides, and other factors including serotonin, tachykinins, and bradykinins in the systemic circulation.[14,15,21] Due to the liver's ability to deactivate serotonin, carcinoid syndrome typically occurs when liver metastases are present. However, retroperitoneal disease, significant tumor burden, and liver dysfunction without metastases can also result in carcinoid syndrome. Of note is that 15% of the time, preoperative imaging fails to demonstrate the liver metastases because they appear as small miliary lesions that go undetected even at laparotomy (**Fig. 5**). It is therefore important that general surgeons be aware of this mode of spread when assessing patients at laparotomy.

The most common symptom is flushing, occurring in up to 94% of patients.[14,21] Flushing has been linked to several factors including serotonin, tachykinins, and

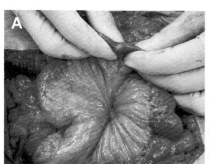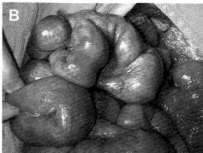

Fig. 1. (*A, B*) Desmoplastic reaction around mesenteric nodal metastases, which causes contraction of the mesentery and kinking of the bowel. The primary tumor is often small (*A*).

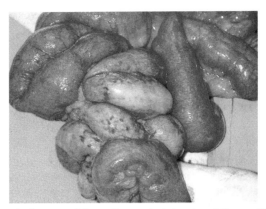

Fig. 2. Chronic ischemic changes of the antimesenteric border of the small bowel in a patient with small bowel carcinoid tumor involving the regional lymph nodes.

histamine. Flushing can be provoked by cheese, wine, nuts, and stress. Diarrhea is the next most common manifestation of carcinoid syndrome, occurring in 80% of patients. Other symptoms include bronchial constriction and wheezing, abdominal pain, and pellagra (niacin deficiency). Carcinoid heart disease develops in 40% to 50% of patients with the syndrome. It is characterized by plaquelike deposits of fibrous tissue on the tricuspid and pulmonary valves and the endocardium (**Fig. 6**).[14,21,26] Plaque formation causes endocardial thickening, which in turn causes retraction and fixation of the valves, leading to valvular dysfunction. The disease predominantly affects the right side of the heart, as the lungs are able to deactivate the serotonin before entering the left atrium. However, left-sided disease has been reported.[21,26–28]

Urinary 5-hydroxyindoleacetic acid (5-HIAA) and CgA levels should be measured to diagnose excessive serotonin secretion, and are useful in monitoring disease response and progression. Diagnostic procedures include computed tomography (CT) (see **Fig. 3**), magnetic resonance imaging (MRI) (see **Fig. 4**), somatostatin-receptor

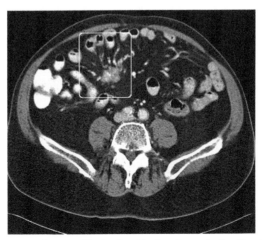

Fig. 3. Computed tomography scan illustrating the "spoke and wheel" pattern of mesenteric involvement, classic for small bowel carcinoids.

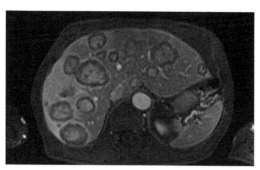

Fig. 4. Incidentally discovered liver metastases on magnetic resonance imaging.

scintigraphy (SRI) (**Fig. 7**), and positron emission tomography (PET) with radiolabeled 5-HTP.[6,16] Characteristic CT findings of a mesenteric mass with radiating densities, the so-called spoke and wheel, is considered pathognomonic for midgut carcinoids mesenteric involvement (see **Fig. 3**). CT and MRI are equally effective at demonstrating regional and distant metastases with a sensitivity of 77% and 80%, respectively, yet underestimate the extent of the disease 25% of the time.[29] SRI has a diagnostic accuracy and positive predictive value of 83% and 100% and has been shown to complement anatomic imaging in assessing the extent of disease.[6] 5-HTP PET has recently been shown to be more sensitive than SRI and CT, although this modality is presently not widely available.[16,30,31]

Surgical treatment

Surgery plays an important role in the management of patients with small bowel carcinoids even in the presence of metastatic disease. Resection of the primary tumor and mesenteric nodal disease is effective in relieving symptoms of gastrointestinal obstruction and ischemic symptoms associated with these tumors.[25,32–34] Resection of mesenteric nodal disease has also been associated with a survival benefit. In a study by Hellman and colleagues, complete resection of mesenteric nodal disease was associated with a significantly improved survival compared with patients in whom

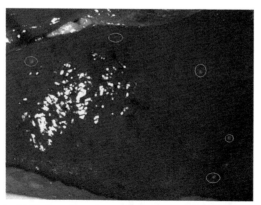

Fig. 5. Small, nonpalpable lesions found intraoperatively in the liver in a patient with clinical carcinoid syndrome and negative imaging preoperatively. These small lesions were histologically proven to be metastatic NETs.

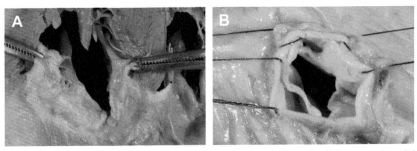

Fig. 6. Plaquelike deposits of fibrous tissue on the tricuspid (*A*) and pulmonary values (*B*) in a patient who suffered from carcinoid heart disease.

this could not be achieved (mean survival 7.9 vs 6.2 years). This improvement was seen in patients with and without hepatic metastases.[33] It has been postulated that resection of the primary in the face of hepatic metastases improves survival and leads to a greater median progression-free survival. Givi and colleagues,[32] in their retrospective review of GI-NET with liver metastases, found that those patients who underwent resection of their primary had a longer median survival (159 months) compared with 47 months in the nonresected group. Although retrospective, this study

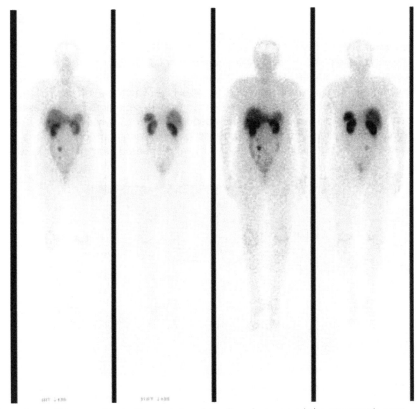

Fig. 7. Octreotide scan illustrating uptake of the liver lesions and the mesenteric mass.

suggested that resection of the primary is important not only in relief of intestinal symptoms but may also deprive the liver metastases of a constant source of hormones and growth factors that could be accelerating their proliferation.

Cytoreduction surgery for hepatic metastases also has an important role in the management of these patients. Resection or ablation of hepatic metastases has been associated with improvement of symptoms of carcinoid syndrome in 67% to 96% of patients by reducing the release of serotonin and other hormones into the systemic circulation.[25,35–37] Cytoreduction surgery for hepatic metastases has also been associated with an improvement in survival and seems to be superior to embolization alone.[33–36,38]

Hepatic artery embolization is another means of debulking the tumor burden in the liver. Embolization with particles, microspheres, and gel foam powder have all been used and produce an overall objective response in 50% to 80% of patients.[9,16,38] Chemoembolization, utilizing doxorubicin in Lipiodol, immediately followed by particle embolization or the use of spheres embedded with cytotoxic drugs such as cisplatin, streptozotocin, or doxorubicin have a theoretical advantage over bland embolization. To date there is no conclusive evidence that demonstrates a superior advantage with one particular technique or agent.[9,21] In a recent study, particle embolization was shown to be more effective in midgut carcinoids whereas chemoembolization was better for pancreatic NETs.[39] Objective response rates for particle embolization were 81% in the carcinoid patients and only 25% in the pancreatic NET patients, whereas chemoembolization had an objective response in only 44% of the carcinoids and 50% response was seen in the pancreatic NETs.

Radiotherapy

External beam radiation has demonstrated little benefit in the treatment of small bowel carcinoid tumors except for pain relief from bone metastases. Radionuclide therapy is a novel approach that has demonstrated benefit in NETs.[6] Coupling a radioisotope to a molecule that is taken up by the tumor cells allows for the delivery of an effective radiation dose to the tumor without damaging healthy tissues. Between 60% and 70% of carcinoid tumors actively take up meta-iodobenzylguanidine (mIBG), thus allowing the use of ^{131}I-mIBG therapy in patients with disseminated disease.[21,40–42] The cumulative experience has demonstrated a tumor and biochemical response of only 15%; however, a symptomatic response of greater than 65% is consistently seen.[6] In one study, improved quality of life was reported in 60% of patients with progressive NETs receiving radionuclide therapy.[40] Leukopenia and thrombocytopenia are the main significant side effects with this treatment. Myelosuppression in patients with extensive bone metastases has been reported.[40,42]

The use of target-labeled somatostatin analogue therapy was inhibited until recently with the inability to achieve a stable compound between the analogue and an effective isotope. [111]Indium-pentreotide initially showed some effect, yet the benefit appeared to be limited.[6,21,40,43] This short-term effect is likely related to the fact that ^{111}In is a γ-emitter and radionuclides emitting β-irradiation have a greater therapeutic effect. Two somatostatin analogues, Sandostatin (Novartis, Basel, Switzerland) and Lanreotide (Ipen, Berkshire, UK) have been coupled to a chelating agent (DOTA) that has allowed for the formation of stable compounds when bound to β-emitters [90]Y (yttrium) or [177]Lu (lutetium). Early reports indicate a higher response rate than seen with mIBG therapy and therefore these modalities may prove to be beneficial not only for palliation but also as adjuvant therapy in the future.[6,9,21,44–46]

Medical therapy

Somatostatin analogues remain the mainstay of symptomatic therapy in patients with carcinoid syndrome. To date the most effective formulations Sandostatin and Lanreotide have demonstrated a symptomatic response of 50% to 75% and biochemical response in 40% to 60% of patients.[6,9,21] A true tumor response (>50% reduction in tumor volume) is rarely seen; however, tumor stability is reported in up 50% of patients.[6,9] The median duration of response is 12 months, at which time the patients start to develop tachyphylaxis.[6] Newer somatostatin analogues, such as SOM 230, have a different binding affinity to the somatostatin receptors and this may provide an alternative therapy once tachyphylaxis develops.

Interferon-α (IFN) has been shown to produce symptomatic and biochemical response rates ranging from 8% to 70%.[6] Many of the studies are plagued with small numbers and many of these patients have the addition of other therapeutic modalities that confound the results. IFN was first introduced as a treatment modality in 1982, yet its exact mechanism of action is still not fully understood. Possible mechanisms include inhibition of angiogenesis, increased number of natural killer cells, inhibition of cell proliferation, and blocking of the cell cycle.[47] Early reports claimed that there was a synergistic benefit in the antiproliferative effects when used in combination with somatostatin analogues.[6] However, a recently published prospective study demonstrated no difference in response rates with the combined use of octreotide and IFN or either therapy alone.[48]

Cytotoxic therapies are considered the first-line therapy for the rare, poorly differentiated midgut carcinoid. The combination of etoposide and cisplatin has demonstrated a response rate of greater than 60%, albeit of short duration (median duration 2–6 months).[6,9] In most small bowel carcinoid with low proliferation capacity (Ki67 <2%) the use of systemic chemotherapy has not been beneficial. In 2 randomized trials the combination of 5-fluorouracil and streptozotocin produced response rates of only 33% and 22%, with no evidence of improved survival.[49,50] Recent interest has revolved around the overexpression of vascular endothelial growth factors and their receptors on NETs, and the related signaling pathways of such epithelial growth factors and mammalian target of rapamycin (mTOR). Tyrosine kinase inhibitors, mTOR inhibitors, and inhibitors of vascular endothelial growth factor look promising and have been shown to stabilize progressive disease in phase II trials.[9,21,51,52]

Prognosis

The prognosis of midgut carcinoids is generally unfavorable compared with the type 1 and 2 gastric carcinoids and rectal carcinoids. As with all NETs, midgut carcinoids are stage-dependent. Using SEER data the overall 5- and 10-year survival rates for well-differentiated small bowel carcinoids in localized disease was 73% and 65%; for regional disease, 71% and 46%; for distant disease, 54% and 30%, respectively.[12] Treatment of these patients involves a multidisciplinary approach. Survival data from centers of excellence that lend themselves to this multidisciplinary approach have demonstrated an improve median survival in stage IV patients over historical controls.[25,37] Kaplan-Meier estimates of 5-year survival exceeds 65% to 75% in Stage IV carcinoid patients compared with 33% from historical controls. Although surgery is the first-line treatment option in small bowel carcinoids, additional therapies are necessary as very few patients are cured from surgery alone.

Appendiceal Carcinoid

The incidence of appendiceal carcinoids has decreased and only comprise 8% of GI-NETs.[12,25,53] Appendiceal carcinoids are still the most common neoplasm of the appendix, compromising 32% to 57% of all appendiceal tumors.[53] It is unclear whether reported epidemiology studies reflect a change in diagnostic or therapeutic behavior rather than a real change in the in the prevalence of the disease. In autopsy series from 26,294 specimens in Malmo, the prevalence of appendiceal carcinoids was 8.4 per 100,000 compared with reported SEER data of 4.5 per 100,000.[53] Most appendiceal carcinoids are found incidentally (1 per 300 appendectomies). The overall rate of metastases is 4% with distant disease in 0.7%.[15] Unlike small bowel carcinoids, the size of the primary is predictive of metastatic potential with tumors smaller than 1 cm rarely demonstrating metastatic disease, whereas lymph node metastases are found in up to 30% of those tumors larger than 2 cm in size. In a Mayo Clinic series, 21% of tumors 2 to 3 cm and 44% of tumors larger than 3 cm in size demonstrated metastases.[54] It is on the basis of these findings that a prognosticating right hemicolectomy should be done in appendiceal tumors larger than 2 cm. Tumors fully resected and smaller than 1 cm can be adequately treated by an appendectomy. Although the evidence is lacking, treatment of lesions between 1 and 2 cm should be individualized based on the pathologic criteria of the tumor itself. Prognostic features that indicate a more aggressive tumor are listed in **Box 2**. Lesions between 1 and 2 cm that have aggressive features should be considered for a right hemicolectomy to assess their lymph node status. Those patients that prove to have lymph node involvement will require ongoing follow-up, whereas those without have been cured.

Fortunately, most tumors (90%) are <1 cm in size, situated at the tip of the appendix, and therefore are invariably cured with appendectomy alone.[15] A rare variant, the goblet-cell or adenocarcinoid, now classified as a mixed endocrine/exocrine tumor, is an exception to the excellent prognosis that most appendiceal carcinoids exhibit. These tumors are aggressive, often displaying peritoneal disease at presentation. Adenocarcinoids do not express somatostatin receptors and therefore do not localize on SRI, nor can radionuclide therapy be used. This tumor, regardless of size, should be treated with a right hemicolectomy, lymph node clearance, and consideration of systemic chemotherapy.[15,53] Disseminated tumors have been treated with peritoneal stripping. The 10-year survival for these lesions is only 60%.[15,53]

HINDGUT CARCINOIDS
Colonic Carcinoids

Colonic carcinoids are rare, accounting for only 8% of GI-NETs. As mentioned earlier, 50% of colonic carcinoids occur in the right colon (embryologic midgut). These lesions differ from the small bowel lesions in that they rarely secrete serotonin and only 5% of

---

Box 2
Pathologic criteria that should influence the need for a prognosticating right hemicolectomy in appendiceal carcinoids 1 to 2 cm in size

Invasion into the mesoappendix

Lymphovascular invasion

Serosal involvement

Involved margins

Positive lymph nodes in appendectomy specimen

High *Ki67* index (>2%)

Goblet-cell variant

the time are they associated with carcinoid syndrome.[15,17] Right colon carcinoids more frequently are poorly differentiated neuroendocrine cancers and have generally metastasized at the time of diagnosis. The remaining carcinoids of the colon usually present as large (>5 cm) exophitic lesions. Radical resection with lymph node clearance should be attempted, although often only debulking is possible.[15] Overall the 5-year survival is slightly worse than that of adenocarcinoma of the colon, at 40%.

Rectal Carcinoids

The incidence of rectal carcinoids is increasing, accounting for 11% of all GI-NETs and 1.5% of rectal neoplasms.[12,13,15] Rectal carcinoids are more common in African Americans and occur most often at 55 years of age or older. Sixty percent are small (<1 cm) and incidentally detected on endoscopy. Like the appendiceal carcinoids prognosis for these lesions is also size-dependent. Tumors smaller than 1 cm have a low incidence of lymph node involvement (0%–3%) and no distant spread; tumors of 1 to 2 cm in size have regional or distant disease in 7% to 34% whereas tumors larger than 2 cm (found in 15%) have regional and distant spread 67% to 100% of the time.[17] Carcinoid syndrome is rare. Both urinary 5-HIAA and CgA are rarely elevated even in the face of disseminated disease.[15]

Surgical excision of the tumor with histologically clear margins and no evidence of invasion into the muscularis is the treatment of choice. Rectal carcinoids smaller than 1 cm can be safely excised endoscopically. Lesions of 1 to 2 cm should be evaluated with transanal ultrasound or MRI to look for evidence of invasion or regional disease. Absence of muscularis invasion and regional lymph node involvement justifies a transanal excision for these intermediate lesions. However, evidence of invasion or regional disease warrants total mesorectal excision, which is also the recommended treatment for all rectal carcinoids larger than 2 cm.

SUMMARY

GI-NETs are a diverse group of tumors that arise from the enterochromaffin cells of the GI tract. Although termed carcinoids—carcinoma-like, because of their indolent behavior—these neoplasms are no longer thought to be benign. Although surgery remains the first-line treatment for most GI-NETs, a multidisciplinary approach is needed, as most patients require multimodality therapy. The rarity of these tumors has led to a lack of randomized trials addressing treatment options, but has led to the development of centers of excellence in this area. It is from the experience and collective knowledge of these centers that one hopes to gain a better understanding of the natural history and best treatment modalities for each of these lesions.

REFERENCES

1. Oberndorfer S. Karzinoid tumore des Dunndarms. Frankf Z Pathol 1907;1:426–30 [in German].
2. Ransom W. A case of primary carcinoma of the ileum. Lancet 2009;2:1020–3.
3. Gosset A, Masson P. Tumeurs endocrines se l'appendice. Presse Med 2009;25: 237–40 [in Italian].
4. Arnold R. Endocrine tumours of the gastrointestinal tract. Introduction: definition, historical aspects, classification, staging, prognosis and therapeutic options. Best Pract Res Clin Gastroenterol 2005;19:491–505.
5. Lembeck F. [Current status of carcinoid research; pharmacological report.]. Krebsarzt 1958;13:196–202 [in German].

6. Oberg K. Diagnosis and treatment of carcinoid tumors. Expert Rev Anticancer Ther 2003;3:863–77.
7. Dayal Y. GI-NETs—uniform but also diverse. Endocr Pathol 2007;18:135–40.
8. Van Eeden S, Quaedvlieg PF, Taal BG, et al. Classification of low-grade neuroendocrine tumors of midgut and unknown origin. Hum Pathol 2002;33:1126–32.
9. Modlin IM, Oberg K, Chung DC, et al. Gastroenteropancreatic neuroendocrine tumours. Lancet Oncol 2008;9:61–72.
10. Baudin E, Bidart JM, Backelot A, et al. Impact of chromogranin A measurement in the work-up of neuroendocrine tumors. Ann Oncol 2001;12:S79–82.
11. Stivanello M, Berruti A, Torta M, et al. Circulating chromogranin A in the assessment of patients with neuroendocrine tumours. A single institution experience. Ann Oncol 2001;12:S73–7.
12. Yao JC, Hassan M, Phan A, et al. One hundred years after "carcinoid": epidemiology of and prognostic factors for neuroendocrine tumors in 35,825 cases in the United States. J Clin Oncol 2008;26:3063–72.
13. Modlin IM, Lye KD, Kidd M. A 5-decade analysis of 13,715 carcinoid tumors. Cancer 2003;97:934–59.
14. de Herder WW. Tumours of the midgut (jejunum, ileum and ascending colon, including carcinoid syndrome). Best Pract Res Clin Gastroenterol 2005;19:705–15.
15. Akerstrom G, Hellman P. Surgery on neuroendocrine tumours. Best Pract Res Clin Endocrinol Metab 2007;21:87–109.
16. Granberg D, Oberg K. Neuroendocrine tumours. Cancer Chemother Biol Response Modif 2005;22:471–83.
17. Kloppel G, Anlauf M. Epidemiology, tumour biology and histopathological classification of neuroendocrine tumours of the gastrointestinal tract. Best Pract Res Clin Gastroenterol 2005;19:507–17.
18. Delle Fave G, Capurso G, Milione M, et al. Endocrine tumours of the stomach. Best Pract Res Clin Gastroenterol 2005;19:659–73.
19. Bordi C, Caruana P, D'Adda T, et al. Smooth muscle cell abnormalities associated with gastric ECL cell carcinoids. Endocr Pathol 1995;6:103–13.
20. Ruszniewski P, Delle Fave G, Cadiot G, et al. Well-differentiated gastric tumors/carcinomas. Neuroendocrinology 2006;84:158–64.
21. Bendelow J, Apps E, Jones LE, et al. Carcinoid syndrome. Eur J Surg Oncol 2008;34:289–96.
22. Woodside KJ, Townsend CM, Mark EB. Current management of gastrointestinal carcinoid tumors. J Gastrointest Surg 2004;8:742–56.
23. Schindl M, Kaserer K, Niederle B. Treatment of gastric neuroendocrine tumors: the necessity of a type-adapted treatment. Arch Surg 2001;136:49–54.
24. Rindi G, Luinetti O, Cornaggia M, et al. Three subtypes of gastric argyrophil carcinoid and the gastric neuroendocrine carcinoma: a clinicopathologic study. Gastroenterology 1993;104:994–1006.
25. Chambers AJ, Pasieka JL, Dixon E, et al. The palliative benefit of aggressive surgical intervention for both hepatic and mesenteric metastases from neuroendocrine tumors. Surgery 2008;144:645–51.
26. Bernheim AM, Connolly HM, Pellikka PA. Carcinoid heart disease. Curr Treat Options Cardiovasc Med 2007;9:482–9.
27. Bhattacharyya S, Davar J, Dreyfus G, et al. Carcinoid heart disease. Circulation 2007;116:2860–5.
28. Bhattacharyya S, Toumpanakis C, Caplin ME, et al. Analysis of 150 patients with carcinoid syndrome seen in a single year at one institution in the first decade of the twenty-first century. Am J Cardiol 2008;101:378–81.

29. Chambers AP, Pasieka JL, Dixon E, et al. The role of imaging studies in the staging of midgut neuroendocrine tumors. J Am Coll Surg 2009;207:S18.

30. Orlefors H, Sundin A, Garske U, et al. Whole-body (11)C-5-hydroxytryptophan positron emission tomography as a universal imaging technique for neuroendocrine tumors: comparison with somatostatin receptor scintigraphy and computed tomography. J Clin Endocrinol Metab 2005;90:3392–400.

31. Pacak K, Eisenhofer G, Goldstein DS. Functional imaging of endocrine tumors: role of positron emission tomography. Endocr Rev 2004;25:568–80.

32. Givi B, Pommier SJ, Thompson AK, et al. Operative resection of primary carcinoid neoplasms in patients with liver metastases yields significantly better survival. Surgery 2006;140:891–7.

33. Hellman P, Lundstrom T, Ohrvall U, et al. Effect of surgery on the outcome of midgut carcinoid disease with lymph node and liver metastases. World J Surg 2002;26:991–7.

34. Boudreaux JP, Putty B, Frey DJ, et al. Surgical treatment of advanced-stage carcinoid tumors: lessons learned. Ann Surg 2005;241:839–45.

35. Chamberlain RS, Canes D, Brown KT, et al. Hepatic neuroendocrine metastases: does intervention alter outcomes? J Am Coll Surg 2000;190:432–45.

36. Sarmiento JM, Heywood G, Rubin J, et al. Surgical treatment of neuroendocrine metastases to the liver: a plea for resection to increase survival. J Am Coll Surg 2003;197:29–37.

37. Eriksson J, Stalberg P, Nilsson A, et al. Surgery and radiofrequency ablation for treatment of liver metastases from midgut and foregut carcinoids and endocrine pancreatic tumors. World J Surg 2008;32:930–8.

38. Osborne DA, Zervos EE, Strosberg J, et al. Improved outcome with cytoreduction versus embolization for symptomatic hepatic metastases of carcinoid and neuroendocrine tumors. Ann Surg Oncol 2006;13:572–81.

39. Gupta S, Johnson MM, Murthy R, et al. Hepatic arterial embolization and chemoembolization for the treatment of patients with metastatic neuroendocrine tumors: variables affecting response rates and survival. Cancer 2005;104:1590–602.

40. Pasieka JL, McEwan A, Rorstad O. The palliative role of [131]I mIBG and ^{111}In-octreotide in patients with metastatic progressive neuroendocrine tumors. Surgery 2004;136:1218–26.

41. Sywak MS, Pasieka JL, McEwan A, et al. [131]I mIBG in the management of metastatic midgut carcinoid tumors. World J Surg 2004;28:1157–62.

42. Taal BG, Hoefnagel CA, Valdes Olmos RA, et al. Palliative effect of metaiodobenzylguanidine in metastatic carcinoid tumors. J Clin Oncol 1996;14:1829–38.

43. Buscombe JR, Caplin ME, Hilson AJ. Long-term efficacy of high-activity[111] In-pentetreotide therapy in patients with disseminated neuroendocrine tumors. J Nucl Med 2003;44:1–6.

44. Frilling A, Weber F, Saner F, et al. Treatment with (90)Y- and (177)Lu-DOTATOC in patients with metastatic neuroendocrine tumors. Surgery 2006;140:968–76.

45. Kwekkeboom DJ, Mueller-Brand J, Paganelli G, et al. Overview of results of peptide receptor radionuclide therapy with 3 radiolabeled somatostatin analogs. J Nucl Med 2005;46(Suppl 1):62S–6S.

46. Waldherr C, Pless M, Maecke HR, et al. Tumor response and clinical benefit in neuroendocrine tumors after 7.4 GBq (90)Y-DOTATOC. J Nucl Med 2002;43:610–6.

47. Zuetenhorst JM, Taal BG. Metastatic carcinoid tumors: a clinical review. Oncologist 2005;10:123–31.

48. Faiss S, Pape UF, Bohmig M, et al. Prospective, randomized, multicenter trial on the antiproliferative effect of lanreotide, interferon alfa, and their combination for

therapy of metastatic neuroendocrine gastroenteropancreatic tumors—the International Lanreotide and Interferon Alfa Study Group. J Clin Oncol 2003;21: 2689–96.

49. Engstrom PF, Lavin PT, Moertel CG, et al. Streptozocin plus fluorouracil versus doxorubicin therapy for metastatic carcinoid tumor. J Clin Oncol 1984;2:1255–9.
50. Bukowski RM, Johnson KG, Peterson RF, et al. A phase II trial of combination chemotherapy in patients with metastatic carcinoid tumors. A Southwest Oncology Group Study. Cancer 1987;60:2891–5.
51. Delaunoit T, Neczyporenko F, Rubin J, et al. Medical management of pancreatic neuroendocrine tumors. Am J Gastroenterol 2008;103:475–83.
52. Papouchado B, Erickson LA, Rohlinger AL, et al. Epidermal growth factor receptor and activated epidermal growth factor receptor expression in gastrointestinal carcinoids and pancreatic endocrine carcinomas. Mod Pathol 2005;18: 1329–35.
53. Stinner B, Rothmund M. Neuroendocrine tumours (carcinoids) of the appendix. Best Pract Res Clin Gastroenterol 2005;19:729–38.
54. Moertel CG, Lefkopoulo M, Lipsitz S, et al. Streptozocin-doxorubicin, streptozocin-fluorouracil, or chlorozotocin in the treatment of advanced islet cell carcinoma. N Engl J Med 1992;326:519–23.

Molecular Markers in Thyroid Cancer Diagnostics

Meredith A. Kato, MD*, Thomas J. Fahey III, MD

KEYWORDS

- Thyroid cancer diagnostics • Thyroid FNA • Thyroid cancer
- Galectin-3 • HBME-1 • Microarray

Approximately 37,340 cases of thyroid cancer were projected for 2008 with resultant 1590 deaths, making it the most common endocrine malignancy in the United States. Thyroid cancer accounts for 2.5% of cancer incidence, but only 0.28% of cancer deaths.[1] Clinically evident thyroid nodules are found in approximately 4.2% of the general population,[2] but the number found on autopsy is much higher, ranging from 8% to 65%.[3] Nodules are more common in women and in patients with a history of radiation exposure.[4] The incidence of thyroid cancer has more than doubled in the last 30 years. This increase is largely due to better radiographic detection of subclinical nodules rather than a truly increased incidence of the disease.[5]

Fine-needle aspiration biopsy (FNA) was adopted into widespread use in the 1970s and 1980s and greatly enhanced the ability to diagnose thyroid nodules preoperatively. Indeed, preoperative FNA reduced the number of thyroid surgeries by at least 25% and doubled the yield for cancer.[6]

Unfortunately, thyroid nodules present clinicians with a diagnostic conundrum as cytologic interpretations of FNAs are limited. Diagnostic outcomes of FNAs fall into 3 broad categories: benign, malignant, and indeterminate. The indeterminate group includes lesions with cellular atypia, suspicious lesions, and follicular lesions, all of which have some concerning features, but fail to meet criteria for diagnosis of cancer.[4] Between 60% and 80% of FNAs are benign, 4% to 7% are malignant, and 10% to 20% are indeterminate.[7,8] The standard of care for indeterminate lesions is surgery to enable a histologic diagnosis. Unfortunately, only 4% to 30% are found to be malignant on histopathology, ultimately rendering many of these operations unnecessary.[7–10] Furthermore, considerable interobserver variability is reported in the cytologic interpretation of FNA specimens.[11,12]

One of the greatest challenges in thyroid cancer research is to develop an adjunct to FNA to clarify the indeterminate lesions as benign or malignant. Such a marker would

Division of Endocrine Surgery, Department of Surgery, New York Presbyterian Hospital, Weill Cornell Medical Center, 525 East 68th Street, F-2024, New York, NY 10068, USA
* Corresponding author.
E-mail address: mek2002@med.cornell.edu (M.A. Kato).

Surg Clin N Am 89 (2009) 1139–1155
doi:10.1016/j.suc.2009.06.012
0039-6109/09/$ – see front matter © 2009 Elsevier Inc. All rights reserved.
surgical.theclinics.com

improve preoperative prognostication and prevent risks associated with surgery in patients with benign lesions. Unfortunately, no one marker has proven the panacea. Nonetheless, several areas of research show great promise in the molecular diagnosis of these lesions.

IMMUNOCYTOCHEMICAL MARKERS
Galectin-3

Galectins are a family of animal lectins defined by their ability to bind β-galactosides and by their consensus amino acid sequences. Galectins have an affinity for a wide variety of glycoproteins and glycolipids. These lectins exert effects in the cytoplasm and at the cell surface where they mediate interactions among cells, and between the cells and extracellular matrices. Some members can induce apoptosis whereas others, including galectin-3, transform cells in culture to a malignant phenotype. Galectins modulate the behavior of cells including cell adhesion and migration, and thus affect metastatic capabilities of tumors.[13]

Galectin-3 seems to play a large role in the pathogenesis of papillary thyroid cancer (PTC). Yoshii and colleagues transfected a PTC cell line with antisense galectin-3 cDNA and saw a significant suppression of anchorage-independent cell proliferation. These investigators concluded that galectin-3 was necessary to maintain the malignant phenotype in the PTC cell line.[14] In another study, the same group transfected human fetal follicular cells with plasmids containing galectin-3 and transformed them into a malignant phenotype. The transformation was demonstrated by increased saturation density, serum-independent growth and clonogenic potential.[15] Several groups established galectin-3 expression in follicular cell malignancies but not in benign lesions or normal thyroid tissue. Expression was detectable in specimens from tissue as well as by FNA, and separated benign from malignant lesions of the thyroid.[16–20] This work opened the door to the possibility of galectin-3 being used as a diagnostic marker for thyroid cancers.

Saussez and colleagues looked at the differential serum levels of galectin-3 in patients with benign lesions and malignant tumors versus controls. The median serum level of galectin-3 was significantly different between the control and malignant groups, between control and benign groups and, most importantly, between the benign and malignant groups. Using a cutoff level of 3.2 ng/mL, the investigators calculated 74% sensitivity, 73% specificity, a positive predictive value of 57%, and a negative predictive value of 85% for detecting a thyroid malignancy among multinodular goiters.[21] However, another group led by Inohara did not detect differences in serum galectin-3 between patients with benign and malignant lesions.[22]

The greatest hope for galectin-3 is as an adjunct to traditional cytopathology of FNA biopsies. Several groups have looked at the diagnostic feasibility of using immunocytochemistry for galectin-3 in FNA specimens.[17,23–27] Sensitivities in these studies ranged from 75% to 100% with specificities from 75% to 100%. In the largest study to date, a prospective multicenter trial, Bartolazzi and colleagues looked at galectin-3 levels in 465 FNA cytology specimens and compared them to final pathology of the surgical specimens. These investigators found a 78% sensitivity and 93% specificity. Of note, 29 of 130 (22%) cancers were missed using the galectin-3 test.[23]

Several investigators issue caveats about using galectin-3 in thyroid nodule diagnostics. Mehrotra and colleagues[28] did not find that galecin-3 distinguished benign from malignant tissue samples, but were sharply criticized for their methods.[29] In a systematic review of the available data on FNA and galectin-3, Sanabria and colleagues[30] concluded that many of the studies had important methodological weaknesses and were not designed to properly evaluate galectin-3 as a diagnostic test. Those that they considered appropriate did not suggest that galectin-3 was a powerful enough marker to be used as a single entity.

Whereas it probably does not have utility as a single marker for thyroid carcinoma, available data suggest that galectin-3 does have potential when used in conjunction with cytology and other markers currently under study (see later discussion).

HBME-1

Hector Battifora mesothelial cell antibody (HBME-1) is a mouse monoclonal antibody originally developed to stain malignant mesothelioma.[31] Early studies found that it also stained thyroid cancers of follicular origin, particularly PTC, with a much greater affinity than benign thyroid lesions.[21–25]

Subsequent work established that the antibody also stained cells from FNA biopsies.[26,32–34] Van Hoeven and colleagues evaluated HBME-1 as a diagnostic test and found 100% sensitivity and 76% specificity for thyroid malignancy in a small patient sample ($n = 29$). Larger-scale studies found sensitivities of 80% to 90%, but specificities varied widely, from 60% to 96%.[26,33] Although encouraging, HBME-1 has not demonstrated utility as a single test for thyroid nodule diagnostics. Many investigators have looked at HBME-1 in combination with other markers as part of a panel.

IMMUNOCYTOCHEMICAL COMBINATIONS
HBME-1 and Galectin-3

Perhaps the greatest potential for these markers is when they are used in combination with each other. Several groups looked at HBME-1 and galectin-3 in concert. Using tissue microarray, Wiseman and colleagues[35] assembled a panel of 7 immunohistochemical markers, including HBME-1, galectin-3, and CK-19, and calculated 87.9% sensitivity and 94% specificity for cancer. Rossi and colleagues[36] looked at the combination of HBME-1 and galectin-3 in tissue samples and found 95% sensitivity and \100% specificity for cancer. Similar results were found on testing FNA samples. Saggiorato and colleagues[26] calculated a sensitivity of 97% and specificity of 91% for cancer after testing 125 FNA specimens.

HBME-1 and Cytokeratin-19

Scognamiglio and colleagues[37] found that HBME-1 together with CK-19 had 83% sensitivity and 100% specificity for malignancy when staining tissue samples. Nga and colleagues[38] applied HBME-1 and CK-19 to FNA specimens and found a 100% sensitivity and 100% specificity, but the sample population was small ($n = 22$).

hTERT and Telomerase

DNA polymerases are unable to replicate the complete sequence of a chromosome. To ensure that functional components of the genome are replicated, the ends of chromosomes are capped with telomeres, repeats of the nonsense sequence TTAGGG. With each cycle of DNA replication, the telomeres at the end of chromosomes shorten. Telomerase is a ribonucleoprotein that functions to lengthen the telomeres and ensure seamless duplication of DNA. Without it, chromosomes can become unstable and enter senescence; with it, cells can gain immortality. Telomerase is not found in healthy somatic cells, except stem cells, lymphocytes, and germline cells. Telomerase activity is also sharply increased in most malignancies.[39]

Many groups have looked at activity of telomerase in thyroid tissues. Whereas most groups detected higher levels in malignant thyroid tumors compared with benign lesions,[40–43] the authors' group did not.[44] Higher activity correlated to higher stage on diagnosis, tall-cell variant of PTC, undifferentiated cancers, extrathyroidal extension, recurrence, distant metastasis, and older age.[45–51] Not surprisingly, high activity levels were found in specimens with background thyroiditis[48–50] and in one case of thyroid lymphoma.[52]

The catalytic subunit of telomerase is hTERT. Some groups have looked into hTERT expression as a potential marker for thyroid malignancy. As with telomerase activity, they found higher expression levels of hTERT in malignant specimens than benign ones.[53–56] Wang and colleagues[57] looked at splice variants of hTERT and found that malignant tumors exhibited a greater proportion of the active variant when compared with benign lesions.

Whereas every study save one found higher activity or expression levels in malignant nodules, nearly every one also found some activity in benign lesions, such as follicular adenomas and thyroiditis. This result limits the diagnostic potential for these markers by lowering specificity. Nonetheless, several groups have explored the diagnostic usefulness of telomerase and hTERT in FNA.[58–60] Two groups concluded that these markers had no diagnostic utility.[61,62] Lerma and colleagues looked at FNAs with suspicious findings but which lacked criteria for a malignant diagnosis. Telomerase activity was positive in 6 of 18 specimens, but only 5 of those 6 were malignant on histology. Of note, they excluded samples with an abundance of lymphocytes.[63] In contrast, Guerra and colleagues[64] found that telomerase testing clarified the diagnosis in 5 of 11 FNAs with indeterminate cytology. Despite these findings, the variation of expression within a given tumor type and the consistent positivity among benign lesions renders telomerase and hTERT short of the sensitivity and specificity needed for them to be useful diagnostically.

GENETIC MARKERS
BRAF

The RAF protein is a serine-threonine kinase along the MAP kinase cascade. The RAF protein has 3 isoforms, ARAF, BRAF, and CRAF, with BRAF being the most common found in thyroid follicular cells.[65] All forms of RAF activate MEK in the MAP kinase cascade, but BRAF does so much more avidly than the other forms.[66] The most common BRAF mutation, occurring in more than 95% of cases, is the $BRAF^{T1799A}$. Here an A → T transversion at position 1799 results in a valine to glutamate substitution at residue 600 (V600E). This occurrence destabilizes the inactive form of the protein, resulting in its constitutive action.[67]

The BRAF mutation is the most common mutation in PTC, occurring in 35% to 69%.[68–71] This mutation is specific to classic and tall-cell variants of PTC; it is rarely found in other types of differentiated thyroid cancer.[68] The BRAF mutation occurs early and plays an important role in the pathogenesis of PTC. In one study, Knauf and colleagues[72] showed thyroid-specific expression of the mutation in mice induced invasive PTC. The mutation confers a worse clinical prognosis as it is associated with older age at diagnosis, tall-cell histology, extrathyroidal extension, lymph node metastasis, recurrence, and advanced tumor stage.[73–75]

Many groups have looked into adding BRAF testing as an adjunct to cytology on FNAs. Knowing BRAF status preoperatively could be reassuring for lesions with benign cytology and could indicate more aggressive surgery in malignant ones. Because of its prevalence and specificity in PTC, testing FNA samples for the BRAF mutation could theoretically classify some indeterminate or follicular lesions as malignant. The majority of studies show that BRAF testing of FNA specimens was highly concordant with BRAF results derived from tissue. Most found BRAF mutations among the indeterminate group of FNAs, but the numbers varied widely and tended to be small; BRAF status clarified between 5% and 43% of indeterminate lesions.[70,76–83] Of note, 2 studies found no BRAF mutations among their indeterminate lesions.[84,85]

BRAF is an extremely important marker in PTC, and there may be a role for preoperative testing to prognosticate and to guide surgical decisions. BRAF testing in FNA specimens is highly specific. However, it lacks the sensitivity necessary to clarify a large proportion of indeterminate or follicular lesions and is unlikely to come into widespread use for this purpose.

RET/PTC

Another derangement along the MAP kinase cascade associated with differentiated thyroid cancer is the RET/PTC rearrangement. RET is the signaling subunit of the receptor for the glial-derived neurotrophic factor family of genes. Although it is normally expressed in c-cells of the thyroid, it is not highly expressed in follicular cells. In the rearrangement, the 3' end of RET fuses with the 5' end of an unrelated gene. There are at least 11 RET/PTC rearrangements described to date, the 2 most common being RET/PTC1 and RET/PTC3. The resulting RET/PTC oncogene constitutively activates the MAP kinase cascade.[65,86]

RET/PTC oncogene is found in approximately 20% of PTC and is not commonly seen in other thyroid cancers.[87] The rearrangement is associated with a younger presentation, classic PTC histology, and an increased risk for lymph node metastasis.[88,89] Early studies showed that transgenic mice expressing the RET/PTC1 or RET/PTC3 oncogene developed papillary carcinoma.[90–92]

RET/PTC rearrangements are associated with childhood and radiation induced PTC. Among post-Chernobyl children with PTC, RET/PTC1 was found in 16% and RET/PTC3 in 58%. In sporadic childhood PTC, RET/PTC1 was found in 47% and RET/PTC 3 in 18%.[93] RET/PTC rearrangements were significantly more frequent among Japanese adult survivors of the atomic bombings during World War II compared patients not exposed to radiation.[94] Further studies conducted in Japan explored the direct relationship between radiation and PTC. Ito and colleagues[95] induced RET/PTC rearrangements in undifferentiated thyroid cells by exposing them to 50 Gy of radiation. Mizuno and colleagues induced PTC in human thyroid tissue transplanted into nude mice. This group found that the rearrangement was present as early as day 2 of exposure to 50 Gy.[96]

As with BRAF mutations, RET/PTC rearrangements have been explored as a possible adjunct to FNA cytology. In most of the studies, RET/PTC testing helped to classify few if any indeterminate lesions.[76,84,85] Cheung and colleagues[97] tested 45 indeterminate or insufficient FNA specimens for RET/PTC 1, 2, and 3, and reached a malignant diagnosis in 11 of them or 24%. As a caveat, however, Elisei and colleagues[98] found RET/PTC rearrangements in the benign lesions of 52% of post-Chernobyl, 38% medically irradiated and sporadic patients. Domingues and colleagues[84] found rearrangements in FNA specimens from benign lesions as well. Like BRAF, RET/PTC rearrangements offer opportunities to study the pathogenesis of PTC, but offer little in the way of diagnostics.

PAX8-PPARγ

The PAX8-PPARγ oncogene is the result of the interchromosomal translocation t(2,3)(q13;p25) joining paired box 8 (PAX8) and peroxisome proliferator-activated receptor gamma (PPARγ).[99] The PAX8-PPARγ oncogene was originally thought to be unique to follicular carcinoma of the thyroid (FTC), but has since been detected in follicular adenoma as well. The oncogene is found in 29% to 56% of FTC and in

4% to 13% follicular adenomas, and is not seen in PTC, anaplastic thyroid carcinoma (ATC), goiters, Hurthle cell adenomas, Hurthle cell carcinomas, or poorly differentiated thyroid cancers.[100–103] One study found the oncogene in 55% of adenomas, but sampled only 11 cases.[102] Another study in Japan found no rearrangements in FTC, suggesting possible regional variation.[104] This oncogene is associated with more favorable prognostic indicators such as female sex, improved tumor differentiation, and lower risk of metastasis.[105]

The mechanism of the PAX8-PPARγ oncogene is incompletely understood. The authors do know that PAX8-PPARγ is near mutually exclusive with RAS mutations and thus is likely to constitute a distinct molecular pathway.[106] The PAX8-PPARγ fusion oncoprotein transforms human thyrocytes in vitro to a malignant phenotype and likely exerts its action by interfering with the transcriptional function of the wild-type PPARγ protein.[107,108] The wild-type PPARγ is upregulated in tumors with the PAX8-PPARγ rearrangement.[109] Several groups have used gene expression microarray to better characterize transcriptional changes specific to PAX8-PPARγ mutants. Functions of differentially expressed genes run the gamut from lipid/glucose/amino acid metabolism, tumorigenesis, angiogenesis, signal transduction, cell growth, and translational control.[110,111] Of note, Giordano and colleagues[112] found that PAX8-PPARγ mutants had upregulated expression of known wild-type PPARγ targets.

Only one group has pursued PAX8-PPARγ testing as a diagnostic adjunct. Sahin and colleagues[105] found that performing PPARγ immunohistochemistry, as a surrogate for PAX8-PPARγ, improved the sensitivity of intraoperative frozen section from 84% to 96%, but lowered specificity from 100% to 90%.

MicroRNA

First described by Lee and colleagues in 1993, microRNAs (miRNA) are short sequences of noncoding RNA that negatively regulate posttranscriptional gene expression. MiRNAs are 19 to 25 base pairs long and are relatively few in number; there are currently 695 listed on the miRBase database maintained by the Sanger Institute (http://microrna.sanger.ac.uk/sequences/). Changes in the expression levels of miRNAs are seen in every cancer studied to date, including lymphomas, colorectal carcinoma, breast cancer, lung cancer, hepatocellular carcinoma, and thyroid cancer. MiRNA regulation has been implicated in the control of metastasis, invasion, proliferation, cell cycle, and apoptosis.[29] As such, they have generated much interest in the diagnosis, prognosis, and treatment of cancer.

Several groups have explored the expression of miRNA in PTC. Early studies used array techniques to test a broad range of known miRNAs in benign and malignant thyroid specimens.[113,114] This early work revealed that miR-221, miR-222, and miR-146b were upregulated in PTC samples in several studies.[113–115] Pallante and colleagues[114] observed that overexpression of miR-221 caused increased proliferation and knockdown caused growth arrest. In the same study, the group transfected a normal differentiated rat thyroid cell line with mutations implicated in PTC such as RAF and RET/PTC, and saw a corresponding increase in miR-221 with each new malignant phenotype. Using bioinformatic analysis they identified p27^{kip1}, an important regulator of cell cycle, as the target for miR-221 and miR-222.[116] Nikiforova and colleagues showed there was a strong relationship between miRNA expression and mutation status in thyroid tumors. These investigators found that miRNA expression levels could accurately cluster tumor specimens by mutation.[113]

Work into other cancers of the thyroid is under way as well. Weber and colleagues found that both miR-197 and miR-346 were overexpressed in follicular thyroid cancer when compared with follicular adenomas. In vitro overexpression induced proliferation whereas knockdown led to growth arrest. This group showed that the likely targets for these miRNAs were the genes ACVR1 and TSPAN3 for miR-197 and EFEMP2, and CFLAR for miR-346. Of note, they were able to accurately identify FTC in 87% of thyroid specimens based on the expression profile of ACVR1, TSPAN3, and EFEMP2.[117] Visone and colleagues[118] looked at the miRNA expression in anaplastic thyroid cancer and found decreased levels of miR-30d, miR-125b, miR-26a, and miR-30a-5p.

The distinct patterns of expression noted among the miRNAs have led some groups to explore the use of miRNA in thyroid nodule diagnostics. Chen and colleagues used reverse transcription-polymerase chain reaction (RT-PCR) to determine the expression levels of miR-221, miR-222, and miR-146b in thyroid FNAs from PTC and benign lesions. All 3 miRNAs were upregulated in malignant specimens, and miR-222 and miR-146b were statistically significant between malignant and benign samples.[115] Nikiforova and colleagues compiled a panel of 7 miRNAs differentially expressed between differentiated cancers of the thyroid and benign lesions and then tested its utility against 13 FNAs. This group found that when one marker was overexpressed more than 2-fold, the sensitivity for malignancy was 100% with a specificity of 94% and accuracy 94%. When 3 or more markers were overexpressed the sensitivity dropped to 88%, but the specificity and accuracy jumped to 100% and 98%, respectively.[113]

MICROARRAY

As applicability of single gene or single protein markers in the diagnosis of thyroid nodules has proven to be disappointing, many groups have turned to high-throughput methods such as microarray. Distinct expression profiles have been identified for many diseased and normal tissues, including thyroid. This technology has been used to explore tumor biology and pathogenesis as well as tumor diagnostics.

A microarray chip contains probe sets to measure quantitatively the expression profiles of thousands of genes. Powerful statistical tools are able to separate accurately the expression profiles according to disease state, and produce a list of genes differentially expressed between tissues carrying various diagnoses. Differential expression of specific genes in an unknown sample can be used to make a diagnosis. Many academic and commercial groups are currently working to create and test gene lists with utility in the clinical realm.

The authors' group has explored microarray technology in thyroid disease for the last 7 years. Early on it was shown that microarray accurately separated benign from specific malignant lesions including PTC, FTC, and Hurthle cell carcinoma.[119–123] In hopes of separating malignant from benign lesions in a broader sense, the authors compared expression between a mix of malignancies and a mix of benign lesions. The resulting expression profile was able to detect malignancy with a sensitivity of 90.9% and a specificity of 96.2%.[124] Encouraged by these results, the authors explored the application of microarray in FNA specimens. Clustering analysis of the expression profiles generated from a mix of benign and malignant FNA specimens resulted in 3 distinct groups, malignant (n = 10), benign (n = 7), and indeterminate (n = 5; 3 benign, 2 FVPTC). The classification of malignant or benign was 100% concordant with the histologic diagnosis. In contrast, the cytologic diagnosis of these 17 FNA specimens was only 76% concordant (13 out of 17).[125] All 5 in the indeterminate cluster had suspicious findings on cytologic evaluation.

Others have explored the application of microarray to distinguish benign from malignant thyroid lesions as well.[126–134] In one of the earliest studies, Mazzanti and

Table 1
Comparison of molecular markers for thyroid carcinoma currently under study

Method	Marker Description	Sensitivity (%)	Specificity (%)	References	Comments
Immunocytochemistry	HBME-1 and Galectin-3	95	100	Rossi[36]	Experiments done on paraffin-embedded tissue blocks, no validation set (n = 95)
Immunocytochemistry	HBME-1 and Galectin-3	97	91	Saggiorato[26]	Experiments done on preoperative FNAs classified as follicular neoplasms, no validation set (n = 125)
Immunocytochemistry	HBME-1 and CK-19	83	100	Scognamiglio[37]	Experiments done on tissue from paraffin-embedded blocks, only follicular adenomas and PTC, no validation set (n = 127)
Immunocytochemistry	HBME-1 and CK-19	100	100	Nga[38]	Validation done on FNAs collected ex vivo (n = 22)
MicroRNA	Three of the following more than 2-fold overexpressed: miR-187, miR-221, miR-222, miR-146b, miR-155, miR-224, miR-197	88	100	Nikiforova[113]	Validation done on RNA from preoperative FNA (n = 13)
Microarray	627 genes more than 2-fold differentially expressed	91	96	Finley[124]	Validation done on RNA from snap-frozen tissue (n = 14)
Microarray/Multigene assay	Differential expression of G3PDH, SYNGR2, LSM7, KIT, Hs.296031, c21orf4 and Hs24183	75	100	Rosen[135]	Validation done on RNA from snap-frozen tissue (n = 10)
Multigene assay	Differential expression of MCM5, MCM7 and RAD9	98	66	Kebebew[141]	Experiments done on RNA from snap frozen tissue, no validation set (n = 95)
Multigene assay	Differential expression of ECM1, TMPRSS4, ANGPT2 and TIMP1	91	95	Kebebew[144]	validation done on RNA from intraoperative FNAs (n = 31)

colleagues used a teaching set of 63 samples to generate a gene list to define benign and malignant within the group. These investigators built 6-gene and 10-gene models from this list and tested them using 10 unknown samples. Using the analysis of variance test with Bonferroni correction and the leave-one-out method of cross-validation, both the 6- and 10-gene models separated benign from malignant with 100% accuracy.[127] In a subsequent study, the group used expression from 41 tumor specimens to build an expression-ratio model based on the 6 genes. The model was tested using 10 unknown samples, and 75% sensitivity and 100% specificity for malignancy were calculated.[135] In one of the largest studies, Prasad and colleagues generated a 75 gene list from 94 samples (50 benign, 44 malignant) and validated it using RT-PCR and Western blot on a new set of 31 thyroid tumors. This group documented differential expression of 6 of the 75 genes between benign and malignant as predicted by microarray.[128]

Multigene Assays

An interesting offshoot from microarray studies is the development of gene panels to distinguish benign from malignant thyroid lesions.[136–140] The group led by McMillan and Kebebew has been especially active in this area. This group developed several smaller arrays with 96 genes to determine expression of a more targeted group of genes. One array tested the differential expression of cell cycle regulatory genes and isolated 3 (MCM5, MCM7, and RAD9), which separated malignancies with a 98.2% sensitivity and a 65.7% specificity.[141] In similar studies, Kebebew and colleagues put extracellular matrix and adhesion molecule and angiogenesis-modulating gene probes on 2 separate 96-gene arrays.[142,143] In this study they used the expression profiles of at least 100 tumors on each array to generate a list of 4 differentially expressed genes with diagnostic potential (ECM1, TMPRSS4, ANGPT2, and TIMP1). In a separate study, Kebebew and colleagues tested the panel against 31 FNA specimens and developed a scoring model for expression. The panel had a sensitivity of 91% and a specificity of 95%.[144]

SUMMARY

Although FNA biopsy is an important preoperative test for thyroid nodules, it does not provide a diagnosis in up to 20% of patients with indeterminate lesions. These patients undergo surgery with its incumbent risks, but a low percentage of them carry a diagnosis of cancer. Early explorations into single markers showed promise, but ultimately lacked either the sensitivity or specificity necessary for wide adoption. Assays testing several markers show the greatest promise in this conundrum (**Table 1**). Immunocytochemistry testing for 2 or more markers has shown a great improvement on single-marker tests. The recent application of miRNAs and the powerful analysis enabled by microarray are also exciting. Future work will determine how many markers (panels of 6, 10 or 100?) measured by what technique (immunocytochemistry, microarray, RT-PCR, enzyme-liked immunosorbent assay?) will ultimately solve this diagnostic dilemma.

REFERENCES

1. Jemal A, Siegel R, Ward E, et al. Cancer statistics, 2008. CA Cancer J Clin 2008; 58(2):71–96.
2. Vander JB, Gaston EA, Dawber TR. The significance of nontoxic thyroid nodules. Final report of a 15-year study of the incidence of thyroid malignancy. Ann Intern Med 1968;69(3):537–40.

3. Wang C, Crapo LM. The epidemiology of thyroid disease and implications for screening. Endocrinol Metab Clin North Am 1997;26(1):189–218.

4. Mazzaferri EL. Management of a solitary thyroid nodule. N Engl J Med 1993; 328(8):553–9.

5. Davies L, Welch HG. Increasing incidence of thyroid cancer in the United States, 1973–2002. JAMA 2006;295(18):2164–7.

6. Gharib H, Goellner JR. Fine-needle aspiration biopsy of the thyroid: an appraisal. Ann Intern Med 1993;118(4):282–9.

7. Yang GC, Liebeskind D, Messina AV. Ultrasound-guided fine-needle aspiration of the thyroid assessed by Ultrafast Papanicolaou stain: data from 1135 biopsies with a two- to six-year follow-up. Thyroid 2001;11(6):581–9.

8. Yang J, Schnadig V, Logrono R, et al. Fine-needle aspiration of thyroid nodules: a study of 4703 patients with histologic and clinical correlations. Cancer 2007; 111(5):306–15.

9. Baloch ZW, Fleisher S, LiVolsi VA, et al. Diagnosis of "follicular neoplasm": a gray zone in thyroid fine-needle aspiration cytology. Diagn Cytopathol 2002;26(1):41–4.

10. Yang GC, Liebeskind D, Messina AV. Should cytopathologists stop reporting follicular neoplasms on fine-needle aspiration of the thyroid? Cancer 2003; 99(2):69–74.

11. Stelow EB, Bardales RH, Crary GS, et al. Interobserver variability in thyroid fine-needle aspiration interpretation of lesions showing predominantly colloid and follicular groups. Am J Clin Pathol 2005;124(2):239–44.

12. Greaves TS, Olvera M, Florentine BD, et al. Follicular lesions of thyroid: a 5-year fine-needle aspiration experience. Cancer 2000;90(6):335–41.

13. Liu FT, Rabinovich GA. Galectins as modulators of tumour progression. Nat Rev Cancer 2005;5(1):29–41.

14. Yoshii T, Inohara H, Takenaka Y, et al. Galectin-3 maintains the transformed phenotype of thyroid papillary carcinoma cells. Int J Oncol 2001;18(4):787–92.

15. Takenaka Y, Inohara H, Yoshii T, et al. Malignant transformation of thyroid follicular cells by galectin-3. Cancer Lett 2003;195(1):111–9.

16. Xu XC, el-Naggar AK, Lotan R. Differential expression of galectin-1 and galectin-3 in thyroid tumors. Potential diagnostic implications. Am J Pathol 1995;147(3): 815–22.

17. Inohara H, Honjo Y, Yoshii T, et al. Expression of galectin-3 in fine-needle aspi-rates as a diagnostic marker differentiating benign from malignant thyroid neoplasms. Cancer 1999;85(11):2475–84.

18. Fernandez PL, Merino MJ, Gomez M, et al. Galectin-3 and laminin expression in neoplastic and non-neoplastic thyroid tissue. J Pathol 1997;181(1):80–6.

19. Orlandi F, Saggiorato E, Pivano G, et al. Galectin-3 is a presurgical marker of human thyroid carcinoma. Cancer Res 1998;58(14):3015–20.

20. Giannini R, Faviana P, Cavinato T, et al. Galectin-3 and oncofetal-fibronectin expression in thyroid neoplasia as assessed by reverse transcription-poly-merase chain reaction and immunochemistry in cytologic and pathologic spec-imens. Thyroid 2003;13(8):765–70.

21. Saussez S, Glinoer D, Chantrain G, et al. Serum galectin-1 and galectin-3 levels in benign and malignant nodular thyroid disease. Thyroid 2008;18(7):705–12.

22. Inohara H, Segawa T, Miyauchi A, et al. Cytoplasmic and serum galectin-3 in diagnosis of thyroid malignancies. Biochem Biophys Res Commun 2008; 376(3):605–10.

23. Bartolazzi A, Orlandi F, Saggiorato E, et al. Galectin-3-expression analysis in the surgical selection of follicular thyroid nodules with indeterminate fine-needle

aspiration cytology: a prospective multicentre study. Lancet Oncol 2008;9(6): 543–9.

24. Collet JF, Hurbain I, Prengel C, et al. Galectin-3 immunodetection in follicular thyroid neoplasms: a prospective study on fine-needle aspiration samples. Br J Cancer 2005;93(10):1175–81.

25. Rossi ED, Raffaelli M, Minimo C, et al. Immunocytochemical evaluation of thyroid neoplasms on thin-layer smears from fine-needle aspiration biopsies. Cancer 2005;105(2):87–95.

26. Saggiorato E, De Pompa R, Volante M, et al. Characterization of thyroid 'follicular neoplasms' in fine-needle aspiration cytological specimens using a panel of immunohistochemical markers: a proposal for clinical application. Endocr Relat Cancer 2005;12(2):305–17.

27. Kim MJ, Kim HJ, Hong SJ, et al. Diagnostic utility of galectin-3 in aspirates of thyroid follicular lesions. Acta Cytol 2006;50(1):28–34.

28. Mehrotra P, Okpokam A, Bouhaidar R, et al. Galectin-3 does not reliably distinguish benign from malignant thyroid neoplasms. Histopathology 2004;45(5): 493–500.

29. Bartolazzi A, Bussolati G. Galectin-3 does not reliably distinguish benign from malignant thyroid neoplasms. Histopathology 2006;48(2):212–3.

30. Sanabria A, Carvalho AL, Piana de Andrade V, et al. Is galectin-3 a good method for the detection of malignancy in patients with thyroid nodules and a cytologic diagnosis of "follicular neoplasm"? A critical appraisal of the evidence. Head Neck 2007;29(11):1046–54.

31. Sheibani K, Esteban JM, Bailey A, et al. Immunopathologic and molecular studies as an aid to the diagnosis of malignant mesothelioma. Hum Pathol 1992;23(2):107–16.

32. Sack MJ, Astengo-Osuna C, Lin BT, et al. HBME-1 immunostaining in thyroid fine-needle aspirations: a useful marker in the diagnosis of carcinoma. Mod Pathol 1997;10(7):668–74.

33. de Micco C, Savchenko V, Giorgi R, et al. Utility of malignancy markers in fine-needle aspiration cytology of thyroid nodules: comparison of Hector Battifora mesothelial antigen-1, thyroid peroxidase and dipeptidyl aminopeptidase IV. Br J Cancer 2008;98(4):818–23.

34. van Hoeven KH, Kovatich AJ. Immunohistochemical staining for proliferating cell nuclear antigen, BCL2, and Ki-67 in vulvar tissues. Int J Gynecol Pathol 1996; 15(1):10–6.

35. Wiseman SM, Melck A, Masoudi H, et al. Molecular phenotyping of thyroid tumors identifies a marker panel for differentiated thyroid cancer diagnosis. Ann Surg Oncol 2008;15(10):2811–26.

36. Rossi ED, Raffaelli M, Mule A, et al. Simultaneous immunohistochemical expression of HBME-1 and galectin-3 differentiates papillary carcinomas from hyperfunctioning lesions of the thyroid. Histopathology 2006;48(7):795–800.

37. Scognamiglio T, Hyjek E, Kao J, et al. Diagnostic usefulness of HBME1, galectin-3, CK19, and CITED1 and evaluation of their expression in encapsulated lesions with questionable features of papillary thyroid carcinoma. Am J Clin Pathol 2006; 126(5):700–8.

38. Nga ME, Lim GS, Soh CH, et al. HBME-1 and CK19 are highly discriminatory in the cytological diagnosis of papillary thyroid carcinoma. Diagn Cytopathol 2008; 36(8):550–6.

39. Kirkpatrick KL, Mokbel K. The significance of human telomerase reverse transcriptase (hTERT) in cancer. Eur J Surg Oncol 2001;27(8):754–60.

40. Brousset P, Chaouche N, Leprat F, et al. Telomerase activity in human thyroid carcinomas originating from the follicular cells. J Clin Endocrinol Metab 1997; 82(12):4214–6.
41. Umbricht CB, Saji M, Westra WH, et al. Telomerase activity: a marker to distinguish follicular thyroid adenoma from carcinoma. Cancer Res 1997;57(11): 2144–7.
42. Kammori M, Takubo K, Nakamura K, et al. Telomerase activity and telomere length in benign and malignant human thyroid tissues. Cancer Lett 2000; 159(2):175–81.
43. Saji M, Westra WH, Chen H, et al. Telomerase activity in the differential diagnosis of papillary carcinoma of the thyroid. Surgery 1997;122(6):1137–40.
44. Yashima K, Vuitch F, Gazdar AF, et al. Telomerase activity in benign and malignant thyroid diseases. Surgery 1997;122(6):1141–5 [discussion: 5–6].
45. Bornstein-Quevedo L, Garcia-Hernandez ML, Camacho-Arroyo I, et al. Telomerase activity in well-differentiated papillary thyroid carcinoma correlates with advanced clinical stage of the disease. Endocr Pathol 2003;14(3):213–9.
46. Cheng AJ, Lin JD, Chang T, et al. Telomerase activity in benign and malignant human thyroid tissues. Br J Cancer 1998;77(12):2177–80.
47. Onoda N, Ishikawa T, Yoshikawa K, et al. Telomerase activity in thyroid tumors. Oncol Rep 1998;5(6):1447–50.
48. Haugen BR, Nawaz S, Markham N, et al. Telomerase activity in benign and malignant thyroid tumors. Thyroid 1997;7(3):337–42.
49. Okayasu I, Osakabe T, Fujiwara M, et al. Significant correlation of telomerase activity in thyroid papillary carcinomas with cell differentiation, proliferation and extrathyroidal extension. Jpn J Cancer Res 1997;88(10):965–70.
50. Trulsson LM, Velin AK, Herder A, et al. Telomerase activity in surgical specimens and fine-needle aspiration biopsies from hyperplastic and neoplastic human thyroid tissues. Am J Surg 2003;186(1):83–8.
51. Straight AM, Patel A, Fenton C, et al. Thyroid carcinomas that express telomerase follow a more aggressive clinical course in children and adolescents. J Endocrinol Invest 2002;25(4):302–8.
52. Lo CY, Lam KY, Chan KT, et al. Telomerase activity in thyroid malignancy. Thyroid 1999;9(12):1215–20.
53. Ito Y, Yoshida H, Tomoda C, et al. Telomerase activity in thyroid neoplasms evaluated by the expression of human telomerase reverse transcriptase (hTERT). Anticancer Res 2005;25(1B):509–14.
54. Asaad NY, Abd El-Wahed MM, Mohammed AG. Human telomerase reverse transcriptase (hTERT) gene expression in thyroid carcinoma: diagnostic and prognostic role. J Egypt Natl Canc Inst 2006;18(1):8–16.
55. Saji M, Xydas S, Westra WH, et al. Human telomerase reverse transcriptase (hTERT) gene expression in thyroid neoplasms. Clin Cancer Res 1999;5(6): 1483–9.
56. Hoang-Vu C, Boltze C, Gimm O, et al. Expression of telomerase genes in thyroid carcinoma. Int J Oncol 2002;21(2):265–72.
57. Wang Y, Kowalski J, Tsai HL, et al. Differentiating alternative splice variant patterns of human telomerase reverse transcriptase in thyroid neoplasms. Thyroid 2008;18(10):1055–63.
58. Mora J, Lerma E. Telomerase activity in thyroid fine needle aspirates. Acta Cytol 2004;48(6):818–24.
59. Kammori M, Nakamura K, Hashimoto M, et al. Clinical application of human telomerase reverse transcriptase gene expression in thyroid follicular tumors by

fine-needle aspirations using in situ hybridization. Int J Oncol 2003;22(5): 985–91.

60. Liou MJ, Chan EC, Lin JD, et al. Human telomerase reverse transcriptase (hTERT) gene expression in FNA samples from thyroid neoplasms. Cancer Lett 2003;191(2):223–7.

61. Matthews P, Jones CJ, Skinner J, et al. Telomerase activity and telomere length in thyroid neoplasia: biological and clinical implications. J Pathol 2001;194(2):183–93.

62. Sebesta J, Brown T, Williard W, et al. Does telomerase activity add to the value of fine needle aspirations in evaluating thyroid nodules? Am J Surg 2001;181(5): 420–2.

63. Lerma E, Mora J. Telomerase activity in "suspicious" thyroid cytology. Cancer 2005;105(6):492–7.

64. Guerra LN, Miler EA, Moiguer S, et al. Telomerase activity in fine needle aspiration biopsy samples: application to diagnosis of human thyroid carcinoma. Clin Chim Acta 2006;370(1–2):180–4.

65. Fagin JA, Mitsiades N. Molecular pathology of thyroid cancer: diagnostic and clinical implications. Best Pract Res Clin Endocrinol Metab 2008;22(6):955–69.

66. Peyssonnaux C, Eychene A. The Raf/MEK/ERK pathway: new concepts of activation. Biol Cell 2001;93(1–2):53–62.

67. Dhillon AS, Kolch W. Oncogenic B-Raf mutations: crystal clear at last. Cancer Cell 2004;5(4):303–4.

68. Kimura ET, Nikiforova MN, Zhu Z, et al. High prevalence of BRAF mutations in thyroid cancer: genetic evidence for constitutive activation of the RET/PTC-RAS-BRAF signaling pathway in papillary thyroid carcinoma. Cancer Res 2003;63(7):1454–7.

69. Cohen Y, Xing M, Mambo E, et al. BRAF mutation in papillary thyroid carcinoma. J Natl Cancer Inst 2003;95(8):625–7.

70. Cohen Y, Rosenbaum E, Clark DP, et al. Mutational analysis of BRAF in fine needle aspiration biopsies of the thyroid: a potential application for the preoperative assessment of thyroid nodules. Clin Cancer Res 2004;10(8):2761–5.

71. Fugazzola L, Mannavola D, Cirello V, et al. BRAF mutations in an Italian cohort of thyroid cancers. Clin Endocrinol (Oxf) 2004;61(2):239–43.

72. Knauf JA, Ma X, Smith EP, et al. Targeted expression of BRAFV600E in thyroid cells of transgenic mice results in papillary thyroid cancers that undergo dedifferentiation. Cancer Res 2005;65(10):4238–45.

73. Nikiforova MN, Kimura ET, Gandhi M, et al. BRAF mutations in thyroid tumors are restricted to papillary carcinomas and anaplastic or poorly differentiated carcinomas arising from papillary carcinomas. J Clin Endocrinol Metab 2003; 88(11):5399–404.

74. Kim TY, Kim WB, Rhee YS, et al. The BRAF mutation is useful for prediction of clinical recurrence in low-risk patients with conventional papillary thyroid carcinoma. Clin Endocrinol (Oxf) 2006;65(3):364–8.

75. Xing M, Westra WH, Tufano RP, et al. BRAF mutation predicts a poorer clinical prognosis for papillary thyroid cancer. J Clin Endocrinol Metab 2005;90(12): 6373–9.

76. Pizzolanti G, Russo L, Richiusa P, et al. Fine-needle aspiration molecular analysis for the diagnosis of papillary thyroid carcinoma through BRAF V600E mutation and RET/PTC rearrangement. Thyroid 2007;17(11):1109–15.

77. Jo YS, Huang S, Kim YJ, et al. Diagnostic value of pyrosequencing for the BRAF V600E mutation in ultrasound-guided fine-needle aspiration biopsy samples of thyroid incidentalomas. Clin Endocrinol (Oxf) 2009;70(1):139–44.

78. Jin L, Sebo TJ, Nakamura N, et al. BRAF mutation analysis in fine needle aspiration (FNA) cytology of the thyroid. Diagn Mol Pathol 2006;15(3):136–43.

79. Chung KW, Yang SK, Lee GK, et al. Detection of BRAFV600E mutation on fine needle aspiration specimens of thyroid nodule refines cyto-pathology diagnosis, especially in BRAF600E mutation-prevalent area. Clin Endocrinol (Oxf) 2006; 65(5):660–6.

80. Salvatore G, Giannini R, Faviana P, et al. Analysis of BRAF point mutation and RET/PTC rearrangement refines the fine-needle aspiration diagnosis of papillary thyroid carcinoma. J Clin Endocrinol Metab 2004;89(10):5175–80.

81. Xing M, Tufano RP, Tufaro AP, et al. Detection of BRAF mutation on fine needle aspiration biopsy specimens: a new diagnostic tool for papillary thyroid cancer. J Clin Endocrinol Metab 2004;89(6):2867–72.

82. Kim SK, Kim DL, Han HS, et al. Pyrosequencing analysis for detection of a BRAFV600E mutation in an FNAB specimen of thyroid nodules. Diagn Mol Pathol 2008;17(2):118–25.

83. Rowe LR, Bentz BG, Bentz JS. Utility of BRAF V600E mutation detection in cytologically indeterminate thyroid nodules. Cytojournal 2006;3:10.

84. Domingues R, Mendonca E, Sobrinho L, et al. Searching for RET/PTC rearrangements and BRAF V599E mutation in thyroid aspirates might contribute to establish a preoperative diagnosis of papillary thyroid carcinoma. Cytopathology 2005;16(1):27–31.

85. Sapio MR, Posca D, Raggioli A, et al. Detection of RET/PTC, TRK and BRAF mutations in preoperative diagnosis of thyroid nodules with indeterminate cytological findings. Clin Endocrinol (Oxf) 2007;66(5):678–83.

86. Nikiforov YE. Thyroid carcinoma: molecular pathways and therapeutic targets. Mod Pathol 2008;21(Suppl 2):S37–43.

87. Santoro M, Carlomagno F, Hay ID, et al. Ret oncogene activation in human thyroid neoplasms is restricted to the papillary cancer subtype. J Clin Invest 1992;89(5):1517–22.

88. Adeniran AJ, Zhu Z, Gandhi M, et al. Correlation between genetic alterations and microscopic features, clinical manifestations, and prognostic characteristics of thyroid papillary carcinomas. Am J Surg Pathol 2006;30(2):216–22.

89. Jhiang SM, Caruso DR, Gilmore E, et al. Detection of the PTC/retTPC oncogene in human thyroid cancers. Oncogene 1992;7(7):1331–7.

90. Santoro M, Chiappetta G, Cerrato A, et al. Development of thyroid papillary carcinomas secondary to tissue-specific expression of the RET/PTC1 oncogene in transgenic mice. Oncogene 1996;12(8):1821–6.

91. Jhiang SM, Sagartz JE, Tong Q, et al. Targeted expression of the ret/PTC1 oncogene induces papillary thyroid carcinomas. Endocrinology 1996;137(1): 375–8.

92. Powell DJ Jr, Russell J, Nibu K, et al. The RET/PTC3 oncogene: metastatic solid-type papillary carcinomas in murine thyroids. Cancer Res 1998;58(23): 5523–8.

93. Nikiforov YE, Rowland JM, Bove KE, et al. Distinct pattern of ret oncogene rearrangements in morphological variants of radiation-induced and sporadic thyroid papillary carcinomas in children. Cancer Res 1997;57(9):1690–4.

94. Hamatani K, Eguchi H, Ito R, et al. RET/PTC rearrangements preferentially occurred in papillary thyroid cancer among atomic bomb survivors exposed to high radiation dose. Cancer Res 2008;68(17):7176–82.

95. Ito T, Seyama T, Iwamoto KS, et al. In vitro irradiation is able to cause RET oncogene rearrangement. Cancer Res 1993;53(13):2940–3.

96. Mizuno T, Kyoizumi S, Suzuki T, et al. Continued expression of a tissue specific activated oncogene in the early steps of radiation-induced human thyroid carcinogenesis. Oncogene 1997;15(12):1455–60.
97. Cheung CC, Carydis B, Ezzat S, et al. Analysis of ret/PTC gene rearrangements refines the fine needle aspiration diagnosis of thyroid cancer. J Clin Endocrinol Metab 2001;86(5):2187–90.
98. Elisei R, Romei C, Vorontsova T, et al. RET/PTC rearrangements in thyroid nodules: studies in irradiated and not irradiated, malignant and benign thyroid lesions in children and adults. J Clin Endocrinol Metab 2001;86(7):3211–6.
99. Kroll TG, Sarraf P, Pecciarini L, et al. PAX8-PPARgamma1 fusion oncogene in human thyroid carcinoma [corrected]. Science 2000;289(5483):1357–60.
100. Dwight T, Thoppe SR, Foukakis T, et al. Involvement of the PAX8/peroxisome proliferator-activated receptor gamma rearrangement in follicular thyroid tumors. J Clin Endocrinol Metab 2003;88(9):4440–5.
101. Nikiforova MN, Biddinger PW, Caudill CM, et al. PAX8-PPARgamma rearrangement in thyroid tumors: RT-PCR and immunohistochemical analyses. Am J Surg Pathol 2002;26(8):1016–23.
102. Cheung L, Messina M, Gill A, et al. Detection of the PAX8-PPAR gamma fusion oncogene in both follicular thyroid carcinomas and adenomas. J Clin Endocrinol Metab 2003;88(1):354–7.
103. Marques AR, Espadinha C, Catarino AL, et al. Expression of PAX8-PPAR gamma 1 rearrangements in both follicular thyroid carcinomas and adenomas. J Clin Endocrinol Metab 2002;87(8):3947–52.
104. Hibi Y, Nagaya T, Kambe F, et al. Is thyroid follicular cancer in Japanese caused by a specific t(2; 3)(q13; p25) translocation generating Pax8-PPAR gamma fusion mRNA? Endocr J 2004;51(3):361–6.
105. Sahin M, Allard BL, Yates M, et al. PPARgamma staining as a surrogate for PAX8/PPARgamma fusion oncogene expression in follicular neoplasms: clinicopathological correlation and histopathological diagnostic value. J Clin Endocrinol Metab 2005;90(1):463–8.
106. Nikiforova MN, Lynch RA, Biddinger PW, et al. RAS point mutations and PAX8-PPAR gamma rearrangement in thyroid tumors: evidence for distinct molecular pathways in thyroid follicular carcinoma. J Clin Endocrinol Metab 2003;88(5):2318–26.
107. Gregory Powell J, Wang X, Allard BL, et al. The PAX8/PPARgamma fusion oncoprotein transforms immortalized human thyrocytes through a mechanism probably involving wild-type PPARgamma inhibition. Oncogene 2004;23(20):3634–41.
108. Au AY, McBride C, Wilhelm KG Jr, et al. PAX8-peroxisome proliferator-activated receptor gamma (PPARgamma) disrupts normal PAX8 or PPARgamma transcriptional function and stimulates follicular thyroid cell growth. Endocrinology 2006;147(1):367–76.
109. Marques AR, Espadinha C, Frias MJ, et al. Underexpression of peroxisome proliferator-activated receptor (PPAR)gamma in PAX8/PPARgamma-negative thyroid tumours. Br J Cancer 2004;91(4):732–8.
110. Lacroix L, Lazar V, Michiels S, et al. Follicular thyroid tumors with the PAX8-PPARgamma1 rearrangement display characteristic genetic alterations. Am J Pathol 2005;167(1):223–31.
111. Lui WO, Foukakis T, Liden J, et al. Expression profiling reveals a distinct transcription signature in follicular thyroid carcinomas with a PAX8-PPAR(gamma) fusion oncogene. Oncogene 2005;24(8):1467–76.

112. Giordano TJ, Au AY, Kuick R, et al. Delineation, functional validation, and bioinformatic evaluation of gene expression in thyroid follicular carcinomas with the PAX8-PPARG translocation. Clin Cancer Res 2006;12(7 Pt 1):1983–93.

113. Nikiforova MN, Tseng GC, Steward D, et al. MicroRNA expression profiling of thyroid tumors: biological significance and diagnostic utility. J Clin Endocrinol Metab 2008;93(5):1600–8.

114. Pallante P, Visone R, Ferracin M, et al. MicroRNA deregulation in human thyroid papillary carcinomas. Endocr Relat Cancer 2006;13(2):497–508.

115. Chen YT, Kitabayashi N, Zhou XK, et al. MicroRNA analysis as a potential diagnostic tool for papillary thyroid carcinoma. Mod Pathol 2008;21(9):1139–46.

116. Visone R, Russo L, Pallante P, et al. MicroRNAs (miR)-221 and miR-222, both overexpressed in human thyroid papillary carcinomas, regulate p27Kip1 protein levels and cell cycle. Endocr Relat Cancer 2007;14(3):791–8.

117. Weber F, Teresi RE, Broelsch CE, et al. A limited set of human MicroRNA is deregulated in follicular thyroid carcinoma. J Clin Endocrinol Metab 2006;91(9):3584–91.

118. Visone R, Pallante P, Vecchione A, et al. Specific microRNAs are downregulated in human thyroid anaplastic carcinomas. Oncogene 2007;26(54):7590–5.

119. Finley DJ, Lubitz CC, Wei C, et al. Advancing the molecular diagnosis of thyroid nodules: defining benign lesions by molecular profiling. Thyroid 2005;15(6):562–8.

120. Lubitz CC, Gallagher LA, Finley DJ, et al. Molecular analysis of minimally invasive follicular carcinomas by gene profiling. Surgery 2005;138(6):1042–8 [discussion: 8–9].

121. Barden CB, Shister KW, Zhu B, et al. Classification of follicular thyroid tumors by molecular signature: results of gene profiling. Clin Cancer Res 2003;9(5):1792–800.

122. Finley DJ, Arora N, Zhu B, et al. Molecular profiling distinguishes papillary carcinoma from benign thyroid nodules. J Clin Endocrinol Metab 2004;89(7):3214–23.

123. Finley DJ, Zhu B, Fahey TJ 3rd. Molecular analysis of Hurthle cell neoplasms by gene profiling. Surgery 2004;136(6):1160–8.

124. Finley DJ, Zhu B, Barden CB, et al. Discrimination of benign and malignant thyroid nodules by molecular profiling. Ann Surg 2004;240(3):425–36 [discussion: 36–7].

125. Lubitz CC, Ugras SK, Kazam JJ, et al. Microarray analysis of thyroid nodule fine-needle aspirates accurately classifies benign and malignant lesions. J Mol Diagn 2006;8(4):490–8, quiz 528.

126. Weber F, Shen L, Aldred MA, et al. Genetic classification of benign and malignant thyroid follicular neoplasia based on a three-gene combination. J Clin Endocrinol Metab 2005;90(5):2512–21.

127. Mazzanti C, Zeiger MA, Costouros NG, et al. Using gene expression profiling to differentiate benign versus malignant thyroid tumors. Cancer Res 2004;64(8):2898–903.

128. Prasad NB, Somervell H, Tufano RP, et al. Identification of genes differentially expressed in benign versus malignant thyroid tumors. Clin Cancer Res 2008;14(11):3327–37.

129. Fujarewicz K, Jarzab M, Eszlinger M, et al. A multi-gene approach to differentiate papillary thyroid carcinoma from benign lesions: gene selection using support vector machines with bootstrapping. Endocr Relat Cancer 2007;14(3):809–26.

130. Jarzab B, Wiench M, Fujarewicz K, et al. Gene expression profile of papillary thyroid cancer: sources of variability and diagnostic implications. Cancer Res 2005;65(4):1587–97.

131. Fontaine JF, Mirebeau-Prunier D, Franc B, et al. Microarray analysis refines classification of non-medullary thyroid tumours of uncertain malignancy. Oncogene 2008;27(15):2228–36.

132. Aldred MA, Huang Y, Liyanarachchi S, et al. Papillary and follicular thyroid carcinomas show distinctly different microarray expression profiles and can be distinguished by a minimum of five genes. J Clin Oncol 2004;22(17):3531–9.

133. Yano Y, Uematsu N, Yashiro T, et al. Gene expression profiling identifies platelet-derived growth factor as a diagnostic molecular marker for papillary thyroid carcinoma. Clin Cancer Res 2004;10(6):2035–43.

134. Yukinawa N, Oba S, Kato K, et al. A multi-class predictor based on a probabilistic model: application to gene expression profiling-based diagnosis of thyroid tumors. BMC Genomics 2006;7:190.

135. Rosen J, He M, Umbricht C, et al. A six-gene model for differentiating benign from malignant thyroid tumors on the basis of gene expression. Surgery 2005; 138(6):1050–6 [discussion: 6–7].

136. Foukakis T, Gusnanto A, Au AY, et al. A PCR-based expression signature of malignancy in follicular thyroid tumors. Endocr Relat Cancer 2007;14(2):381–91.

137. Denning KM, Smyth PC, Cahill SF, et al. A molecular expression signature distinguishing follicular lesions in thyroid carcinoma using preamplification RT-PCR in archival samples. Mod Pathol 2007;20(10):1095–102.

138. Cerutti JM, Delcelo R, Amadei MJ, et al. A preoperative diagnostic test that distinguishes benign from malignant thyroid carcinoma based on gene expression. J Clin Invest 2004;113(8):1234–42.

139. Pagedar NA, Chen DH, Wasman JK, et al. Molecular classification of thyroid nodules by cytology. Laryngoscope 2008;118(4):692–6.

140. Shibru D, Hwang J, Khanafshar E, et al. Does the 3-gene diagnostic assay accurately distinguish benign from malignant thyroid neoplasms? Cancer 2008;113(5):930–5.

141. Kebebew E, Peng M, Reiff E, et al. Diagnostic and prognostic value of cell-cycle regulatory genes in malignant thyroid neoplasms. World J Surg 2006;30(5): 767–74.

142. Kebebew E, Peng M, Reiff E, et al. ECM1 and TMPRSS4 are diagnostic markers of malignant thyroid neoplasms and improve the accuracy of fine needle aspiration biopsy. Ann Surg 2005;242(3):353–61 [discussion: 61–3].

143. Kebebew E, Peng M, Reiff E, et al. Diagnostic and prognostic value of angiogenesis-modulating genes in malignant thyroid neoplasms. Surgery 2005; 138(6):1102–9 [discussion: 9–10].

144. Kebebew E, Peng M, Reiff E, et al. Diagnostic and extent of disease multigene assay for malignant thyroid neoplasms. Cancer 2006;106(12):2592–7.

Recurrent Laryngeal Nerve Monitoring: State of the Art, Ethical and Legal Issues

Peter Angelos, MD, PhD, FACS

KEYWORDS

- Recurrent laryngeal nerve monitoring
- Ethical issues in neuromonitoring
- Legal issues in neuromonitoring

Despite many advances in surgical techniques during the last several decades, the risk for recurrent laryngeal nerve (RLN) injury during thyroid and parathyroid surgery has only declined, not disappeared. In the first half of the twentieth century, Lahey[1] and subsequently Riddell[2] independently described a technique for thyroidectomy, in which an attempt was made to find the RLN in every case rather than taking the traditional approach of avoiding even seeing the nerve. The superiority of this approach has been documented by Hermann and colleagues[3] who reviewed thyroidectomies for benign diseases from 1979 to 1990 when nerves were not visualized (n = 15,865) and from 1991 to 1998 when visualization of the RLN was standard practice (n = 10,548). These authors showed that the risk for permanent RLN injury in the former group was 1.1%, but in the latter group, in which visualization of the nerve became standard practice, the risk of permanent RLN injury decreased to 0.4%.

Most surgeons attempt to identify the RLN, thereby minimizing the risk of injuring it. Despite adopting this technique, there are several well-described circumstances that increase the likelihood of RLN injury. Thomusch and colleagues[4] conducted a multivariate analysis that analyzed risk factors for patients undergoing thyroidectomy for benign disease. These investigators found that larger extent of resection and recurrent goiter were independent variables that contribute to the probability of RLN injury. In addition, Dralle and colleagues[5] have identified abnormal anatomy, bulky disease, and surgeon inexperience as additional risk factors for RLN injury. The approach of routinely identifying the RLN has been adopted by most surgeons and has at least partially been credited with the low risk for permanent RLN injury of less than 2%.[6,7]

Despite this low rate of permanent RLN injury, this complication continues to be problematic for patients and surgeons. The morbidity of permanent hoarseness is

---

Section of General Surgery and Surgical Oncology, MacLean Center for Clinical Medical Ethics, University of Chicago, 5841 South Maryland Avenue, MC 4052, Chicago, IL 60637, USA
E-mail address: pangelos@surgery.bsd.uchicago.edu

Surg Clin N Am 89 (2009) 1157–1169
doi:10.1016/j.suc.2009.06.010
0039-6109/09/$ – see front matter © 2009 Elsevier Inc. All rights reserved.

surgical.theclinics.com

readily apparent and has been documented.[8,9] Not surprisingly, RLN injuries continue to be frequent sources of medical malpractice claims against surgeons.[10] Surgeons have therefore sought methods to try to reduce injuries to the RLN. RLN monitoring is an attempt to reduce the risk of nerve injury during thyroid and parathyroid surgery.

OPTIONS FOR RLN MONITORING

Although RLN monitoring has garnered significantly more interest in recent years, there were attempts in prior decades to use technology to minimize the risk of injury to the RLN. As early as the 1960s, some clinicians were exploring the use of electrical stimulation of the RLN as a means of identification and preservation.[11,12] However, only in recent years has the technology become sufficiently user-friendly and commercially available that widespread use of RLN monitoring during thyroid surgery has been undertaken. These changes have led to many studies in the last decade, describing intraoperative nerve monitoring during thyroid surgery.

The basics of RLN monitoring technology involve 2 components: a method of stimulating the RLN intraoperatively and a method of assessing vocal fold response to the stimulation. The stimulation of the RLN is by low-voltage stimulation of tissues on or near the RLN or indirectly by stimulating the vagus nerve. The monitoring of the response to stimulation of the RLN has included several different techniques. Several groups have described finger palpation of the cricoarytenoid muscle during nerve stimulation as a method of demonstrating that the RLN is intact.[13-16] Riddell[17] and later Eltzschig and colleagues[18] described monitoring of RLN function using vocal cord observation by direct or fiberoptic laryngoscopy. Several investigators have described the use of intramuscular vocal cord electrodes, the so-called hook electrodes.[19-26] This technique of RLN monitoring is effective, but does require skill and experience to appropriately place the hook electrodes. Although less common than the use of hook electrodes, the use of postcricoid surface electrodes has also been described and appears to be effective.[27] The most widely used method of RLN monitoring in recent years has been the use of endotracheal tube surface electrodes.[28-40]

The use of endotracheal tube surface electrodes as the sensor for RLN monitoring has become the most popular method worldwide because of the ease of use and commercial availability. No particular skill or experience is required of the surgeon to place the electrode in the correct location. Instead, the electrode is on the endotracheal tube itself. As long as the anesthesiologist accurately places the electrode in contact with the vocal cords, the electrode is in the correct location for neuromonitoring.[41] Usually, getting the correct location for the electrode is not difficult as long as the vocal cords can be seen at the time of intubation. If fiberoptic intubation is required, the positioning of the electrode in contact with the vocal cords is made more difficult because the cords cannot be readily seen from the lumen of the endotracheal tube. In this circumstance, it is necessary to take another look from outside the endotracheal tube with the fiberoptic scope after the patient is intubated to ensure that the electrode is in contact with the cords. With just a little practice, accurately positioning the electrode during intubation rarely adds time to the procedure.

The 2 most commonly used RLN monitoring systems in the United States are the nerve integrity monitor (NIM) system manufactured by Medtronic Xomed (Minneapolis, Minnesota) and the Nerveäna system manufactured by Neurovision Medical (Ventura, California). The NIM system uses a special endotracheal tube with the vocal cord electrodes embedded into the wall of the tube. This system is convenient in that the endotracheal tube is already prepared and simply needs to be placed appropriately in contact with the vocal cords. These special Medtronic endotracheal tubes are reinforced so that they do not often kink at the teeth even when taped in the midline. However, only certain common adult size endotracheal tubes are manufactured, and the use of these tubes in the pediatric population is problematic. The endotracheal tube and the stimulator probe are single-use items, adding to the convenience. The NIM unit that is available in many hospitals is the same unit used for RLN monitoring and also for facial nerve monitoring in parotid surgery.

The Nerveäna system is specifically designed for RLN monitoring and therefore is much less ubiquitous in hospitals than the NIM system at present. However, the Nerveäna system uses an electrode that can be attached to any endotracheal tube. This approach results in a lower cost per case. In addition, the stimulator used by the Nerveäna system is a small dissecting clamp that has been modified to carry the stimulating electric current. The stimulator is therefore a multiuse item. Because any size endotracheal tube can be used (with the appropriately sized electrode), the Nerveäna system can be readily used in pediatric patients. Because it is advantageous to tape the endotracheal tube in the midline to center the electrode in the vocal cords, the tubes often kink at the teeth when directed straight back over the patient's face and away from the operative field. If a nasal Ring, Adair, Elwin (RAE) tube (Mallinckrodt, Inc., St. Louis, Missouri) is used in a trans-oral fashion rather than a trans-nasal fashion, then the permanent curve of the tube can be used so that the end of the endotracheal tube is positioned away from the operative field, and there is much less risk of kinking of the tube.

When RLN monitoring is to be undertaken using any of the electromyography type of sensors or when using laryngeal palpation, neuromuscular blockade is avoided during the induction of general endotracheal anesthesia.[30,42] If neuromuscular blockade is required during induction, a short-acting agent is generally recommended. Marusch and colleagues[43] have reported that RLN monitoring can be undertaken even in the presence of neuromuscular blockade, at least when using needle electrodes in the vocalis muscle to monitor summed action potentials. However, despite this report, the use of neuromuscular blockade when using endotracheal tube surface electrodes should still be avoided.

Almost all the reports examining the use of intraoperative RLN monitoring have described various types of intermittent nerve stimulation. The NIM system uses a fine probe that can be used to precisely stimulate different anatomic structures. The Nerveäna system uses a fine dissecting instrument as the stimulator. A continuous stimulation system has been described whereby a flexible cuff electrode is atraumatically placed around the vagus nerve so that continuous stimulation can be used.[44,45] Thus far, there have not been clear benefits shown with this new technique of continuous rather than intermittent nerve stimulation.

EFFECTIVENESS OF RLN MONITORING

A review of the relevant medical literature on RLN monitoring in the last 10 years shows many articles that explore aspects of RLN monitoring in different settings. Some of the earlier studies were small series designed to show that RLN monitoring was feasible. In 1999, Timon and Rafferty[31] showed in 21 consecutive patients that a nerve monitor could be helpful in RLN localization. Also in 1999, Horn and Rotzscher[30] reported on a series of 96 patients with 167 nerves at risk, in which the endotracheal surface electrode was used for RLN monitoring. These investigators found a rate of RLN palsy of 0.60% of nerves at risk at 3 days postoperatively. They compared this rate with the rates seen in a previous unpublished series of 300 patients with 558 nerves at risk, in which no nerve monitor was used. In this earlier series, the postoperative RLN palsy rate was 4.3% of nerves at risk in cases with visualization of the RLN and 2.87% of nerves at risk in cases of nonvisualization of the RLN. There is no mention of whether these differences are statistically significant, but it is surprising that visualization of the RLN in the earlier series (that is not fully reported) resulted in higher rates of vocal cord dysfunction than did nonvisualization of the nerve.

In subsequent years, several groups reported their single-center experience of series of patients (number of patients ranging from 19 to 97) in which RLN monitoring was used.[21,24,25,27,32–34,36] None of these studies were large enough to draw any statistically significant conclusions about whether RLN monitoring decreased the rates of nerve injury. Yet the authors generally agreed that RLN monitoring was "safe, simple, and effective for intraoperative monitoring."[27] Several groups noted that the monitor sometimes malfunctioned, and just because there was no signal, one could not be certain that there would be no cord movement postoperatively. This type of technical issue is a problem that is revisited later in the article. One group reported a single patient with "rapidly resolving hoarseness … due to extensive electrical stimulation of the nerve."[30] This apparent transient nerve injury caused by the stimulation of neuromonitoring was not described in any of the other series.

Since 2002, several groups have reported series of more than 100 patients in which RLN monitoring was used. These studies helped to point out how RLN monitoring could be used, but they did not compare a monitored group of patients with an unmonitored group. Hamelman and colleagues[23] reported on a series of 238 patients with 431 nerves at risk, which used needle electrodes through the cricothyroid membrane. Dackiw and colleagues[35] reported on 117 patients with 176 nerves at risk who underwent thyroidectomy and parathyroidectomy in which RLN monitoring was done by use of endotracheal tube surface electrodes. Eltzschig and colleagues[18] used a laryngeal mask airway (LMA), with fiberoptic visualization of the cords through the LMA to monitor RLN function during the procedure. Only 90% of the 363 consecutive patients studied could actually have a thyroidectomy successfully performed with LMA anesthesia. Jonas[46] reported on 417 patients with 784 nerves at risk in 2002 in whom the RLN was identified intraoperatively 98.9% of the time. Although there was no comparison group in which neuromonitoring was not used in this study, the investigators clearly recommend stimulating the vagus nerve to increase accuracy of the determination that a nerve injury has occurred. Several additional large series of patients undergoing thyroidectomy with RLN monitoring have been reported. Although these studies have resulted in varying degrees of endorsements to use the neuromonitoring in thyroid surgery, none of the studies provides statistically significant data to support the use of neuromonitoring.[15,47–50]

Five large studies have been published in the last 7 years that compare a monitored group of patients with a nonmonitored group to determine if there is a difference in RLN injuries. Friedrich and colleagues[51] reported in 2002, a prospective study of 116 patients with 223 nerves at risk who underwent thyroid surgery. They compared RLN palsy rates in the group with RLN monitoring with rates in the group without RLN monitoring. The transient RLN palsy rate was 10.7% in the group with RLN monitoring compared with a rate of 9.6% in the group without nerve monitoring. When permanent vocal cord paralysis was compared, a reduction was seen in the monitored group (1.8%) compared with the unmonitored group (3.0%), but this difference did not reach significance.[51]

In 2004, Dralle and colleagues[5] reported a multi-institutional prospective non-randomized study of 16,448 patients with 29,998 nerves at risk who underwent thyroidectomy. The patients were divided into 3 groups: no RLN identification, visual RLN identification, and visual identification combined with neuromonitoring. This study showed that only in cases of surgeons who treated a lesser number of patients (ie, <45 nerves at risk per year) did RLN monitoring decrease the risk of RLN paralysis from 1.4% to 0.9%. However, when specifically examining the impact of RLN monitoring on nerve injury rates, the authors found no statistically significant difference between visual identification alone and combined visualization with RLN monitoring.[5]

In 2005, Witt[52] reported a retrospective review of 136 consecutive patients who underwent thyroidectomy at a single institution. Of the 190 nerves at risk, 107 were unmonitored and 83 were monitored using an endotracheal surface electrode. There was no reduction in transient or permanent vocal cord dysfunction when comparing the monitored and unmonitored patients. The author concluded that although RLN integrity as determined by an electrophysiologic signal does not always translate into clinical postoperative vocal cord mobility, a signal does provide evidence that the RLN was not severed.[52]

In 2006, Chan and colleagues[37] studied 1000 RLNs at risk in 639 consecutive patients who underwent thyroidectomy. Of this group, 501 nerves were dissected with use of neuromonitoring and 499 were operated with the use of routine RLN identification alone without neuromonitoring. These were not randomized groups. The authors found no significant difference in postoperative, transient, and permanent paralysis rates between neuromonitored and control groups. However, in subgroup analysis, the authors found that the postoperative RLN palsy rate was higher for reoperative thyroidectomy patients in the control group but not in the neuromonitoring group.[37] Based on these findings, the authors concluded that RLN monitoring during thyroid surgery cannot be demonstrated to significantly reduce RLN injury compared with routine RLN identification without neuromonitoring. However, for select high-risk operations, the use of neuromonitoring "may be associated with an improved outcome."[37]

The largest retrospective study was performed by Shindo and Chheda[39] in 2007. These authors retrospectively reviewed charts of 684 patients (1043 nerves at risk) who underwent thyroidectomy by a single surgeon. Of this group, 427 patients had the operation performed with neuromonitoring using endotracheal tube surface electrodes, and 257 patients did not have neuromonitoring during their surgery. Although there was a modest reduction in postoperative RLN paresis in the monitored group, this was not a statistically significant difference.[39]

A few additional studies from the literature require separate attention. Several authors have looked at RLN neuromonitoring in pediatric patients who underwent thyroidectomy.[24,53–55] All of these studies are small, single-institution series with no control group. The findings are reminiscent of those in the adult population; RLN neuromonitoring seems to be effective in illustrating nerve integrity, but not in preventing RLN injury. One group studied the use of RLN monitoring to aid in the identification of 14 nonrecurrent laryngeal nerves.[56] Another group explored specifically the benefits of RLN monitoring as an aid in finding the external branch of the superior laryngeal nerve (EBSLN).[16] They concluded that out of 100 nerves at risk, the use of a nerve stimulator was useful in identifying only 1 EBSLN. It should be noted, however, that this group of investigators assessed function by palpation of the posterior cricoarytenoid muscle contraction for RLN stimulation and observation of cricothyroid muscle twitch with EBSLN stimulation.

One of the most important studies of RLN monitoring was by Thomusch and colleagues[26] in 2004. This group prospectively studied 8534 patients from multiple institutions with 15,403 nerves at risk. They compared neuromonitoring results depending on where the nerve was stimulated. Indirect stimulation of the vagus nerve was compared with direct stimulation of the RLN. The results show that indirect (vagal) stimulation excluded postoperative, permanent vocal cord palsy with a specificity of 97.6% and a negative predictive value of 99.6%. In comparison, direct (RLN) stimulation was insufficient to predict permanent RLN palsy with a sensitivity of 45.9% and a positive predictive value of 11.6%.[26] These data emphasize the importance of doing more with the RLN monitor than just stimulating the RLN after it has been clearly identified.

Based on the literature, RLN monitoring can be effective in assisting the surgeon in identifying the RLN, predicting that the nerve is intact, and perhaps even more importantly, predicting when the nerve is not intact. Use of an RLN monitor does not prevent nerve injuries. Nor does it turn an unsafe surgeon into a safe surgeon. The RLN monitor is simply an adjunct that may be helpful, but based on the current data, it should never replace the meticulous technique of the surgeon.

HOW TO USE THE RLN MONITOR FOR INTRAOPERATIVE DECISION MAKING

It is essential for any surgeon contemplating use of the RLN monitor to fully understand how to use the technology to optimize patient care. Many authors have pointed out that there are technology-related issues that can make the use of the RLN monitor problematic. Specifically, when one begins an operation, one does not know that the system is connected correctly or that the electrode is in the correct location in the vocal cords (if the endotracheal surface electrode is being used). It is for these reasons that a systematic approach to RLN monitoring is critical.

Several surgeons have recommended routine stimulation of the vagus nerve as the first step to ensure that the RLN neuromonitoring system is functioning correctly and as the last step to ensure that, at the completion of the operation, the entire RLN is intact.[26,40,57–59] By systematically ensuring that there is a signal when the vagus nerve is stimulated, the surgeon can start the operation knowing that the entire RLN is intact and that the neuromonitor is positioned and connected correctly. If the vagal stimulation step is skipped and the surgeon moves directly into dissection of the RLN adjacent to the thyroid gland, the surgeon does not know if the neuromonitoring system is working correctly. In addition, stimulation of the RLN proves only that there is no injury of the nerve between the point of stimulation and the neuromuscular endplate. For example, if the RLN were injured low in the tracheoesophageal groove but was exposed and stimulated higher in the groove, one would see a positive signal. This would suggest that the RLN is intact, but in fact, it would only be intact from the point of stimulation to the neuromuscular endplate.

If a signal is present with vagal stimulation at the beginning of the operation and it remains present when initially stimulating the RLN, the subsequent loss of signal should not be ignored. Initially, stimulation of the nerve with finger palpation of the posterior cricoarytenoid muscle can help ensure that the patient is not paralyzed. A careful examination of the course of the nerve should be undertaken to look for any potential cause of injury. Sometimes excessive traction can result in loss of signal. If this is the case, releasing the traction will often result in return of signal. Sometimes stimulation along different points of the RLN can help to pinpoint the site of injury. Once potential sources of false loss of signal are ruled out, the surgeon should go back and stimulate the vagus again. If there remains no signal with stimulation of the vagus nerve when there had initially been a good signal, the surgeon should assume that the nerve has been injured. Based on the very high specificity and negative predictive value of signal loss from the vagus,[26] careful consideration should be given to converting a bilateral operation into a staged operation or to performing a near-total or subtotal thyroidectomy on the contralateral side. Above all, it is important to minimize the chances of bilateral vocal cord palsy, which can be life threatening.

CONTEMPORARY USE OF RLN MONITORING

One of the central questions that a practicing surgeon often faces is whether what he or she is doing in the operating room is similar to or different from what other surgeons are doing. A major source of discussion when surgeons who perform significant volumes of thyroid and parathyroid surgery meet relates to neuromonitoring. All surgeons who do these operations know the risks of RLN injury, and most can remember patients who have been affected by a nerve injury either transiently or permanently. Despite this interest, it has been difficult for most surgeons to understand the rates at which RLN monitoring is done nationwide and whether the rates are increasing or decreasing. Until recently, there were few data to address these questions. However, in the last 2 years, 2 studies have explored issues in the use of RLN monitoring.

In 2007, Horne and colleagues[60] mailed a questionnaire to 1685 randomly selected otolaryngologists representing approximately half of the practicing otolaryngologists in the United States. A total of 685 (40.7%) of those surveyed completed the questionnaires, of which 81% (555) reported performing thyroidectomy in their practices. Most respondents who performed thyroidectomy in their practices reported performing less than 25 thyroidectomies per year. The respondents not performing thyroidectomy were excluded from the analysis. About 44.9% of respondents reported using RLN monitoring during thyroidectomy in their current practice. A smaller group, 23% of respondents, reported using neuromonitoring for all cases of thyroidectomy. The investigators solicited responses in the questionnaires as to why the surgeon did or did not use RLN monitoring. The top 6 responses for each group are noted in **Table 1**. These reasons provide important insights into why these surgeons made the choice to either use or not use the RLN monitor.

In 2009, Sturgeon and colleagues[61] reported on a different survey of neuromonitoring use among registrants of the 2006 annual meeting of the American Association of Endocrine Surgeons (AAES). Several important similarities and differences are

Table 1 Reasons for using or not using RLN monitor	
Reasons for not using RLN monitor	
Rely on anatomy	25%
Not needed	25%
Too many false positives/unreliable	20%
Not available	12%
Cost	11%
Not used in training; never tried	8%
Reasons for using RLN monitor	
Improves safety of the procedure	34%
Helpful in revision surgery/large goiters	33%
Medical-legal protection	22%
It is available; no reason not to use it	22%
It provides additional help in surgery	15%
Believe it to be the standard of care	12%[60]

immediately apparent when this survey is compared with that of Horne and colleagues. First of all, the registrants of the AAES meeting were overwhelmingly general surgeons with a particular clinical interest in endocrine surgery. There were only a few otolaryngologists at the meeting because at the time of the 2006 meeting, otolaryngologists were not eligible for membership, although they were welcome to attend the meeting. (Since that time, the AAES has changed its bylaws so that otolaryngologists may become members.) Second, this is a much smaller study that was Internet based rather than having questionnaires mailed. A total of 117 surveys were completed, giving a response rate of 41%, which is virtually identical to the response rate of the other study. However, the respondents to the AAES survey reported themselves to be 81% in academic practice, 16% in private practice, and only 3% managed care.[61] This result is in marked contrast to the otolaryngology group where 15.5% of respondents practiced in an academic setting, and 84.5% were in private practice or a health maintenance organization.[60] These differences undoubtedly reflect the differences in surveying registrants to a surgical meeting as compared with surveying members of a specialty society. In addition, the respondents to the survey conducted by Sturgeon and colleagues reported a higher volume of thyroid surgery, with 58% stating that they performed more than 100 thyroidectomies per year.

Sturgeon and colleagues[61] found that a total of 37.1% of respondents described themselves as users of neuromonitoring. This percentage is less than that seen among the otolaryngologists. The "user group" could be further broken down to the 13.8% of surgeons who were "routine users" and the 23.3% who were "selective users." Surgeons who treated a large number of patients were most likely to always use neuromonitoring and, not surprisingly, they were least likely to have never tried neuromonitoring.[61]

These 2 studies are all of the data that is available to try to understand the current rates of RLN monitoring in the United States. Based on the data from these 2 studies, one of them involving primarily private practice otolaryngologists with low-volume thyroid surgery practices and the other involving primarily academic general surgeons with high-volume endocrine practices, it can be inferred that most of the thyroidectomies performed in the United States seem to be done without RLN monitoring. This issue is certainly a moving target and will inevitably change in the future.

POTENTIAL LEGAL ISSUES IN RLN MONITORING

Kern[10] examined jury verdict reports in malpractice cases involving endocrine surgery between 1985 and 1991 and found that surgical injuries, mostly recurrent nerve injuries, accounted for the greatest number of cases and the highest cost of litigation. Therefore, some attention must be given to the legal issues surrounding RLN monitoring. Among respondents to the AAES survey described earlier, 10% of the users of neuromonitoring and 12% of the nonusers had been named in a lawsuit due to RLN injury.[61] In the otolaryngology survey, Horne and colleagues[60] reported that 22% of the respondents mentioned "medical-legal protection" as a reason for using RLN monitoring during thyroid surgery.[60]

The central question with respect to the malpractice issues related to RLN monitoring is whether the use of the monitor intraoperatively is considered "standard of care" with respect to thyroid surgery. The legal definition of the "standard of care" is the attention, caution, or prudence that another comparable physician would provide in caring for a patient in a similar circumstance. Failure to meet the standard of care results in negligence. If, therefore, RLN monitoring were the standard of care in thyroid surgery, a surgeon who failed to use neuromonitoring would be negligent. The determination that something is standard of care should take into account the outcomes as reported in the surgical literature concerning a particular technique and the actual practice of comparable and prudent physicians. At present, because there is no statistically significant evidence that RLN monitoring results in lower rates of RLN injury, even if most surgeons were to use RLN monitoring, it would not constitute the standard of care for thyroid surgery.

Some surgeons have the mistaken belief that use of the RLN monitor will somehow be beneficial in a lawsuit if an injury were to occur. However, if an injury to the nerve occurs, whether the RLN monitor is used or not, the surgeon is at risk of being named in a malpractice suit because the use of the RLN monitor would not be considered standard of care. There are scenarios in which a plaintiff's attorney could argue that using the RLN monitor is worse than not using the monitor. For example, if the surgeon claims that no negligence occurred because RLN monitoring was used, the plaintiff's attorney might argue that the surgeon was so negligent that even with RLN monitoring he or she injured the RLN. There are also scenarios in which a plaintiff's attorney could be critical of not using the RLN monitor. For example, if there is a nerve injury and the RLN monitor was not used, the plaintiff's attorney might claim that an injury would not have occurred, had the RLN monitor been used. Of course, there is no basis to support either of these claims. Therefore, whether RLN monitoring is used or not during thyroidectomy, the determining factor that brings a lawsuit is whether the nerve is injured. Because the literature shows no difference in rates of RLN injury whether neuromonitoring is used or not, the most prudent approach for the surgeon is to use the techniques that have been shown to minimize RLN injury, that is, careful, meticulous dissection with the attempt to visualize the RLN in every case possible.

POTENTIAL ETHICAL ISSUES IN RLN MONITORING

The biggest ethical issues that arise with respect to neuromonitoring in thyroid surgery surround informed consent and advertising by surgeons or medical facilities. Based on the data in the literature, neuromonitoring does not result in lower rates of RLN injury. Despite this, there are many surgeons who will be tempted to tell patients that using the RLN monitor will make the operation safer. Because patients present to surgeons seeking accurate medical information, surgeons have a responsibility to honestly disclose the risks of surgery. In this context, any suggestion that RLN monitoring will reduce the low risk of RLN injury is misleading to patients and is unethical. In addition, any surgeon or medical facility that advertises that neuromonitoring will make thyroid surgery more "safe" is misleading the public. It is all too frequent that claims are made on the Internet that thyroid surgery is made safer by use of the RLN monitor. Although a marketing department cannot be expected to know that such a claim runs counter to the medical literature, it is incumbent on surgeons to ensure that misleading claims are not presented to patients.

SUMMARY

Does the analysis of the literature along with the legal and ethical issues discussed earlier suggest that RLN neuromonitoring should *not* be used? The answer is unquestionably "No." Quite the contrary—although there is no increase in documented safety of RLN monitoring during thyroid surgery, there may be other reasons why a surgeon might choose to use monitoring. Some of these issues have been suggested in the questionnaire study by Horne and colleagues.[60] Some surgeons believe that RLN monitoring might help even in less than statistically significant ways. Some investigators have noted that neuromonitoring can aid in dissection in some cases, is easy to use, aids in anatomic identification of the RLN, and aids in resident training.[48] Some surgeons report that it is reassuring to know that one RLN is intact before embarking on dissection of the other side.[58]

As with so much in surgery, decisions must be made without sufficient evidence to give a clear answer. When it comes to RLN monitoring during thyroid surgery, as long as the principles of safe thyroid surgery are not compromised, use of the neuromonitor would seem to provide few negative results. If the device is available and not overly expensive, surgeons should use individual judgment to decide whether to use the device. Much as gastrointestinal surgeons individually decide whether to perform bowel anastamoses in a stapled or hand-sewn fashion, thyroid surgeons must decide whether to use neuromonitoring. Just as cost, time saved, resident education, and other ill-defined issues have an impact on the controversy of stapled versus hand sewn methods, so also numerous individual concerns will have an impact on whether a surgeon decides to use RLN monitoring during thyroid surgery. Regardless of the ultimate decision that each surgeon makes, he or she should fully understand the technology of RLN monitoring and how to best use the technology to gain the greatest amount of useful intraoperative information.

REFERENCES

1. Lahey F. Routine dissection and demonstration of the recurrent laryngeal nerve in subtotal thyroidectomy. Surg Gynecol Obstet 1938;66:775–7.
2. Riddell V. Injury to recurrent laryngeal nerves during thyroidectomy—a comparison between the results of identification and non-identification in 1022 nerves exposed to risk. Lancet 1956;29:638–41.
3. Hermann M, Alk G, Roka R, et al. Laryngeal recurrent nerve injury in surgery for benign thyroid diseases—effect of nerve dissection and impact of individual surgeon in more than 27,000 nerves at risk. Ann Surg 2002;235:261–8.
4. Thomusch O, Machens A, Sekulla C, et al. Multivariate analysis of risk factors for postoperative complications in benign goiter surgery: prospective multicenter study in Germany. World J Surg 2000;24(11):1335–41.
5. Dralle H, Sekulla C, Haerting J, et al. Risk factors of paralysis and functional outcome after recurrent laryngeal nerve monitoring in thyroid surgery. Surgery 2004;136(6):1310–22.
6. Holt GR, McMurray GT, Joseph DJ. Recurrent laryngeal nerve injury following thyroid operations. Surg Gynecol Obstet 1977;144(4):567–70.
7. Wagner HE, Seiler C. Recurrent laryngeal nerve palsy after thyroid gland surgery. Br J Surg 1994;81(2):226–8.
8. Smith E, Taylor M, Mendoza M, et al. Spasmodic dysphonia and vocal fold paralysis: outcomes of voice problems on work-related functioning. J Voice 1998;12(2):223–32.
9. Smith E, Verdolini K, Gray S, et al. Effect of voice disorders on the quality of life. J Med Speech Lang Pathol 1996;4:223–44.
10. Kern KA. Medicolegal analysis of errors in diagnosis and treatment of surgical endocrine disease. Surgery 1993;114(6):1167–73 [discussion: 1173–4].
11. Flisberg K, Lindholm T. Electrical stimulation of the human recurrent laryngeal nerve during thyroid operation. Acta Otolaryngol Suppl 1969;263:63–7.
12. Shedd DP, Durham C. Electrical identification of the recurrent laryngeal nerve. I. Response of the canine larynx to electrical stimulation of the recurrent laryngeal nerve. Ann Surg 1966;163(1):47–50.
13. James AG, Crocker S, Woltering E, et al. A simple method for identifying and testing the recurrent laryngeal nerve. Surg Gynecol Obstet 1985;161(2):185–6.

14. Randolph GW, Kobler JB, Wilkins J. Recurrent laryngeal nerve identification and assessment during thyroid surgery: laryngeal palpation. World J Surg 2004;28(8): 755–60.
15. Tomoda C, Hirokawa Y, Uruno T, et al. Sensitivity and specificity of intraoperative recurrent laryngeal nerve stimulation test for predicting vocal cord palsy after thyroid surgery. World J Surg 2006;30(7):1230–3.
16. Loch-Wilkinson TJ, Stalberg PL, Sidhu SB, et al. Nerve stimulation in thyroid surgery: is it really useful? ANZ J Surg 2007;77(5):377–80.
17. Riddell V. Thyroidectomy: prevention of bilateral recurrent nerve palsy. Results of identification of the nerve over 23 consecutive years (1946–69) with a description of an additional safety measure. Br J Surg 1970;57(1):1–11.
18. Eltzschig HK, Posner M, Moore FD Jr. The use of readily available equipment in a simple method for intraoperative monitoring of recurrent laryngeal nerve function during thyroid surgery: initial experience with more than 300 cases. Arch Surg 2002;137(4):452–6 [discussion: 456–7].
19. Lipton RJ, McCaffrey TV, Litchy WJ. Intraoperative electrophysiologic monitoring of laryngeal muscle during thyroid surgery. Laryngoscope 1988;98(12):1292–6.
20. Rice DH, Cone-Wesson B. Intraoperative recurrent laryngeal nerve monitoring. Otolaryngol Head Neck Surg 1991;105(3):372–5.
21. Tschopp KP, Gottardo C. Comparison of various methods of electromyographic monitoring of the recurrent laryngeal nerve in thyroid surgery. Ann Otol Rhinol Laryngol 2002;111(9):811–6.
22. Tschopp K, Probst R. [New aspects in surgery of the thyroid gland with intraoperative monitoring of the recurrent laryngeal nerve]. Laryngorhinootologie 1994; 73(11):568–72 [in German].
23. Hamelmann WH, Meyer T, Timm S, et al. [A Critical Estimation of Intraoperative Neuromonitoring (IONM) in Thyroid Surgery]. Zentralbl Chir 2002;127(5):409–13 [in German].
24. Brauckhoff M, Gimm O, Thanh PN, et al. First experiences in intraoperative neurostimulation of the recurrent laryngeal nerve during thyroid surgery of children and adolescents. J Pediatr Surg 2002;37(10):1414–8.
25. Yarbrough DE, Thompson GB, Kasperbauer JL, et al. Intraoperative electromyographic monitoring of the recurrent laryngeal nerve in reoperative thyroid and parathyroid surgery. Surgery 2004;136(6):1107–15.
26. Thomusch O, Sekulla C, Machens A, et al. Validity of intra-operative neuromonitoring signals in thyroid surgery. Langenbecks Arch Surg 2004;389(6):499–503.
27. Marcus B, Edwards B, Yoo S, et al. Recurrent laryngeal nerve monitoring in thyroid and parathyroid surgery: the University of Michigan experience. Laryngoscope 2003;113(2):356–61.
28. Eisele DW. Intraoperative electrophysiologic monitoring of the recurrent laryngeal nerve. Laryngoscope 1996;106(4):443–9.
29. Barwell J, Lytle J, Page R, et al. The NIM-2 nerve integrity monitor in thyroid and parathyroid surgery. Br J Surg 1997;84(6):854.
30. Horn D, Rotzscher VM. Intraoperative electromyogram monitoring of the recurrent laryngeal nerve: experience with an intralaryngeal surface electrode. A method to reduce the risk of recurrent laryngeal nerve injury during thyroid surgery. Langenbecks Arch Surg 1999;384(4):392–5.
31. Timon CI, Rafferty M. Nerve monitoring in thyroid surgery: is it worthwhile? Clin Otolaryngol Allied Sci 1999;24(6):487–90.
32. Lamade W, Meyding-Lamade U, Buchhold C, et al. [First continuous nerve monitoring in thyroid gland surgery]. Chirurg 2000;71(5):551–7 [in German].

33. Hemmerling TM, Schurr C, Dern S, et al. [Intraoperative electromyographic recurrent laryngeal nerve identification as a routine measure]. Chirurg 2000;71(5): 545–50 [in German].

34. Brennan J, Moore EJ, Shuler KJ. Prospective analysis of the efficacy of continuous intraoperative nerve monitoring during thyroidectomy, parathyroidectomy, and parotidectomy. Otolaryngol Head Neck Surg 2001;124(5):537–43.

35. Dackiw AP, Rotstein LE, Clark OH. Computer-assisted evoked electromyography with stimulating surgical instruments for recurrent/external laryngeal nerve identification and preservation in thyroid and parathyroid operation. Surgery 2002; 132(6):1100–6 [discussion: 1107–8].

36. Djohan RS, Rodriguez HE, Connolly MM, et al. Intraoperative monitoring of recurrent laryngeal nerve function. Am Surg 2000;66(6):595–7.

37. Chan WF, Lang BH, Lo CY. The role of intraoperative neuromonitoring of recurrent laryngeal nerve during thyroidectomy: a comparative study on 1000 nerves at risk. Surgery 2006;140(6):866–72 [discussion: 872–3].

38. Chan WF, Lo CY. Pitfalls of intraoperative neuromonitoring for predicting postoperative recurrent laryngeal nerve function during thyroidectomy. World J Surg 2006;30(5):806–12.

39. Shindo M, Chheda NN. Incidence of vocal cord paralysis with and without recurrent laryngeal nerve monitoring during thyroidectomy. Arch Otolaryngol Head Neck Surg 2007;133(5):481–5.

40. Chiang FY, Lu IC, Kuo WR, et al. The mechanism of recurrent laryngeal nerve injury during thyroid surgery–the application of intraoperative neuromonitoring. Surgery 2008;143(6):743–9.

41. Lu IC, Chu KS, Tsai CJ, et al. Optimal depth of NIM EMG endotracheal tube for intraoperative neuromonitoring of the recurrent laryngeal nerve during thyroidectomy. World J Surg 2008;32(9):1935–9.

42. Hemmerling TM, Schmidt J, Bosert C, et al. Intraoperative monitoring of the recurrent laryngeal nerve in 151 consecutive patients undergoing thyroid surgery. Anesth Analg 2001;93(2):396–9, 3rd contents page.

43. Marusch F, Hussock J, Haring G, et al. Influence of muscle relaxation on neuromonitoring of the recurrent laryngeal nerve during thyroid surgery. Br J Anaesth 2005;94(5):596–600.

44. Lamade W, Ulmer C, Seimer A, et al. A new system for continuous recurrent laryngeal nerve monitoring. Minim Invasive Ther Allied Technol 2007;16(3): 149–54.

45. Ulmer C, Koch KP, Seimer A, et al. Real-time monitoring of the recurrent laryngeal nerve: an observational clinical trial. Surgery 2008;143(3):359–65.

46. Jonas J. [Reliabilty of intraoperative recurrent laryngeal nerve monitoring in thyroid surgery]. Zentralbl Chir 2002;127(5):404–8 [in German].

47. Beldi G, Kinsbergen T, Schlumpf R. Evaluation of intraoperative recurrent nerve monitoring in thyroid surgery. World J Surg 2004;28(6):589–91.

48. Snyder SK, Hendricks JC. Intraoperative neurophysiology testing of the recurrent laryngeal nerve: plaudits and pitfalls. Surgery 2005;138(6):1183–91 [discussion: 1191–2].

49. Kunath M, Marusch F, Horschig P, et al. [The value of intraoperative neuromonitoring in thyroid surgery–a prospective observational study with 926 patients]. Zentralbl Chir 2003;128(3):187–90 [in German].

50. Hermann M, Hellebart C, Freissmuth M. Neuromonitoring in thyroid surgery: prospective evaluation of intraoperative electrophysiological responses for the prediction of recurrent laryngeal nerve injury. Ann Surg 2004;240(1):9–17.

51. Friedrich T, Staemmler A, Hansch U, et al. [Intraoperative electrophysiological monitoring of the recurrent laryngeal nerve in thyroid gland surgery–a prospective study]. Zentralbl Chir 2002;127(5):414–20 [in German].
52. Witt RL. Recurrent laryngeal nerve electrophysiologic monitoring in thyroid surgery: the standard of care? J Voice 2005;19(3):497–500.
53. Meyer T, Hamelmann W, Timmermann W, et al. The advantages and disadvantages of nerve monitoring during thyroid surgery in childhood. Eur J Pediatr Surg 2006;16(6):392–5.
54. Meyer T, Hocht B. Recurrent laryngeal nerve monitoring during thyroid surgery in childhood. Eur J Pediatr Surg 2006;16(3):149–54.
55. White WM, Randolph GW, Hartnick CJ, et al. Recurrent laryngeal nerve monitoring during thyroidectomy and related cervical procedures in the pediatric population. Arch Otolaryngol Head Neck Surg 2009;135(1):88–94.
56. Brauckhoff M, Walls G, Brauckhoff K, et al. Identification of the non-recurrent inferior laryngeal nerve using intraoperative neurostimulation. Langenbecks Arch Surg 2002;386(7):482–7.
57. Timmermann W, Hamelmann WH, Thomusch O, et al. [Effectiveness and results of intraoperative neuromonitoring in thyroid surgery. Statement of the Interdisciplinary Study Group on Intraoperative Neuromonitoring of Thyroid Surgery]. Chirurg 2004;75(9):916–22 [in German].
58. Dralle H, Sekulla C, Lorenz K, et al. Intraoperative monitoring of the recurrent laryngeal nerve in thyroid surgery. World J Surg 2008;32(7):1358–66.
59. Dionigi G. Use of a single bipolar electrode in the posterior arytenoids muscles for bilateral monitoring of the recurrent laryngeal nerves in thyroid surgery: standardization of the technique [comment]. Eur Arch Otorhinolaryngol 2008;265(11):1431–2.
60. Horne SK, Gal TJ, Brennan JA. Prevalence and patterns of intraoperative nerve monitoring for thyroidectomy. Otolaryngol Head Neck Surg 2007;136(6):952–6.
61. Sturgeon C, Sturgeon T, Angelos P. Neuromonitoring in thyroid surgery: attitudes, usage patterns, and predictors of use among endocrine surgeons. World J Surg 2009;33:417–25.

Surgical Management of Well-Differentiated Thyroid Cancer: State of the Art

James Suliburk, MD[a], Leigh Delbridge, MD, FRACS[b],*

KEYWORDS

• Thyroid cancer • Lymph nodes • Thyroidectomy
• Papillary • Follicular

When the subject of the extent surgery for well-differentiated thyroid cancer (WDTC) was last reviewed in *Surgical Clinics of North America*, Dackiw and Zeiger noted that it continued to be an area of controversy.[1] At that time the major issue related to the optimal extent of thyroidectomy, with the reviewers making a strong case for total thyroidectomy being the treatment of choice. The subject continues to be controversial; however, the last 5 years has seen a major change in focus in relation to the long-term goals of therapy and the surgical management of cervical lymph nodes. The American Thyroid Association (ATA) guidelines for the management of thyroid cancer were last published in 2006 and updated in 2009. They list several goals of therapy.[2] The major goal of initial surgical therapy is "to remove the primary tumor, disease that has extended beyond the thyroid capsule, and involved cervical lymph nodes." Furthermore, the major goal of long-term management is "accurate surveillance for possible recurrence in patients thought to be free of disease."[2] Because more than 85% of patients with WDTC will have low-risk papillary cancer, a principal aim of therapy has now become to assure these patients that they are free of disease, with a negative cervical ultrasound and undetectable serum thyroglobulin level.

This approach is based on an appreciation of 4 main issues: firstly that residual metastases in cervical lymph nodes represent the most common site of recurrent disease;[3] secondly that metastatic involvement of cervical lymph nodes does indeed impact survival;[4] thirdly that prophylactic surgical clearance of the central lymph node compartment can facilitate long-term follow-up with reduction of thyroglobulin levels;[5]

[a] Michael E. DeBakey Department of Surgery, Baylor College of Medicine, Houston, TX, USA
[b] Department of Endocrine & Oncology Surgery, Royal North Shore Hospital, St Leonards, 2065, Sydney, NSW, Australia
* Corresponding author.
E-mail address: leighd@med.usyd.edu.au (L. Delbridge).

Surg Clin N Am 89 (2009) 1171–1191
doi:10.1016/j.suc.2009.06.013
surgical.theclinics.com
0039-6109/09/$ – see front matter © 2009 Elsevier Inc. All rights reserved.

and finally that long-term follow-up with cervical ultrasound and serum thyroglobulin is highly sensitive in the detection of recurrent disease.[6]

Nonmedullary WDTC comprises a group of tumors including papillary thyroid carcinoma (PTC) and follicular thyroid carcinoma (FTC), with Hürthle cell carcinoma being a subtype of follicular carcinoma.[7] Anaplastic thyroid cancer and the poorly differentiated subtypes of PTC (insular, tall cell variant, columnar cell) are not discussed in this review.

EPIDEMIOLOGY

Thyroid cancer, although relatively rare (2% of all cancers), is the most common endocrine malignancy and there has been a steady increase in its incidence over the past 15 to 20 years. The incidence of thyroid cancer has risen faster in women than any other cancer over the last decade and the rising incidence in men exceeds that of all but 2 cancers.[8] In the United States, the incidence is increasing fastest in the northeast as well as in southern parts of the country.[9] The distribution of the disease remains two-thirds in women and one-third in men, and approximately 1 in 100 men and women will be diagnosed with cancer of the thyroid during their lifetime. Although thyroid cancer can occur at any age, it is most commonly found in those older than 30 years of age with the median age of diagnosis being 47 years. The overall 5-year relative survival rate for 1996 to 2004 from 17 SEER (Surveillance Epidemiology and End Results) geographic areas was 96.9%.

It is clear that the vast majority (87%) of the excess thyroid cancers detected in the past 15 years are attributed to an increase in small cancers (less than 2 cm in diameter).[10] Thus although the incidence has more than doubled over the time period the mortality has remained the same, and the increased amount of small cancers does not contribute to mortality for the disease. Increased detection is almost certainly the result of improved pathologic sectioning and incidental detection of clinically occult nodules on imaging ordered for reasons other than thyroid disease.[11–13]

RISK FACTORS

The most pronounced environmental risk factor for thyroid cancer is exposure to ionizing radiation (energy from the high-frequency electromagnetic spectrum such as gamma rays or x-rays). Ionizing radiation is either due to medical treatment (childhood radiation therapy for benign or malignant disease, adult treatment of malignancies) or nuclear fallout (atomic bomb/testing survivors, nuclear energy accidents). Ionizing radiation may exert this effect through several changes to the cell, including genomic instability.[14,15] The effects of ionizing radiation are most pronounced in children, especially those younger than 10 years old at the time of exposure. The latency period of developing cancer from this exposure is approximately 10 years for patients having external beam radiation exposure to less than 5 years for victims of the Chernobyl accident, and the increased risk persists for 30 to 40 years.[16,17] Exposure to ionizing radiation has been shown to increase the risk of malignancy for a thyroid nodule to 30% to 40%. Furthermore, this risk of malignancy is increased regardless of nodule number and size, and multifocal malignancy is found more than half of the time.[18] A history of prior radiation exposure mandates initial total thyroidectomy.

Patients presenting with benign thyroid disease may also be at higher risk of harboring a malignant nodule. Cold nodules found on radionuclide scanning in patients with Graves disease may be malignant 15% to 38% of the time and complex cysts in thyroid disease may also have within them a malignancy approximately 17% of the time. Patients with a nodule of 4 cm or larger have been shown to have up to a 34% false negative rate on fine-needle aspiration (FNA), and 40% of indeterminate lesions on FNA were later found on histologic section to be malignant.[19]

The sex-specific distribution is equal in those older than 65 and given that overall two-thirds of cancer cases are women, there would seem to be a link between reproductive hormones and the development of thyroid cancer. Estrogen has been linked as a stimulus for genomic instability and this may be how it exerts its mutagenic effects on the thyroid.[20] Studies have yet to conclusively link traditional carcinogens such as alcohol and tobacco to the development of WDTC. Data are conflicting as to what role iodine-rich versus iodine-deficient diets play in the development of thyroid cancer. Countries with iodine-rich diets such as the United States and Sweden have slightly increased incidence of PTC, and countries with iodine-deficient diets such as Switzerland and Australia have slightly increased incidence of FTC.[21]

GENETIC SUSCEPTIBILITY AND MOLECULAR PATHOGENESIS

Although not well defined, there most certainly exists a genetic component to WDTC. In fact a family history of thyroid carcinoma may increase an individual's risk 3-fold when a parent has the disease and up to 6-fold if a sibling has the disease.[22] Thyroid cancer may be associated with germline mutation syndromes such as familial adenomatous polyposis/Gardner syndrome (*APC* gene mutation), Cowden disease (*PTEN* gene mutation), Carney syndrome (*PRKAR1A* gene), and Werner Syndrome (*WRN* gene mutation), although it is a small percentage of each of these patients that will develop thyroid carcinoma.[23]

PTC and FTC have distinct genomic and proteomic signatures. Pathways are now emerging that demonstrate how these differences play a role in governing tumor biology. Mutations that involve *RET*, *NTRK1*, *BRAF*, *PPARγ*, or *Ras* can be detected in almost 70% of cases.[24] There are at least 12 different *RET* mutations, known as PTC/Ret chimeric oncoproteins, which seem to be an early event in thyroid tumorigenesis, with series showing a high prevalence in papillary microcarcinomas and also a high proportion of the post-Chernobyl childhood-induced papillary thyroid carcinomas.[25,26] *BRAF* mutations are seldom found in radiation-induced cancer. These mutations are postulated to produce a more aggressive phenotype of PTC as they are found in many of the more poorly differentiated subtypes of PTC.[27–29] Follicular carcinomas have mutations in PPARγ (rarely found in PTC), AKT pathways, and *Ras*.[30,31] Future treatments will formulate surgical and molecular therapies tailored to the patient's pathologic molecular signature.

NATIONAL AND INTERNATIONAL GUIDELINES FOR TREATMENT

The surgical management of WDTC continues to be controversial in the absence of prospective randomized trials of treatment to guide the clinician. Because of the overall good prognosis and indolent course of the disease, such trials would take decades to complete. As such, clinicians must use the best available evidence that generally consists of retrospective reviews of large case series.

Well-established evidenced-based guidelines for the treatment of thyroid cancer in North America come from the National Comprehensive Cancer Network (NCCN) Practice Guidelines in Oncology (www.nccn.org, 2007), as well as from the ATA (www.thyroid.org, 2009) and the National Cancer Institute (NCI) (www.cancer.gov).[2] Prior guidelines published jointly by the American Association of Clinical Endocrinologists (http://www.aace.com/pub/pdf/guidelines/thyroid_carcinoma.pdf) and the American Association of Endocrine Surgeons (http://www.endocrinesurgery.org/practice_guidelines/practice_guidelines.cfm) were also published in 2001.[32] Internationally, the European Thyroid Cancer Taskforce has issued guidelines that were published in 2006[33] and the British Thyroid Association/Royal College of Physicians published guidelines in 2007 (http://www.british-thyroid-association.org/Guidelines).

For the most part the guidelines are in agreement with regard to the treatment of thyroid cancer; however, there are several areas of controversy due to the lack of prospective trials. Areas of surgical controversy include preoperative laryngoscopy, total thyroidectomy for noninvasive follicular cancer, and indications for prophylactic central lymph node dissection. This review addresses the authors' opinion in these areas.

PREOPERATIVE EVALUATION
Clinical Presentation

Evaluation of the patient with a suspected thyroid cancer first begins with thorough history taking to evaluate what risk factors the patient may have for malignancy. In general, patients commonly self-diagnose a lump in their neck found during palpation. Other patients may present with a thyroid nodule detected incidentally on imaging ordered for a different medical reason (thyroid incidentaloma). Key aspects of the history include the presence of symptoms (dysphagia, voice change, coughing, choking, dyspnea, pain, sudden increase in size, and so forth) as well as exposure to ionizing radiation and family history of thyroid or parathyroid disease. Physical examination should assess for features of the nodule(s) as well as any cervical lymphadenopathy. Suspicious or worrisome features include nodules that are hard, fixed, irregular, 4 cm or larger, or those lesions with associated lymphadenopathy. **Box 1** lists high-risk as well as moderate-risk characteristics that may be associated with

---

Box 1
Clinical characteristics of thyroid nodules adapted from Hegedus et al[34]

Suspicious clinical characteristics of thyroid nodules

High risk

   Family history of thyroid cancer or multiple endocrine neoplasia syndrome

   Rapid growth, especially during levothyroxine therapy

   Hard or firm nodule

   Fixation of nodule to adjacent structures

   Cervical lymphadenopathy

   History of head or neck irradiation

Moderate risk

   Age <20 or > 60 years

   Male sex

   Nodule >4 cm

   Complex cystic nodule

   Mass effect symptoms: dysphagia, voice change, dyspnea, cough

Data from Hegedus L. Clinical practice. The thyroid nodule. N Engl J Med 2004;351:1764–71.

thyroid cancer. A general rule to follow is that any lesion with 2 or more associated high-risk characteristics may have a malignancy rate greater than 80%.[34]

DIAGNOSTIC EVALUATION
Laboratory

The initial investigation required in all patients with a thyroid lesion is biochemical assessment of thyroid function, as clinical assessment of thyroid function is not a reliable indicator of thyroid status. Ideally the thyrotropin level should be known before FNA, as an aspirate from a hyperfunctioning nodule may lead to confounding results. If the nodule is simply a hyperfunctioning one, the risk of malignancy may be so low that excision to rule out malignancy is rarely if ever warranted.

Fine-Needle Aspiration

FNA biopsy (or FNB—fine-needle biopsy) is the gold standard for preoperative evaluation of a suspected thyroid cancer. Effective use of FNA is operator dependent and requires an experienced multidisciplinary group including allied health technologists, radiologists, cytopathologists, endocrinologists, and surgeons. When correctly applied and interpreted it provides quick and specific information about the cytology of a nodule from which the histology may be inferred. FNA is best performed with image guidance via ultrasound which increases the accuracy, sensitivity, and specificity.[35] Contraindications are few and complications rare. When targeting cystic lesions with solid components, ultrasound should be used to obtain a sample from the solid component.[36] Controversy exists over whether the best samples are obtained with passage of the needle through the lesion with or without continuous suction. Obtaining insufficient specimen for diagnosis is minimized by having immediate cytopathologic interpretation of the results. In 2007 a consensus conference hosted by the NCI proposed further classification of FNA results based on a 6-tiered system.[37] Those categories and their risk of malignancy are listed in **Table 1**. The main feature of this system is that it serves to further classify the atypical lesions by risk of malignancy and potentially spare unnecessary surgery to patients with "low-risk" atypical lesions. In this manner, surgeon and patient may discuss risk and benefit of surgical excision of the atypical lesion. There is no test to differentiate malignancy from benign disease in follicular lesions, as the diagnosis rests solely on the demonstration of follicular cells outside the capsule or within blood vessels on histologic specimen. If the specimen is inadequate, FNA should be repeated and if again inadequate the patient should proceed with surgical excision. In addition, if the lesion is cystic and recurs after aspiration then the lesion should be excised, as FNA has an accuracy of only 80% in this case and these cysts may degenerate or harbor an occult carcinoma.[38] FNA should generally be performed on nodules larger than 1 cm, as any nodule harboring a carcinoma smaller than 1 cm is clinically insignificant with the exception being those associated with clinical symptoms, lymphadenopathy, or in patients with a history of ionizing radiation exposure.

IMAGING
Ultrasound

It cannot be overemphasized that manual palpation of thyroid nodules is extremely variable between even experienced clinicians and as such imaging with ultrasound, especially surgeon-performed ultrasound, has become essential to the evaluation of the thyroid gland. Surgeon-performed ultrasound is rapidly becoming an extension of the physical examination, adding images containing objective information to the

Table 1
Cytopathologic diagnosis and risk of malignancy adapted from Baloch and colleagues,[37] combining the traditional classification of FNA results with the classification as proposed by the NCI consensus conference in 2007

	Cytopathologic Diagnosis and Risk of Malignancy		
Traditional FNA Category	NCI 2007 Conference FNA Category	Alternate Category Terms	Risk of Malignancy
Benign	Benign		<1%
Atypical or indeterminate	Follicular lesion of undetermined significance	Atypia of undetermined significance, Atypical follicular lesion, Cellular follicular lesion	5%–10%
	Neoplasm - Follicular Neoplasm - Hürthle Cell Neoplasm	Suspicious for neoplasm - Suspicious for follicular neoplasm - Suspicious for Hürthle cell neoplasm	20%–30%
	Suspicious for malignancy		50%–75%
Malignant	Malignant		100%
Inadequate	Nondiagnostic	Unsatisfactory Inadequate	

Data from Baloch ZW, LiVolsi VA, Asa SL, et al. Diagnostic terminology and morphologic criteria for cytologic diagnosis of thyroid lesions: a synopsis of the National Cancer Institute Thyroid Fine-Needle Aspiration State of the Science Conference. Diagn Cytopathol 2008;36:425–37.

subjective palpation by the surgeon's hands. Whereas there are some ultrasound characteristics that may indicate a higher risk of malignancy (intrinsic calcification, blurred or ill-defined margin, hypervascularity, or hypoechoic features), none so far have proven reliable enough to surpass FNA as a method of detecting malignant pathology within the suspicious nodule.[35] When a diagnosis of cancer is made (on FNA), neck ultrasound performed by an individual with experience in thyroid cancer is mandatory to evaluate for lymphadenopathy that may not be detected by physical examination.[39] This procedure focuses on the level II to IV jugular chain nodes. Ultrasound is not reliable in detecting lymphadenopathy in the level V and superior mediastinal lymph node basins. Level VI lymphadenopathy is not always seen due to acoustic distortion. Surrounding structures including bone, tracheal air, and the overlying thyroid tissue prevent detailed imaging in these substernal, retroclavicular, intrathoracic, paratracheal, and retrotracheal positions where computed tomography (CT) scanning is the best imaging modality. However, ultrasound facilitates detection of locoregional disease that is otherwise clinically occult, which may change the operative procedure thus theoretically allowing for a more complete resection, minimizing the potential for local recurrence and the need for reoperative surgery. Preoperative ultrasound examination of the cervical nodes also provides a baseline study, because guidelines for long-term follow-up all now recommend routine cervical ultrasound examination.

Computed Tomography and Magnetic Resonance Imaging

Whereas ultrasound is the imaging study of choice in evaluation of the thyroid gland, CT also has an important role. CT is best used as an adjunct modality in imaging advanced thyroid pathology when there is substernal, intrathoracic, or retrotracheal pathology/extension of the gland suspected. As noted earlier, these are areas in which ultrasound imaging is limited as a result of acoustic distortion because of bone or air. In these situations, a CT scan can be very helpful in the preoperative assessment, discerning the development of lymphadenopathy as well as determining invasion/compression of the aerodigestive tracts. Magnetic resonance imaging can perform the same imaging as CT although at a much higher cost.

Laryngoscopy

Laryngoscopy is increasingly being advocated for routine use before thyroid surgery whether for benign or malignant disease. Flexible laryngoscopy is easily performed in the office setting with topical nasal anesthetics and a fiber-optic scope. In the case of a patient with preexisting voice changes, or in the presence of a thyroid cancer, it is essential to determine the status of the vocal cords preoperatively.[40]

STAGING

The historical stage distribution and corresponding 5-year survival based on SEER data is summarized in **Table 2**.[8] There are other multiple staging and prognostic systems for WDTC. Some of the most commonly used systems include the sixth edition of the American Joint Committee on Cancer (AJCC) TNM (Tumor, Node, Metastasis) system, AMES (Age, Metastases, Extent, Size), AGES (Age, Grade, Extent, Size), EORTC (European Organization for Research and Treatment of Cancer), and MACIS (Metastasis, Age, Completeness of Resection, Invasion, and Size) with most authorities now using the sixth edition AJCC system as summarized in **Table 3**.[41–45]

Table 2
Historic stage of disease with percent presentation of each case and corresponding 5-year survival, from SEER Web site[8]

Percent Total Cases (%)	Historic Stage at Diagnosis	5-Year Survival (%)
59	Tumor confined to thyroid	99.7
34	Tumor spread to locoregional lymph nodes	96.9
5	Distant metastasis	57.8
3	Unknown	89.5

Data from Ries LAG, Krapcho M, Stinchcomb DG, et al, eds. SEER Stat fact Sheet—Cancer of the Thyroid. In: SEER Database. Bethesda, MD: NCI; 2008; with permission.

Although the aforementioned staging systems are valuable, it is important to realize that these systems were developed principally to predict death from metastatic disease, not local recurrence. However, the main aim of long-term surveillance for most patients with WDTC is the detection of possible local recurrence in those thought to be free of disease. There are numerous systems proposed for assessment of recurrence risk. The most useful is that based on the ATA guidelines, which propose a 3-level stratification determined after initial surgery and remnant ablation.[2]

- *Low risk*: Patients will have complete tumor resection at surgery with no locoregional invasion, absence of aggressive histology (eg, tall-cell, insular, or columnar cell carcinoma), absence of vascular invasion, and absence of uptake outside the thyroid bed on remnant ablation.
- *Intermediate risk*: Patients will have either microscopic invasion of tumor into perithyroidal tissues, aggressive histology, or vascular invasion.
- *High risk*: Patients will have either macroscopic tumor invasion, incomplete tumor resection, uptake outside the thyroid bed on remnant ablation, or distant metastases.

Papillary Thyroid Carcinoma

PTC is the most common cancer of the thyroid. PTC occurs in all age groups and is 3 times more common in women than in men, although this predominance does not exist in those younger than 20 and older than 60 years. PTC typically presents as a firm nodule, and may be gray with indistinct borders and adherence to surrounding structures. PTC may occur in any part of the thyroid gland with the most ominous location being posterior on the gland, as growth and extension here will be into the larynx and trachea thus making local disease difficult to control. More than half the time it is multifocal (multiple tumors within the gland).

The World Health Organization recognizes multiple variants of papillary carcinoma, with some of the more poorly differentiated variants especially noteworthy for their poorer prognosis including insular, tall cell, and columnar.[46,47] The most common variant is the follicular. The follicular variant has a follicular architecture that predominates, although with careful search the nuclear features of classic papillary carcinoma are found. The follicular variant represents a diagnostic challenge even for experienced cytopathologists due to features that overlap with follicular adenoma and carcinoma.[48,49] The prognosis of the follicular variant is similar to that of classic PTC.

In relation to surgical management of the thyroid gland, initial total thyroidectomy is clearly the operation of choice for PTC diagnosed preoperatively. Total thyroidectomy is associated with longer disease-free survival, ability to use

Table 3
TNM system for papillary and follicular thyroid cancer, from AJCC Cancer Staging Manual[43]

TNM system for papillary and follicular thyroid cancer

PTC & PTC <45 Years	5-Year Survival
Any T, N, M0	100%
Any T, N, M1	100%

Tumor (T)

Tx	Primary Tumor unable to be assessed
T0	No evidence of primary tumor
T1	Tumor ≤ 2 cm and limited to thyroid
T2	Tumor >2 cm, <4 cm limited to thyroid
T3	Tumor > 4 cm limited to thyroid or minimal extension
T4a	Tumor invading subcutaneous tissue, larynx, trachea, esophagus, or recurrent laryngeal nerve
T4b	Tumor invading prevertebral fascia, encasing carotid artery or mediastinal vessels

Sixth edition AJCC TNM System for Papillary and Follicular Thyroid Cancer

Stage	PTC & FTC ≥45 Years	5-Year Survival
I	T1 N0 M0	100%
II	T2 N0 M0	100%
III	T3 N0 M0 / T1–3 N1a M0	95.8%
IVa	T4a N0 M0 / T4a N1a M0 / T1–4a N1b M0	45.3%
IVb	T4b, any N, M0	
IVc	Any T, any N, M1	

Regional lymph nodes (N)

Nx	Regional nodes unable to be assessed
N0	No regional node disease
N1a	Regional nodes involved in level VI only (central compartment)
N1b	Regional nodes involved in cervical or superior mediastinal basins (unilateral or bilateral)

Distant metastasis (M)

Mx	Distant metastasis cannot be assessed
M0	No evidence of distant metastasis
M1	Distant metastasis present

From Greene FL, Page DL, Fleming ID, et al, eds. AJCC Cancer Staging Manual, 6th edition. New York: Springer-Verlag; 2002; with permission.

radioiodine to detect and treat residual normal thyroid tissue or disease, ability to monitor serum thyroglobulin, reduced need for reoperative surgery, and improved survival in tumors greater than 1 cm.[1,50–53] This progress represents a small but important evolution over the past 5 to 10 years in surgical therapy for papillary thyroid cancer. An additional reason to perform total thyroidectomy is the fact that more than half of thyroid cancer specimens will have foci of PTC in the contralateral lobe. It is debatable whether these particular foci are of clinical significance, as some studies would indicate they are not whereas others indicate a higher incidence of metastatic or persistent disease.[42,54] However, these patients are clearly at higher risk for recurrence when only lobectomy is performed and when recurrence occurs, 30% to 50% of patients will die of thyroid cancer.[55,56]

The more recent area of controversy relates to the role of elective or "prophylactic" central compartment lymph node dissection. The 2007 NCCN guidelines recommend to perform central lymph node dissection in a compartment-oriented fashion if diseased lymph nodes are identified either preoperatively or at the time of surgery. The ATA recommendations are for routine central lymph node dissection for PTC and Hürthle cell cancers in presence of disease. While prophylactic central compartment lymphadenectomy is advocated the ATA does not mandate it. With a surgeon experienced in thyroid cancer resection, morbidity of unilateral central node dissection concomitant with total thyroidectomy should be minimal. The authors' practice is to perform routine prophylactic central (level VI) lymph node dissection on the ipsilateral side of the tumor. The authors have demonstrated significantly lower thyroglobulin levels in patients undergoing prophylactic unilateral central node dissection compared with those who did not, supporting a role for improved local disease control and reduced recurrence.[5] Furthermore, a unilateral dissection reduces the risk of permanent hypoparathyroidism compared with bilateral central neck dissection, given that only one inferior parathyroid gland will require removal and autotransplantation. For lateral neck disease determined by FNA biopsy, clinical examination, or imaging, resection of all diagnosed disease should be completed in a compartment-oriented fashion.[2,57] "Berry picking" or removal of only what the surgeon deems enlarged lymph nodes is no longer regarded as appropriate surgical therapy in a compartment that has never been formally cleared.[58,59] The same principles apply in patients undergoing completion thyroidectomy following diagnostic lobectomy whereby cancer has subsequently been demonstrated. The authors have recently demonstrated that central neck dissection in that situation is equally safe compared with initial surgery.[60]

One issue not well defined is what actually constitutes the anatomic borders of a "central node dissection." The authors' practice is to dissect inferiorly to the thoracic inlet at the level of the innominate artery and brachiocephalic vein, medially to the anterior surface of trachea using the contralateral thymus as a boundary thus encompassing any pretracheal nodes, laterally to the carotid sheath, and superiorly to the level of the hyoid. With extensive disease, the dissection may continue further caudally incorporating Level VII, removing retromanubrial nodes down to the innominate vein. The inferior parathyroid on the side of the unilateral central node dissection is identified and routinely autotransplanted by mincing the parathyroid in balanced salt solution and injecting it via a blunt needle into the sternocleidomastoid. If that parathyroid is not identified and autotransplanted, then by definition either an appropriate dissection has not been performed or it has been inadvertently removed with the specimen.

The selective lateral neck dissection is performed when preoperative imaging, clinical examination, or FNA confirms lateral neck lymphadenopathy and presence of metastatic disease. Borders of the lateral neck dissection are the same as those previously published and described elsewhere.[61] This procedure is a "compartment-oriented" dissection that clears the jugular nodes (level IIa,b through IV) as well as the supraclavicular fossa nodes posterior and inferolateral to the sternocleidomastoid (level Vb) sparing the spinal accessory nerve, the vagus nerve, the phrenic nerve, the carotid artery, the internal jugular vein, and the sternocleidomastoid.

The authors' approach is illustrated in **Fig. 1**. This method for treating thyroid cancer minimizes morbidity (when performed by an experienced thyroid surgeon) and aggressively treats locoregional disease. Routine ipsilateral central compartment lymphadenectomy limits the need to reoperate for recurrent disease in the central compartment, which is perilous and at higher risk of unintentional injury to the recurrent laryngeal nerve as well as hypoparathyroidism.[62–64]

The goal of treatment of thyroid cancer no longer is for 5 or even 10- or 20-year survival. The goal has now shifted to achieving athyroglobulinemia, thus reassuring the patient of absence of disease recurrence and reducing the need for reoperative cervical surgery. Adequately powered randomized prospective trials are unlikely able to be accomplished to provide definitive data to support aggressive lymphadenectomy because of the large number of cases needed and the heterogeneity of descriptions in the extent of lymphadenectomy, but large retrospective case series as well as prospective case control series analyses continue to emerge demonstrating reduced locoregional recurrence and lower thyroglobulin levels with more aggressive surgery.[4,65–67] The risks of aggressive surgery must always be balanced against benefit, hence the need for surgeons experienced in advanced thyroid cancer treatment to perform the operation with minimal morbidity.

Follicular Thyroid Carcinoma

FTC represents about 5% to 10% of thyroid cancer cases. The treatment of follicular carcinoma is much the same as that of papillary carcinoma and staging is identical. A fundamental difference between FTC and PTC is the histology and cytopathology. FTC is not as readily diagnosed on FNA. The FNA will generally be interpreted as follicular lesion or follicular neoplasm (see **Table 1**) of which most are benign. Diagnosis of FTC is generally made after a diagnostic lobectomy has been performed and thus further treatment decisions are based on this. Malignancy depends on the demonstration of either capsular or vascular invasion.[46] The major issue relates to management of low-risk tumors, in this situation defined as minimally invasive follicular carcinoma (MIFC). Regardless of the extent of capsular invasion, any evidence of angioinvasion indicates a propensity to metastasize more so than lesions that have only capsular invasion which rarely metastasize.[49] As such, low-risk tumors that have only capsular invasion and no angioinvasion may be treated with lobectomy and isthmectomy alone, although completion thyroidectomy may be considered to facilitate long-term follow-up in the same way that total thyroidectomy is the preferred treatment in PTC.[68,69] For tumors with angioinvasive characteristics or widely invasive FTC, total thyroidectomy/completion thyroidectomy is the surgical treatment of choice. Routine lymphadenectomy of the central compartment is not practiced in FTC as it metastasizes through vascular channels, as opposed to PTC that spreads through the lymphatics.[70,71] As such there is no place for lymphadenectomy except in the rare case of nodal disease present at the time of initial surgery.

Hürthle cell thyroid carcinoma represents a variant of follicular carcinoma.[46] Also known as an oncocytic cell carcinoma, the Hürthle cell variant seems to be a more aggressive variant of FTC, with a 10-year mortality of 25% compared with

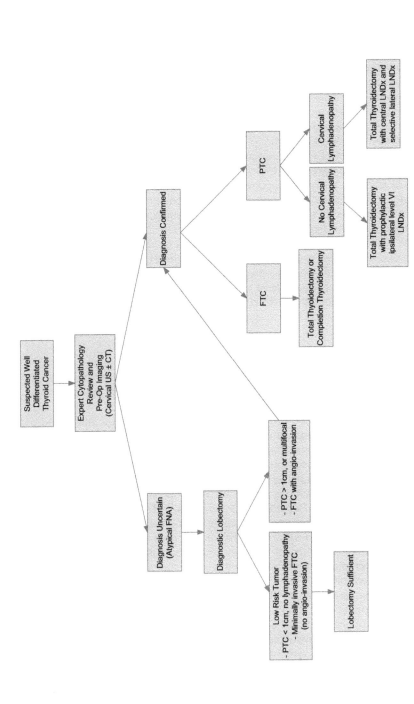

Fig. 1. Surgical decision making in well-differentiated thyroid cancer. CT, computed tomography; FNA, fine-needle aspiration; FTC, follicular thyroid carcinoma; LNDx, lymphadenectomy; PTC, papillary thyroid carcinoma; US, ultrasonography.

a 10 year mortality rate of 15% in FTC.[72] This carcinoma is usually found in an older patient population; it is more likely to present as an advanced tumor and have locoregional metastasis, and is less likely to concentrate [131]I.[73,74] As such, a more aggressive surgical approach of total thyroidectomy with ipsilateral central compartment lymphadenectomy, and lateral neck dissection guided by physical examination and preoperative imaging is warranted.

FOLLOW-UP CARE: THERAPY, SURVEILANCE, AND RECURRENCE

Whereas it is true that the vast majority of patients with WDTC will do very well, treatment still requires a multidisciplinary approach. Treatment of thyroid cancer continues to evolve and now is best done through a team approach to combine surgical therapy, expert pathology review, long-term thyrotropin suppression, radioactive iodine therapy, and in select cases external beam radiotherapy. Ideally, this will involve having experienced thyroid specialists in surgery, pathology, endocrinology, nuclear medicine, and radiation oncology all within the same center. Without this broad-based approach, gaps in care can emerge that may compromise the overall as well as disease-free survival of the patient, who can in today's modern treatment era come to expect to be cured of this cancer.

There exists an ever-growing number of thyroid cancer survivors. On January 1, 2005, in the United States there were approximately 388,386 men and women alive who had a history of cancer of the thyroid: 86,920 men and 301,466 women.[8] The therapy for thyroid cancer in hierarchical order is proper initial surgery, thyrotropin suppression, radioablative iodine therapy, and ongoing lifelong surveillance to detect recurrent disease. For advanced or unresectable cases of disease external beam radiation therapy has shown to be helpful.[75] Recurrence is common in thyroid cancer and may occur in approximately 30% of patients.[56] Most often this occurrence occurs locally and within 10 years of initial surgery. Factors identified as high risk for recurrence include age (<15, >45), male sex, family history, tumor >4 cm, bilateral disease, vascular invasion, and unfavorable histology.[56] The ATA lists guidelines for thyrotropin suppression as well as ongoing surveillance practice for high- and low-risk patients accordingly.[2]

Postoperative surveillance has shifted from a focus on radioiodine scanning to neck ultrasound and thyroglobulin measurement.[2] With the advent of thyroglobulin measurement endocrinologists now have a sensitive and specific biochemical marker of recurrent disease development and burden. Because recurrence most often occurs in the thyroid bed or neck, the advent of high-resolution ultrasound allows the location of recurrence to be defined anatomically. Recurrence that is detected on ultrasound should be surgically resected when possible. This resection should be compartment oriented when the compartment has not been formally cleared. If the recurrence is in a field that has previously had a compartment-oriented dissection, intraoperative ultrasound as well as image-guided wire placements can help define nonpalpable disease to serve as guidance for resection. Recurrence that is not identifiable by high-resolution sonography but shows definitive elevated thyroglobulin may also be identified through whole-body radioiodine scanning. This technique may further be combined with CT or even thyrotropin-stimulated positron emission tomography/CT to identify the anatomic location of disease.[76,77] Again there is now an emphasis on surgical resection of disease when possible while maintaining minimal morbidity to the patient. When disease is not amenable to surgical therapy it is treated with radioidine ablation, with dosing dependent on the degree and organ location of disease burden.[7,78]

SPECIAL CONSIDERATIONS: CHILDREN, FAMILIAL NONMEDULLARY THYROID CANCER, AND PAPILLARY MICROCARCINOMA

Children

Pediatric thyroid cancer accounts for 1% to 2% of malignancies in children and, like that of adult WDTC, is the most common endocrine malignancy.[79,80] SEER data from 1988 to 2000 noted 566 cases of pediatric thyroid carcinoma, with 90% being PTC or follicular variant of PTC, 84% of patients female, and 37% of patients with nodal disease present at diagnosis.[81] Of the histologic subtypes of papillary thyroid cancer, the diffuse sclerosing subtype is more common in young patients, especially children and adolescents, and although the tumor is known for metastasizing early to regional lymph nodes and the lung it has a favorable prognosis.[82] The solid/trabecular variant is found to be more likely to recur than other subtypes.[83] Children with thyroid cancer frequently have cervical and even distant metastasis up to 90% and 25% of the time, respectively, at diagnosis.[84,85] Children do have an overall better prognosis than adults with thyroid cancer, and although children tend to present with larger tumors and more frequent local regional metastasis their 15-year survival is near 100%, underscoring the fact that age is the most important prognosticator in WDTC.[86,87] Because of the very long survival, children are also more likely to have recurrent disease at some point in their lives, and at least one third of pediatric thyroid cancer patients will have recurrence.[88,89]

The authors' approach to pediatric thyroid cancer is much the same as that for adult thyroid cancer. Total thyroidectomy with routine ipsilateral central compartment lymphadenectomy is the operation of choice. Lateral neck dissection is commenced only for physical examination, imaging, or biopsy-verified lateral neck metastasis. This stance is supported by the fact that multivariate analysis clearly shows improved disease-free survival with total thyroidectomy compared with lesser resections, and that children are likely to have locoregional recurrence much the same as adults.[90] Routine unilateral central compartment lymphadenectomy by experienced surgeons is practiced in children with minimal morbidity as it is in adults, minimizes the need for perilous reoperative surgery in the central compartment, and clears the regional nodes most frequently associated with metastasis.[53,91–93] Furthermore, because children are more likely to present with advanced disease and there is an inverse relationship between radioiodine ablative therapy and large volume disease, there is a need to remove as much disease as possible with initial surgery.[94,95] As in adults, the goal of surgery is to remove initial disease using surgery that is tailored to minimizing morbidity while at the same time resecting locoregional disease and minimizing the need for reoperation.

Familial Nonmedullary Thyroid Cancer

Although rare and accounting for less than 5% of cases, familial nonmedullary thyroid cancer (FNMTC) may be diagnosed when 2 first-degree relatives have the disease in the absence of exposure to high-risk radiation or other genetic syndrome.[96,97] FNMTC is mostly always a papillary carcinoma and is present with 95% accuracy when 3 first-degree relatives have thyroid cancer.[98] These patients have a more aggressive local disease compared with those who have nonheritable forms of thyroid cancer; they have a higher rate of multicentric tumors, extrathyroidal invasion, lymph node spread, and higher rates of tumor recurrence.[96,99] It is unclear whether or not patients have a decreased survival compared with nonheritable forms of thyroid cancer, as limited sample sizes and overall good prognosis make statistical prediction difficult. Triponez and colleagues found a decreased disease-free survival in the disease especially in patients who had more than 2 direct relatives, a trend observed by Alsanea and colleagues and Uchino and colleagues as well.[99–101] Given the higher probability of increased local disease burden and higher recurrence rate, the operation of choice is again a total thyroidectomy with routine ipsilateral central compartment lymphadenectomy and indication for lateral neck dissection, guided by preoperative imaging, physical examination, or biopsy.

Papillary Microcarcinoma

Papillary microcarcinoma (PMC) is being increasingly diagnosed, whether by the increased use of cervical ultrasound or by increased pathologic detection, and is reaching epidemic proportions.[102] Papillary microcarcinoma refers to tumors measuring 1 cm or less. The incidence of these tumors is approximately 35% in autopsy series and in general these lesions are not clinically relevant. However, lesions that are symptomatic, show aggressive histology on final pathologic analysis, or are associated with lymphadenopathy must be treated aggressively.

In a recent study from the Mayo Clinic, 900 patients with PMC over a 60-year period were reviewed.[103] Thirty percent had lymph node metastases, 2% had extrathyroidal spread, and 0.3% had distant metastases at the time of diagnosis. The overall survival of patients with PMC did not differ from expected survival of the population such that at 20 years, there was recurrence in regional lymph nodes in 5% and in the thyroid bed in 2%; there was no distant recurrence at 20 years. Overall, the investigators were able to reaffirm the excellent prognosis of PMC. Overall survival is not statistically altered from the general population and 99% of patients are not at risk of distant metastases or cancer-related death, regardless of initial treatment.

As such there is no evidence base for the management of PMC and treatment largely comes down to the philosophical view: if the aim of treatment is to render the patient with no evidence of residual disease and minimize recurrence then total thyroidectomy, central lymph node dissection, and radioactive iodine ablation will be used; however, if the aim of treatment is to minimize intervention and treatment-related morbidity then a more conservative approach can be justified. The ATA guidelines recommend that "thyroid lobectomy alone may be sufficient treatment for small, low-risk, intrathyroidal papillary carcinomas in the absence of cervical metastases" (Level A—recommendation R26). On the other hand, multifocal PMC (≥ 2 tumors), or lymph node metastases are both associated with a recommendation for total thyroidectomy.[2]

SUMMARY

With proper initial surgery planned and performed by experienced thyroid surgeons and follow-up treatment with thyrotropin suppression and radioiodine ablation, patients can now expect to achieve clinical disease-free status. There is, however, a subset of patients who present with advanced disease that must be treated aggressively. There is no accurate method for predicting preoperatively which patient will develop metastatic or recurrent disease. As a result of this an aggressive initial approach, involving total thyroidectomy and routine prophylactic central compartment cervical node dissection, to promote disease-free survival and minimize the need for reoperation in hazardous scarred surgical fields with minimal morbidity to the patient is warranted. Postoperative surveillance with thyroglobulin measurement and neck ultrasound is able to diagnose recurrence before the disease burden becomes excessive. Multidisciplinary care teams are necessary to treat these patients and follow them long term. Interaction within these teams will also form the foundation for translational research efforts to discover the next generation of targeted therapies for thyroid cancer. As such the prognosis will continue to remain good and most patients can expect to be cured of their disease. High-risk patients and those with aggressive disease and worse clinical outcomes with current treatments will have ever more improved outcomes in the future.

REFERENCES

1. Dackiw AP, Zeiger M. Extent of surgery for differentiated thyroid cancer. Surg Clin North Am 2004;84:817–32.
2. Cooper DS, Doherty GM, Haugen BR, et al. Management guidelines for patients with thyroid nodules and differentiated thyroid cancer. Thyroid 2006;16:109–42.
3. Shah MD, Hall FT, Eski SJ, et al. Clinical course of thyroid carcinoma after neck dissection. Laryngoscope 2003;113:2102–7.
4. Lundgren CI, Hall P, Dickman PW, et al. Clinically significant prognostic factors for differentiated thyroid carcinoma: a population-based, nested case-control study. Cancer 2006;106:524–31.
5. Sywak M, Cornford L, Roach P, et al. Routine ipsilateral level VI lymphadenectomy reduces postoperative thyroglobulin levels in papillary thyroid cancer. Surgery 2006;140:1000–5 [discussion: 1005–7].
6. Pacini F, Molinaro E, Castagna MG, et al. Recombinant human thyrotropin-stimulated serum thyroglobulin combined with neck ultrasonography has the highest sensitivity in monitoring differentiated thyroid carcinoma. J Clin Endocrinol Metab 2003;88:3668–73.
7. Mazzaferri EL. Practical management of thyroid cancer: a multidisciplinary approach. London: Springer: 2006.
8. Horner MJ, Ries LAG, Krapcho M, et al, editors. SEER Cancer Statistics Review, 1975–2006, National Cancer Institute. Bethesda (MD). Available at: http://seer.cancer.gov/csr/1975_2006/, based on November 2008 SEER data submission, posted to the SEER web site, 2009.
9. Mitchell I, Livingston EH, Chang AY, et al. Trends in thyroid cancer demographics and surgical therapy in the United States. Surgery 2007;142:823–8 [discussion: 828 e821].
10. Davies L, Welch HG. Increasing incidence of thyroid cancer in the United States, 1973–2002. JAMA 2006;295:2164–7.
11. Burgess JR, Tucker P. Incidence trends for papillary thyroid carcinoma and their correlation with thyroid surgery and thyroid fine-needle aspirate cytology. Thyroid 2006;16:47–53.
12. Grodski S, Brown T, Sidhu S, et al. Increasing incidence of thyroid cancer is due to increased pathologic detection. Surgery 2008;144:1038–43 [discussion: 1043].
13. Leenhardt L, Grosclaude P, Cherie-Challine L. Increased incidence of thyroid carcinoma in france: a true epidemic or thyroid nodule management effects? Report from the French Thyroid Cancer Committee. Thyroid 2004;14:1056–60.
14. Nagar S, Morgan WF. The death-inducing effect and genomic instability. Radiat Res 2005;163:316–23.
15. Snyder AR, Morgan WF. Lack of consensus gene expression changes associated with radiation-induced chromosomal instability. DNA Repair (Amst) 2005;4:958–70.
16. Schneider AB, Sarne DH. Long-term risks for thyroid cancer and other neoplasms after exposure to radiation. Nat Clin Pract Endocrinol Metab 2005;1:82–91.
17. Acharya S, Sarafoglou K, LaQuaglia M, et al. Thyroid neoplasms after therapeutic radiation for malignancies during childhood or adolescence. Cancer 2003;97:2397–403.

18. Mihailescu DV, Schneider AB. Size, number, and distribution of thyroid nodules and the risk of malignancy in radiation-exposed patients who underwent surgery. J Clin Endocrinol Metab 2008;93:2188–93.
19. McCoy KL, Jabbour N, Ogilvie JB, et al. The incidence of cancer and rate of false-negative cytology in thyroid nodules greater than or equal to 4 cm in size. Surgery 2007;142:837–44 [discussion 844, e831–33].
20. Li JJ, Weroha SJ, Lingle WL, et al. Estrogen mediates Aurora-A overexpression, centrosome amplification, chromosomal instability, and breast cancer in female ACI rats. Proc Natl Acad Sci U S A 2004;101:18123–8.
21. Harach HR, Escalante DA, Day ES. Thyroid cancer and thyroiditis in Salta, Argentina: a 40-yr study in relation to iodine prophylaxis. Endocr Pathol 2002; 13:175–81.
22. Hemminki K, Eng C, Chen B. Familial risks for nonmedullary thyroid cancer. J Clin Endocrinol Metab 2005;90:5747–53.
23. Wreesmann VB, Singh B. Clinical impact of molecular analysis on thyroid cancer management. Surg Oncol Clin N Am 2008;17:1–35, vii.
24. Kondo T, Ezzat S, Asa SL. Pathogenetic mechanisms in thyroid follicular-cell neoplasia. Nat Rev Cancer 2006;6:292–306.
25. Nikiforov YE, Rowland JM, Bove KE, et al. Distinct pattern of ret oncogene rearrangements in morphological variants of radiation-induced and sporadic thyroid papillary carcinomas in children. Cancer Res 1997;57:1690–4.
26. Viglietto G, Chiappetta G, Martinez-Tello FJ, et al. RET/PTC oncogene activation is an early event in thyroid carcinogenesis. Oncogene 1995;11:1207–10.
27. Davies H, Bignell GR, Cox C, et al. Mutations of the BRAF gene in human cancer. Nature 2002;417:949–54.
28. Nikiforova MN, Kimura ET, Gandhi M, et al. BRAF mutations in thyroid tumors are restricted to papillary carcinomas and anaplastic or poorly differentiated carcinomas arising from papillary carcinomas. J Clin Endocrinol Metab 2003;88: 5399–404.
29. Quiros RM, Ding HG, Gattuso P, et al. Evidence that one subset of anaplastic thyroid carcinomas are derived from papillary carcinomas due to BRAF and p53 mutations. Cancer 2005;103:2261–8.
30. Cheung L, Messina M, Gill A, et al. Detection of the PAX8-PPAR gamma fusion oncogene in both follicular thyroid carcinomas and adenomas. J Clin Endocrinol Metab 2003;88:354–7.
31. Nikiforova MN, Lynch RA, Biddinger PW, et al. RAS point mutations and PAX8-PPAR gamma rearrangement in thyroid tumors: evidence for distinct molecular pathways in thyroid follicular carcinoma. J Clin Endocrinol Metab 2003;88: 2318–26.
32. Cobin RH, Gharib H, Bergman DA, et al. Thyroid Carcinoma Task Force. AACE/AES AACE/AAES medical/surgical guidelines for clinical practice: management of thyroid carcinoma. American Association of Clinical Endocrinologists. American College of Endocrinology. Endocr Pract 2001;7:202–20.
33. Pacini F, Schlumberger M, Dralle H, et al. European consensus for the management of patients with differentiated thyroid carcinoma of the follicular epithelium. Eur J Endocrinol 2006;154:787–803.
34. Hegedus L. Clinical practice. The thyroid nodule. N Engl J Med 2004;351: 1764–71.
35. Morris LF, Ragavendra N, Yeh MW. Evidence-based assessment of the role of ultrasonography in the management of benign thyroid nodules. World J Surg 2008;32:1253–63.

36. Lundgren CI, Zedenius J, Skoog L. Fines benign thyroid nodules: an evidence-based review. World J Surg 2008;32:1247–52.
37. Baloch ZW, LiVolsi VA, Asa SL, et al. Diagnostic terminology and morphologic criteria for cytologic diagnosis of thyroid lesions: a synopsis of the National Cancer Institute Thyroid Fine-Needle Aspiration State of the Science Conference. Diagn Cytopathol 2008;36:425–37.
38. Delbridge L. Solitary thyroid nodule: current management. ANZ J Surg 2006;76:381–6.
39. Kouvaraki MA, Shapiro SE, Fornage BD, et al. Role of preoperative ultrasonography in the surgical management of patients with thyroid cancer. Surgery 2003;134:946–54 [discussion: 954–945].
40. Shaha AR. Routine laryngoscopy in thyroid surgery: a valuable adjunct. Surgery 2007;142:865–6.
41. Byar DP, Green SB, Dor P, et al. A prognostic index for thyroid carcinoma. A study of the E.O.R.T.C. Thyroid Cancer Cooperative Group. Eur J Cancer 1979;15:1033–41.
42. Cady B, Rossi R. An expanded view of risk-group definition in differentiated thyroid carcinoma. Surgery 1988;104:947–53.
43. Greene FL, Page DL, Fleming ID, et al, editors. AJCC cancer staging manual. 6th edition. New York: Springer-Verlag; 2002. p. 77–87.
44. Hay ID, Bergstralh EJ, Goellner JR, et al. Predicting outcome in papillary thyroid carcinoma: development of a reliable prognostic scoring system in a cohort of 1779 patients surgically treated at one institution during 1940 through 1989. Surgery 1993;114:1050–7 [discussion: 1057–58].
45. Hay ID, Grant CS, Taylor WF, et al. Ipsilateral lobectomy versus bilateral lobar resection in papillary thyroid carcinoma: a retrospective analysis of surgical outcome using a novel prognostic scoring system. Surgery 1987;102:1088–95.
46. DeLellis RA, et al. Pathology and genetics of tumours of endocrine organs. Lyon, France: IARC Press; 2004. p. 320.
47. LiVolsi VA. Unusual variants of papillary thyroid carcinoma. Adv Endocrinol Metab 1995;6:39–54.
48. Lin HS, Komisar A, Opher E, et al. Follicular variant of papillary carcinoma: the diagnostic limitations of preoperative fine-needle aspiration and intraoperative frozen section evaluation. Laryngoscope 2000;110:1431–6.
49. Baloch ZW, LiVolsi VA. Our approach to follicular-patterned lesions of the thyroid. J Clin Pathol 2007;60:244–50.
50. Bilimoria KY, Bentrem DJ, Ko CY, et al. Extent of surgery affects survival for papillary thyroid cancer. Ann Surg 2007;246:375–81 [discussion: 381–374].
51. Hay ID, Grant CS, Bergstralh EJ, et al. Unilateral total lobectomy: is it sufficient surgical treatment for patients with AMES low-risk papillary thyroid carcinoma? Surgery 1998;124:958–64 [discussion: 964–956].
52. Mazzaferri EL. Treating differentiated thyroid carcinoma: where do we draw the line? Mayo Clin Proc 1991;66:105–11.
53. Mazzaferri EL, Jhiang SM. Long-term impact of initial surgical and medical therapy on papillary and follicular thyroid cancer. Am J Med 1994;97:418–28.
54. Massin JP, Savoie JC, Garnier H, et al. Pulmonary metastases in differentiated thyroid carcinoma. Study of 58 cases with implications for the primary tumor treatment. Cancer 1984;53:982–92.
55. DeGroot LJ, Kaplan EL, Straus FH, et al. Does the method of management of papillary thyroid carcinoma make a difference in outcome? World J Surg 1994;18:123–30.

56. Mazzaferri EL, Kloos RT. Clinical review 128: current approaches to primary therapy for papillary and follicular thyroid cancer. J Clin Endocrinol Metab 2001;86:1447–63.
57. Grubbs EG, Evans DB. Role of lymph node dissection in primary surgery for thyroid cancer. J Natl Compr Canc Netw 2007;5:623–30.
58. Doherty GM. Routine central neck lymph node dissection for thyroid carcinoma. Surgery 2006;140:1007–8.
59. Moley JF, Wells SA. Compartment-mediated dissection for papillary thyroid cancer. Langenbecks Arch Surg 1999;384:9–15.
60. Alvarado R, Sywak MS, Delbridge LW, et al. Central lymph node dissection as a secondary procedure for papillary thyroid cancer: is there added morbidity? Surgery 2009;145(5):514–8.
61. Robbins KT, Shaha AR, Medina JE, et al. Consensus statement on the classification and terminology of neck dissection. Arch Otolaryngol Head Neck Surg 2008;134:536–8.
62. Segal K, Friedental R, Lubin E, et al. Papillary carcinoma of the thyroid. Otolaryngol Head Neck Surg 1995;113:356–63.
63. Simon D, Goretzki PE, Witte J, et al. Incidence of regional recurrence guiding radicality in differentiated thyroid carcinoma. World J Surg 1996;20:860–6 [discussion: 866].
64. White ML, Gauger PG, Doherty GM. Central lymph node dissection in differentiated thyroid cancer. World J Surg 2007;31:895–904.
65. Low TH, Delbridge L, Sidhu S, et al. Lymph node status influences follow-up thyroglobulin levels in papillary thyroid cancer. Ann Surg Oncol 2008;15: 2827–32.
66. Tisell LE, Nilsson B, Molne J, et al. Improved survival of patients with papillary thyroid cancer after surgical microdissection. World J Surg 1996;20:854–9.
67. Lundgren CI, Hall P, Dickman PW, et al. Influence of surgical and postoperative treatment on survival in differentiated thyroid cancer. Br J Surg 2007;94:571–7.
68. Delbridge L, Parkyn R, Philips J, et al. Minimally invasive follicular thyroid carcinoma: completion thyroidectomy or not? ANZ J Surg 2002;72:844–5.
69. van Heerden JA, Hay ID, Goellner JR, et al. Follicular thyroid carcinoma with capsular invasion alone: a nonthreatening malignancy. Surgery 1992;112: 1130–6 [discussion: 1136–38].
70. D'Avanzo A, Treseler P, Ituarte PH, et al. Follicular thyroid carcinoma: histology and prognosis. Cancer 2004;100:1123–9.
71. Grebe SK, Hay ID. Follicular thyroid cancer. Endocrinol Metab Clin North Am 1995;24:761–801.
72. Hundahl SA, Fleming ID, Fremgen AM, et al. National Cancer Data Base report on 53,856 cases of thyroid carcinoma treated in the U.S., 1985–1995 [comments]. Cancer 1998;83:2638–48.
73. Herrera MF, Hay ID, Wu PS, et al. Hurthle cell (oxyphilic) papillary thyroid carcinoma: a variant with more aggressive biologic behavior. World J Surg 1992;16: 669–74 [discussion: 774–665].
74. Lopez-Penabad L, Chiu AC, Hoff AO, et al. Prognostic factors in patients with Hurthle cell neoplasms of the thyroid. Cancer 2003;97:1186–94.
75. Brierley JD, Tsang RW. External beam radiation therapy for thyroid cancer. Endocrinol Metab Clin North Am 2008;37:497–509, xi.
76. Palmedo H, Bucerius J, Joe A, et al. Integrated PET/CT in differentiated thyroid cancer: diagnostic accuracy and impact on patient management. J Nucl Med 2006;47:616–24.

77. Zoller M, Kohlfuerst S, Igerc I, et al. Combined PET/CT in the follow-up of differentiated thyroid carcinoma: what is the impact of each modality? Eur J Nucl Med Mol Imaging 2007;34:487–95.
78. Van Nostrand D, Atkins F, Yeganeh F, et al. Dosimetrically determined doses of radioiodine for the treatment of metastatic thyroid carcinoma. Thyroid 2002;12: 121–34.
79. Kuhel WI, Ward RF. Thyroid cancer in children. Lancet 1995;346:719–20.
80. Miller RW, Young JL Jr, Novakovic B. Childhood cancer. Cancer 1995;75:395–405.
81. Shapiro NL, Bhattacharyya N. Population-based outcomes for pediatric thyroid carcinoma. Laryngoscope 2005;115:337–40.
82. Carcangiu ML, Bianchi S. Diffuse sclerosing variant of papillary thyroid carcinoma. Clinicopathologic study of 15 cases. Am J Surg Pathol 1989;13:1041–9.
83. Collini P, Mattavelli F, Pellegrinelli A, et al. Papillary carcinoma of the thyroid gland of childhood and adolescence: morphologic subtypes, biologic behavior and prognosis: a clinicopathologic study of 42 sporadic cases treated at a single institution during a 30-year period. Am J Surg Pathol 2006;30:1420–6.
84. Brink JS, van Heerden JA, McIver B, et al. Papillary thyroid cancer with pulmonary metastases in children: long-term prognosis. Surgery 2000;128:881–6 [discussion: 886–7].
85. Newman KD, Black T, Heller G, et al. Differentiated thyroid cancer: determinants of disease progression in patients <21 years of age at diagnosis: a report from the Surgical Discipline Committee of the Children's Cancer Group. Ann Surg 1998;227:533–41.
86. Collini P, Massimino M, Leite SF, et al. Papillary thyroid carcinoma of childhood and adolescence: a 30-year experience at the Istituto Nazionale Tumori in Milan. Pediatr Blood Cancer 2006;46:300–6.
87. Miccoli P, Minuto MN, Ugolini C, et al. Papillary thyroid cancer: pathological parameters as prognostic factors in different classes of age. Otolaryngol Head Neck Surg 2008;138:200–3.
88. Spinelli C, Bertocchini A, Antonelli A, et al. Surgical therapy of the thyroid papillary carcinoma in children: experience with 56 patients < or = 16 years old. J Pediatr Surg 2004;39:1500–5.
89. Robie DK, Dinauer CW, Tuttle RM, et al. The impact of initial surgical management on outcome in young patients with differentiated thyroid cancer. J Pediatr Surg 1998;33:1134–8 [discussion: 1139–40].
90. Jarzab B, Handkiewicz Junak D, Wloch J, et al. Multivariate analysis of prognostic factors for differentiated thyroid carcinoma in children. Eur J Nucl Med 2000;27:833–41.
91. Harwood J, Clark OH, Dunphy JE. Significance of lymph node metastasis in differentiated thyroid cancer. Am J Surg 1978;136:107–12.
92. Goretzki PE, Simon D, Frilling A, et al. Surgical reintervention for differentiated thyroid cancer. Br J Surg 1993;80:1009–12.
93. Savio R, Gosnell J, Palazzo FF, et al. The role of a more extensive surgical approach in the initial multimodality management of papillary thyroid cancer in children. J Pediatr Surg 2005;40:1696–700.
94. Bal CS, Kumar A, Pant GS. Radioiodine dose for remnant ablation in differentiated thyroid carcinoma: a randomized clinical trial in 509 patients. J Clin Endocrinol Metab 2004;89:1666–73.
95. Rosario PW, Maia FF, Cardoso LD, et al. Correlation between cervical uptake and results of postsurgical radioiodine ablation in patients with thyroid carcinoma. Clin Nucl Med 2004;29:358–61.

96. Lupoli G, Vitale G, Caraglia M, et al. Familial papillary thyroid microcarcinoma: a new clinical entity. Lancet 1999;353:637–9.
97. Sturgeon C, Clark OH. Familial nonmedullary thyroid cancer. Thyroid 2005;15: 588–93.
98. Kebebew E. Hereditary non-medullary thyroid cancer. World J Surg 2008;32: 678–82.
99. Uchino S, Noguchi S, Kawamoto H, et al. Familial nonmedullary thyroid carcinoma characterized by multifocality and a high recurrence rate in a large study population. World J Surg 2002;26:897–902.
100. Alsanea O, Wada N, Ain K, et al. Is familial non-medullary thyroid carcinoma more aggressive than sporadic thyroid cancer? A multicenter series. Surgery 2000;128:1043–50 [discussion: 1050–1041].
101. Triponez F, Wong M, Sturgeon C, et al. Does familial non-medullary thyroid cancer adversely affect survival? World J Surg 2006;30:787–93.
102. Grodski S, Delbridge L. An update on papillary microcarcinoma. Curr Opin Oncol 2009;21:1–4.
103. Hay ID, Hutchinson ME, Gonzalez-Losada T, et al. Papillary thyroid microcarcinoma: a study of 900 cases observed in a 60-year period. Surgery 2008;144: 980–7 [discussion: 987–8].

Sporadic and Familial Medullary Thyroid Carcinoma: State of the Art

Tricia A. Moo-Young, MD[a], Amber L. Traugott, MD[a],
Jeffrey F. Moley, MD[a,b],*

KEYWORDS

- Medullary thyroid cancer • RET tyrosine kinase • Sporadic
- Multiple endocrine neoplasia • Preventative surgery

Medullary thyroid carcinoma (MTC) comprises 5% to 10% of all thyroid cancers. Most cases are sporadic (75%); however, the proportion of patients with MTC with a familial predisposition syndrome is the highest of any hereditary cancer syndrome (approximately 25%), and this possibility should be considered when evaluating any patient with MTC. The familial syndromes include multiple endocrine neoplasia (MEN) 2A, MEN 2B, and familial non-MEN MTC (FMTC). Familial MTC syndromes affect about 1 in 30,000 individuals. MTC develops from the calcitonin-producing parafollicular or C cells. These cells are neuroectodermal in origin and thus belong to the amine precursor uptake decarboxylation cell family. C cells make up only about 1% of the thyroid cell mass and are primarily concentrated in the posterior upper third of the gland.[1] Histologically, MTC is characterized by a solid mass of cells with uniform polygonal shapes and finely granular eosinophilic cytoplasm.[2] Pathologists have described the presence of amyloid deposition as being pathognomonic for MTC, being found in one-third of MTC cases. In 2004, Khurana and colleagues[1] reported that the sole constituent of these amyloid deposits is full-length calcitonin. C-cell hyperplasia may be a precursor to MTC, and it is most commonly seen in familial forms of MTC.[3]

MEN 2A is the most common subtype of familial MTC (80% of hereditary MTC cases). These patients develop multifocal bilateral MTC (nearly 100% penetrance), pheochromocytoma (42% penetrance), and hyperparathyroidism (10%–30% penetrance).[4] Features that are rarer in MEN 2A are cutaneous lichen planus amyloidosis

[a] Department of Surgery, Washington University School of Medicine, 660 South Euclid Avenue, Box 8109, St Louis, MO 63110, USA
[b] St Louis Veterans Administration Medical Center, St Louis, MO, USA
* Corresponding author. Endocrine and Oncologic Surgery, Washington University School of Medicine, 660 South Euclid Avenue, Box 8109, St Louis, MO 63110.
E-mail address: moleyj@wustl.edu (J.F. Moley).

Surg Clin N Am 89 (2009) 1193–1204
doi:10.1016/j.suc.2009.06.021
0039-6109/09/$ – see front matter © 2009 Published by Elsevier Inc.

surgical.theclinics.com

and Hirschsprung disease. MEN2B patients develop MTC (very early onset, also with 100% penetrance) and pheochromocytoma (40% penetrance) but do not have hyper-parathyroidism. These patients also have multiple mucosal neuromas (often visible on the eyelids and lips), ganglioneuromatosis of the gastrointestinal tract, and megacolon (**Fig. 1**). FMTC represents a clinical variant of MEN 2A in which MTC is the only clinical feature.[5] Controversy exists around what familial pattern of inheritance classifies a patient as FMTC versus MEN 2A. The strictest clinical criteria require that the FMTC proband has more than 10 carriers of MTC in the kindred with multiple members older than 50 years, none of whom have been diagnosed with hyperparathyroidism or pheochromocytoma.[6] A less rigid definition characterizes FMTC patients as having at least 4 affected family members with MTC alone.[7] Caution should be exercised in any patient given the diagnosis of FMTC because misclassification of MEN 2A as FMTC may result in failure to screen for pheochromocytoma and hyperparathyroidism.

CLINICAL PRESENTATION AND DIAGNOSIS

Presymptomatic preventative surgery for young patients with familial MTC syndromes is discussed later in this article. In patients who did not undergo preventative surgery, familial MTC usually presents with multifocal bilateral disease. Patients with sporadic MTC (sMTC) more commonly have unifocal tumors, later age of onset, and absence of C cell hyperplasia. Every patient presenting with newly diagnosed MTC should be counseled about the possibility of familial disease and offered genetic testing. Patients with MTC should have a full family history taken at the time of initial consultation, with attention given to thyroid and parathyroid disease, adrenal tumors, hypertension,

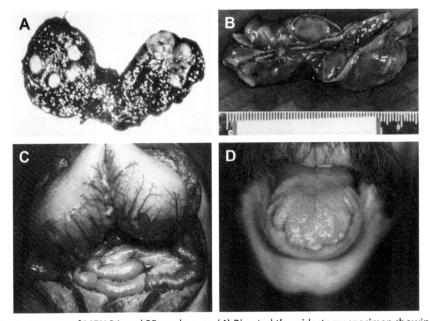

Fig. 1. Features of MEN 2A and 2B syndromes. (*A*) Bisected thyroidectomy specimen showing multifocal, bilateral MTC tumors. (*B*) Adrenalectomy specimen showing pheochromocytoma. (*C*) Megacolon in patient with MEN 2B. (*D*) Tongue nodules in patient with MEN 2B. (*Courtesy of* S.A. Wells [photograph A] and R. Thompson [photographs B, C, and D]. *From* Moley JF. Medullary thyroid cancer. In: Clark OH, Duh Q-Y, editors. Textbook of Endocrine Surgery. Philadelphia: WB Saunders Co; 1997; with permission.)

Hirschsprung disease, and sudden unexplained deaths. Physical examination should take note of the size of palpable neck nodules, fixation to surrounding structures, and the presence of cervical lymphadenopathy. Characteristic features of MEN 2B phenotype, such as tongue nodules, should also be noted. Symptoms of extensive local disease include dysphagia, hoarseness, dyspnea, stridor, and coughing. Direct examination of the vocal cords before surgical intervention may reveal vocal cord paralysis, indicating involvement of the recurrent laryngeal nerve. Patients presenting with elevated levels of calcitonin may exhibit diarrhea as the initial symptom of their disease.

The dominant nodule should be evaluated first for calcitonin, with fine needle aspiration (FNA) aided by immunocytochemical staining. In one study, FNA was successful in diagnosing MTC in more than 80% of patients. In the remaining patients, the pathologic diagnosis was not apparent until the surgical specimen was evaluated histologically.[8]

Serum calcitonin measurement is a sensitive marker for MTC. It is useful in screening at-risk individuals and in monitoring previously treated patients for disease recurrence. Cost analysis in Europe has suggested that routine calcitonin screening in patients undergoing evaluation for thyroid nodules is cost effective; however, this practice has not gained widespread acceptance in the United States.[9] In a screening setting, a basal serum calcitonin level exceeding 20 pg/mL warrants further investigation to rule out MTC. A mildly elevated serum calcitonin level can occur in C-cell hyperplasia, autoimmune thyroiditis, chronic renal failure, and advanced age, and it can be due to variation among commercial assays. Calcitonin may be measured either in a basal state or after stimulation by the secretagogues calcium and pentagastrin. Pentagastrin is no longer available commercially, and basal measurement is commonly followed using highly sensitive commercial assays.

Preoperative evaluation of patients with known or suspected MTC should include measurement of serum calcitonin, carcinogenic embryonic antigen (CEA), and serum calcium and *RET* proto-oncogene analysis. Biochemical screening for pheochromocytoma (plasma metanephrines or 24-hour urine catecholamines) should be conducted for any patient with MTC who is older than 10 years. Preoperative imaging may include a neck ultrasound with lymph node mapping of the cervical nodal compartments (**Fig. 2**). The sensitivity of intraoperative palpation by an experienced surgeon to detect lymph node metastases is only 64%.[10] In patients presenting with a palpable thyroid nodule, cervical lymph node metastases are common (>75%), with 10% to 15% of these patients also having evidence of distant metastases.[10] MTC most commonly metastasizes to the bones, liver, and lungs. Detection of distant disease begins with computed tomography (CT) of neck, chest, and abdomen. CT is the most sensitive test to detect lung and mediastinal lymph node metastases.[11] Contrast-enhanced magnetic resonance imaging (MRI) is most sensitive for the detection of liver metastases, and bone metastases are seen best on either axial MRI or bone scan. In one series, CT has been found to be superior to 2-deoxy-2-[18F]fluoro-D-glucose (FDG) positron emission tomography (PET) for lung, liver, and bone metastases.[12] However, FDG-PET was more sensitive than CT in detecting neck and mediastinal disease. Imaging to identify distant disease is not indicated in every patient with MTC. Imaging is most likely to detect metastatic disease in patients with a basal serum calcitonin level greater than 400 pg/mL.[13]

SURGICAL APPROACH TO MTC: CLINICALLY EVIDENT, FAMILIAL, AND SPORADIC

Differences in survival exist between patients who achieve complete remission, those with biochemical persistent disease, and those with evidence of distant metastatic disease.[14] Patients with MTC who present with clinically apparent disease (palpable

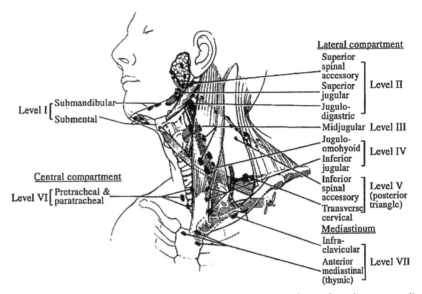

Fig. 2. Anatomic landmarks and lymph node compartments in the neck and upper medias-tinum encountered in surgical reinterventions in medullary thyroid carcinoma. The central compartment is delimited inferiorly by the innominate vein, superiorly by the hyoid bone, laterally by the carotid sheaths, and dorsally by the prevertebral fascia. It comprises lymphatic and soft tissues around the esophagus as well as pretracheal and paratracheal lymph nodes that drain the thyroid bed (level 6). The submandibular nodal group (level 1) is subsumed in the central compartment by some classifications. The lateral compartments span the area between the carotid sheath, the sternocleidomastoid muscle, and the trape-zius muscle. The inferior border is defined by the subclavian vein, and the hypoglossal nerve determines the superior boundary. The lymph node chain adjacent to the jugular vein is divided cranially to caudally in superior jugular nodes (level 2), midjugular nodes (level 3), and inferior jugular nodes (level 4). Lymph nodes situated in the posterior triangle between the dorsolateral sternocleidomastoid muscle, the trapezius muscle, and the subcla-vian vein are classified as level 5 nodes. Mediastinal lymphatic tissue is referred to as level 7 lymph nodes. (*From* Musholt TJ, Moley JF. Management of persistent or recurrent medullary thyroid carcinoma. Prob Gen Surg 1997;14:89–109; with permission.)

mass) are at significant risk of having regional lymph node metastases. At the authors' institution, more than 75% of patients presenting with palpable MTC, hereditary or sporadic, have central cervical lymph node metastases (level 6 nodes), with a similar rate of spread to the ipsilateral lateral neck nodes (levels 2–4), and a 47% rate of involvement of contralateral level 2 to 4 nodes.[10] At a minimum, patients with palpable MTC should undergo total thyroidectomy with central lymph node dissection and unilateral dissection of level 2 to 5 nodes. Ultrasound evaluation of cervical nodes should be done before surgery and is useful in determining whether a contralateral level 2 to 4 dissection is also necessary. Ultrasound evaluation of central and low level 4 nodes may be limited in patients who have short necks or who are unable to extend their neck.

Preoperative calcitonin level should always be obtained. Asymptomatic adult or younger patients, with positive *RET* mutation screening, should have a thyroidectomy and central lymph node dissection (level 6) if the preoperative calcitonin level is elevated (>40 pg/mL). Preoperative ultrasonographic evaluation of neck nodes should be done if calcitonin is elevated, and suspicious nodes should be marked and removed at operation. Patients with codon 634 (level 2) mutations have an increasing risk of lymph node metastasis beginning in the mid-teens, with more than 40% cumulative risk by the age of 20 years.[15] The surgical approach in older RET mutation carriers should be individualized based on calcitonin level, presence of palpable disease, imaging results, RET mutation, and family history.

The likelihood of ipsilateral lateral compartment lymph node involvement (levels 2–4) is related to the presence and extent of nodal disease in the central compartment. In one study, the presence of 0, 1 to 3, or more than 4 central lymph node metastases was correlated with 10.1%, 77%, and 98% risk of metastatic involvement of ipsilateral level 2 to 4 nodes, respectively. For contralateral lateral compartment involvement, the rates were 4.9%, 28%, and 77% with no central lymph node metastases, 1 to 9, and 10 or more, respectively.[16] Thus, in patients with preoperative imaging suggesting central lymph node metastases, serious consideration should be given to doing at least an ipsilateral level 2 to 4 compartment lymph node dissection.

Preservation of parathyroid function in these operations should be a major concern of the surgeon, and expertise in identification and preservation of the glands is essential for optimal outcomes. If a central lymph node dissection is performed, the lower parathyroid glands must be removed and autotransplanted because they are intimately associated with level 6 nodes. It is often possible to preserve one or both upper glands on an intact vascular pedicle, but if it is not possible, they should also be removed and transplanted. Normal parathyroid glands should not be discarded with the specimen, and an effort should be made to leave all normal parathyroid tissue in the patient. MEN 2A patients with primary hyperparathyroidism should undergo either total parathyroidectomy with autotransplantation or subtotal parathyroidectomy, leaving enough viable parathyroid tissue in situ to prevent hypoparathyroidism. For MEN2A patients, the forearm is an excellent autotransplantation site (because of the risk of later graft-dependent hyperparathyroidism), whereas the sternocleidomastoid muscle is usually used for MEN 2B and FMTC patients.

In patients with clinically apparent, palpable sMTC, total thyroidectomy, with compartment-oriented neck dissection, results in long-term local control in most cases and biochemical cure of the disease in about 50% of cases (**Fig. 3**).[17] At present, a rational approach to the surgical management of sMTC should take into account the clinical evidence, the serum calcitonin level, and the preoperative ultrasound evaluation for lymph node metastases. Two reports from a center in Japan

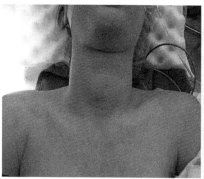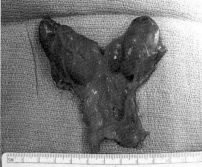

Fig. 3. Total thyroidectomy and central neck dissection in a MEN 2A patient with palpable MTC. (Photos by author.)

described a unilateral approach to some patients with sMTC. In these reports, a small number of patients were treated with lobectomy and unilateral node dissection alone, with good reported biochemical cure rates and no recurrence in the remaining lobe.[18] The authors have found this approach to be useful in palliative situations (bulky unilateral neck disease with distant metastases).

POSTOPERATIVE SURVEILLANCE

A preoperative calcitonin level serves as a marker of disease burden, and postsurgical reduction of basal levels indicates success in eradicating the tumor. Calcitonin levels usually stabilize by 72 hours after surgery but may continue to decrease thereafter. Postoperative surveillance is necessary to monitor for persistent or recurrent disease. Patients with mildly elevated (<150 pg/mL) but stable serum calcitonin levels after adequate primary surgery should be kept under observation. New calcitonin elevation, rapid calcitonin doubling time, or onset of palpable disease should prompt a metastatic workup. Workup for detection of local disease should start with a neck ultrasound. FNA of any suspicious masses may confirm the diagnosis. Evaluation for distant disease should include CT of the neck, chest, and abdomen. FDG-PET imaging may also be helpful in detecting recurrence. Many patients with persistently high levels of calcitonin following surgery will do well for years without radiographic or clinical evidence of disease recurrence.

MANAGEMENT OF PERSISTENT OR RECURRENT DISEASE
Surgical Therapy

Reoperation is usually reserved for patients with elevated calcitonin levels in the setting of inadequate initial operation, imaging evidence of recurrent or persistent disease, and threat of compression or invasion of the trachea and major vessels. In experienced hands, reoperative surgery for locoregional disease can achieve a long-term biochemical cure in up to one-third of patients.[19] Before proceeding with neck reoperation with curative intent, a metastatic workup is necessary to evaluate the lungs, liver, and bones. Patients who have systemic symptoms of the metastatic tumor burden (ie, pain, flushing, and diarrhea) may benefit from a palliative tumor debulking procedure.

Re-exploration of the neck carries a higher risk of complications, including thoracic duct leak, injury to a recurrent laryngeal nerve, and hypoparathyroidism. Central neck reoperations in children are especially dangerous because of the small size of the parathyroid glands and should be avoided unless absolutely necessary. Redo central neck dissection may be facilitated by a "back-door" or lateral approach, where the strap muscles are mobilized laterally off the carotid, and the space between the carotid and the trachea is entered through a previously unoperated tissue plane.[20] The recurrent laryngeal nerve and parathyroid glands may then be identified and preserved. Lateral neck dissections (levels 2–5) are performed as necessary, based on preoperative ultrasound and surgical palpation (**Fig. 4**).

Radiation Therapy

Radioactive iodine ablation has not been shown to be beneficial in MTC, probably because the tumor cells do not take up iodine. A "bystander effect" has been suggested for radioactive iodine treatment of small intrathyroidal tumors, but this has only been reported anecdotally. Currently published studies investigating the role of external beam radiation therapy (EBRT) in MTC have been retrospective series using small patient cohorts. The benefit of EBRT in MTC thus remains controversial. Based

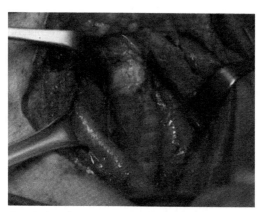

Fig. 4. Photograph of central neck compartment after redo central neck dissection for persistent medullary thyroid carcinoma. Thyroid and central neck lymph nodes have been removed; parathyroids were removed and autotransplanted. (Photo by author.)

on these studies, patients most likely to benefit from postoperative EBRT are those whose pathology demonstrates "high-risk features" such as microscopic residual disease, extraglandular invasion, or lymph node involvement. In the study by Brierley and colleagues,[21] 46 of 73 patients underwent EBRT at a median dose of 40 Gy. Overall, there was no benefit shown for those receiving EBRT. Subgroup analysis of 40 patients with "high-risk features," however, showed a higher local/regional relapse-free rate in irradiated patients compared with nonirradiated ones. Unlike the surgical series, however, none of these studies showed that EBRT reduced calcitonin levels in any patient with MTC. The added disadvantage of EBRT is its effect on tissues (ie, radiation-induced scarring and fibrosis), which makes subsequent surgical intervention more difficult and risky.

Systemic Therapy

The use of immunotherapeutic antibody-based treatments targeted at CEA in selected patients with MTC showed limited promise in clinical trials. A single study using the humanized anti-CEA monoclonal antibody labetuzumab showed significant inhibition of MTC tumor growth in vivo, but in a phase I trial using labetuzumab, there was only limited benefit in patients with advanced MTC.[22] The authors suggested that the lack of a significant treatment response could be related to the relationship between pharmacokinetics and tumor burden, suggesting that the drug was likely to be more successful in patients with early-stage disease.

Previous clinical response rates for chemotherapy in patients with locally advanced or metastatic MTC have been disappointing. The understanding of MTC molecular oncogenesis, however, has resulted in identification of novel molecular targets for treatment. Most current targeted molecular therapies fall under the classification of tyrosine kinase inhibitors (TKIs).[23] Vandetanib (ZD6474, Zactima) is a novel anilinoquinazoline compound engineered to selectively inhibit vascular endothelial growth factor receptor, endothelial growth factor receptor, and RET tyrosine kinases.[24] Several multi-institutional phase II trials are ongoing for MTC patients with unresectable, measurable, and locally advanced MTC. Results have been encouraging but have not been published as of this writing.

Sorafenib (BAY 43-9006) is an orally formulated TKI that selectivity targets RET.[25,26] In the United States, the drug is approved by the Food and Drug Administration (FDA) for the treatment of advanced renal cell cancer and unresectable hepatocellular cancer. Its efficacy in MTC has only been tested in very small pilot studies.[27] The results are promising, with 2 patients exhibiting a response, one of whom had a complete response after just 6 months of treatment. A larger phase II trial is currently under way.

In a phase II trial using sunitinib (SU11248), treatment was associated with disease stabilization in 5 of 6 patients with MTC.[26] The chemotherapeutic agent 17-allylamino-geldanamycin acts as a heat shock protein and a TKI. In vivo, it has been shown to have specific activity against RET protein and MTC cell lines.[23] This drug is currently being tested in patients with advanced medullary and differentiated thyroid carcinomas. Many of these newer targeted therapies have a cytostatic effect on tumor progression, with no complete, durable responses as yet. In the future, new agents and combinatorial therapy will be evaluated.

PROGNOSIS AND LONG-TERM SURVIVAL

The American Joint Committee on Cancer defines 4 stages of disease in MTC. The different stages take into account tumor size, evidence of regional lymph node or distant metastases, and tumor invasion. In one study, 10-year cause-specific survival was 71%. Of the 53 patients with MTC, the mean age at diagnosis was 46, and distribution of familial and sporadic MTC was 17% and 83%, respectively. Prognosis was most influenced by stage, and postoperative basal calcitonin levels correlated most strongly with survival.[28] In a later study of 104 patients, of which 44% had hereditary MTC, cause-specific survival was 89%. By univariate analysis, age, stage, gender, distant metastases, and extent of surgery were all significant prognostic factors. Only age and stage, however, were statistically significant by multivariate analysis.[29] A more recent study by Rendl and colleagues[14] again confirmed that the most sensitive predictors of survival were age at diagnosis and tumor stage. In this series, there was a difference in survival time based on whether patients achieved biochemical and radiographic remission. In those who did not, 10-year survival was slightly reduced to 73%. These observations demonstrate the indolent nature of the disease, the appropriateness of reoperative surgery when technically possible, and the potential usefulness of cytostatic agents that keep clinically occult disease under control.

GENETIC BASIS OF FAMILIAL MTC AND PHENOTYPE CORRELATIONS

The predisposition gene for MEN 2A, 2B, and FMTC is the *RET* proto-oncogene, located on chromosome 10q11.2. This gene encodes a tyrosine kinase receptor protein involved in growth, differentiation, and migration of developing tissues. The full-length protein includes an extracellular cysteine-rich ligand-binding domain, a transmembrane domain, an intracellular juxtamembrane domain, and an intracellular tyrosine kinase domain. The mutations responsible for MTC are missense mutations, which result in amino acid changes that cause "gain-of-function" alterations in the protein.[7] These are inherited in an autosomal dominant fashion. Thus MEN 2 carriers confer a 50% risk of genetic transmission to their offspring.

There are consistent associations between the specific *RET* mutation (genotype) and clinical phenotype of patients with familial forms of MTC (**Table 1**). This includes age of onset, aggressiveness of MTC, and presence or absence of other endocrine neoplasms. MEN 2B patients expressing the M918T mutation have the most aggressive forms of MTC, with evidence of disease often present in early infancy. MEN 2A

Table 1
Genotype-phenotype correlation in hereditary medullary thyroid carcinoma[a]

Codon	Risk Level	MEN 2B	MEN 2A			FMTC	HSCR
			MTC	Pheo	HPT		
533	I		X	X		X	
9-Bp ins	I[b]					X	
606	I[b]		X				
609	II[b]		X	X	X	X	X
611	II		X	X	X	X	X
618	II		X	X	X	X	X
620	II		X	X		X	X
630	II[b]		X		X	X	
631	I[b]		X	X		X	
634	II		X	X	X	X	
768	I		X	X		X	
777	I[b]					X	
790	I		X	X		X	
791	I		X	X	X	X	
804	I		X	X	X	X	
804 +806	III[b]	X					
883	III	X					
891	I		X			X	
912	I[b]					X	
918	III	X					

Abbreviations: HSCR, Hirschsprung disease; HPT, hyperparathyroidism; Pheo, pheochromocytoma.
[a] Risk levels are based on 2001 consensus guidelines.
[b] Mutations not reported at the time of consensus guidelines publication.

patients have a variable course of MTC disease presentation and progression, whereas patients with FMTC demonstrate an indolent form that more often presents in the later decades of life. There is considerable overlap between the RET codons affected in FMTC and those in MEN 2A, which supports the theory that FMTC is a variant of MEN 2A and not a distinct clinical entity.

Pheochromocytoma is detected in about 50% of patients with 634 and 918 mutations but is rarely seen in mutations of exon 10 (codon 609, 611, 620). The specific amino acid change within the codon may also affect expression of features in MEN 2. In MEN 2A patients with amino acid substitutions at codon 618, the penetrance of pheochromocytoma is variable, with C618R showing 41% penetrance; C618G, 24%; and C618Y, 0%.[30] Hyperparathyroidism in MEN 2A is most commonly associated with the C634R mutation.[31]

These genotype-phenotype correlations have important implications for the management of MEN 2 patients and their families. Knowing the specific *RET* codon mutation allows the clinician to stratify patients into specific risk groups that help predict the age of onset and aggressiveness of MTC and the need for biochemical surveillance of the associated endocrine neoplasms. The original consensus guidelines written in 2001 identify 3 risk groups: low (level I), high (level II), and highest (level III).[32]

PREVENTATIVE SURGERY IN MEN 2 PREDISPOSITION GENE CARRIERS

The best chance of cure in familial MTC is provided by complete surgical resection before malignant transformation or spread beyond the thyroid gland. Patients with specific germ-line *RET* mutations are stratified into specific risk groups based on reported age of onset and aggressiveness of the disease. Patients with the highest risk (level III) are MEN 2B and should undergo prophylactic total thyroidectomy as soon as possible within the first year of life. Individuals with MEN 2A mutations (codons 611, 618, 620, and 634) are considered high risk and should undergo thyroidectomy around 5 years of age.[33] In the experience of the authors and others, the risk of nodal metastases in MEN 2A or FMTC patients younger than 8 years is extremely low, and it has not been reported if the calcitonin level is less than 40 pg/mL.[33] Furthermore, there was a 6% to 8% incidence of hypoparathyroidism in children undergoing routine central neck dissection.[33] For these reasons, the authors no longer routinely perform central neck dissections in these young patients, unless indicated by preoperatively elevated serum calcitonin levels (>40 pg/mL in a child >6 months old), radiographic evidence of lymph node metastases, or nodules more than 5 mm in size at any age. In familial MTC patients with level I *RET* codon mutations, the need for prophylactic thyroidectomy before 5 years of age is controversial. If patients are not undergoing surgery, they should be followed closely with annual checks of basal serum calcitonin levels.

More than 50% of sMTCs harbor a RET mutation in the tumor cells only (somatic mutation).[34] The utility of identifying whether a *RET* mutation is present in the tumor cells in sMTC has yet to be defined, but it has been suggested that sMTCs with somatic RET mutations in codon 918 are more aggressive than tumors without the mutation.[35,36]

In the absence of symptoms consistent with catecholamine access or known adrenal mass, routine surveillance for pheochromocytoma is dictated by the familial subtype and the identified *RET* mutation. The incidence of pheochromocytoma in any form of familial MTC before 10 years of age is exceptionally rare, although our group recently removed a 5-cm pheochromocytoma from an 8-year-old girl with MEN 2A (codon 634 mutation). Plasma metanephrines or 24-hour urine catecholamines should be checked annually in patients with MEN 2A and MEN 2B. In MEN 2A patients, surveillance for primary hyperparathyroidism by measurement of serum calcium levels should begin around the age of 10 years in those carrying the *RET* 630 and 634 mutations, and it should begin at the age of 20 years for those carrying mutations in the other codons.

SUMMARY

MTC accounts for 5% to 10% of all thyroid cancers. The high frequency of familial cases mandates screening and genetic testing. The aggressiveness and age of onset of familial MTC differs depending on the specific genetic mutation, and this should determine the timing and extent of surgery. Sporadic MTC can present at any age, and it is usually associated with a palpable mass and the presence of nodal metastases. Surgery is standard treatment for any patient presenting with resectable MTC. Further studies are needed to investigate the role of radiation therapy in the palliation and local control of postresection and advanced-stage MTC. New systemic therapies for metastatic disease are being investigated. Targeted molecular therapies, based on knowledge of the pathways affected by RET mutations, are being tested in multiple clinical trials.

REFERENCES

1. Khurana R, Agarwal A, Bajpai VK, et al. Unraveling the amyloid associated with human medullary thyroid carcinoma. Endocrinology 2004;145(12):5465–70 [Epub 2004 Sep 30].
2. Hazard JB. The C cells (parafollicular cells) of the thyroid gland and medullary thyroid carcinoma. A review. Acta Neurol (Napoli) 1977;32(4):491–519.
3. LiVolsi VA. C cell hyperplasia/neoplasia. J Clin Endocrinol Metab 1997;82(1): 39–41.
4. Howe JR, Norton JA, Wells SJ. Prevalence of pheochromocytoma and hyperparathyroidism in multiple endocrine neoplasia type 2A: results of long-term follow-up. Surgery 1993;114(6):1070–7.
5. Moers AM, Landsvater RM, Schaap C, et al. Familial medullary thyroid carcinoma: not a distinct entity? Genotype-phenotype correlation in a large family. Am J Med 1996;101(6):635–41.
6. Farndon JR, Leight GS, Dilley WG, et al. Familial medullary thyroid carcinoma without associated endocrinopathies: a distinct clinical entity. Br J Surg 1986;73:278–81.
7. Eng C, Clayton D, Schuffenecker I, et al. The relationship between specific RET proto-oncogene mutations and disease phenotype in multiple endocrine neoplasia type 2. International RET mutation consortium analysis. JAMA 1996; 276(19):1575–9.
8. Chang TC, Wu SL, Hsiao YL. Medullary thyroid carcinoma: pitfalls in diagnosis by fine needle aspiration cytology and relationship of cytomorphology to RET proto-oncogene mutations. Acta Cytol 2005;49(5):477–82.
9. Mayr B, Brabant G, von zur Muhlen A. Incidental detection of familial medullary thyroid carcinoma by calcitonin screening for nodular thyroid disease. Eur J Endocrinol 1999;141(3):286–9.
10. Moley JF, DeBenedetti MK. Patterns of nodal metastases in palpable medullary thyroid carcinoma: recommendations for extent of node dissection. Ann Surg 1999;229(6):880–7 [discussion: 7–8].
11. Giraudet AL, Vanel D, Leboulleux S, et al. Imaging medullary thyroid carcinoma with persistent elevated calcitonin levels. J Clin Endocrinol Metab 2007;92(11):4185–90.
12. Oudoux A, Salaun PY, Bournaud C, et al. Sensitivity and prognostic value of positron emission tomography with F-18-fluorodeoxyglucose and sensitivity of immunoscintigraphy in patients with medullary thyroid carcinoma treated with anticarcinoembryonic antigen-targeted radioimmunotherapy. J Clin Endocrinol Metab 2007;92(12):4590–7.
13. Machens A, Schneyer U, Holzhausen HJ, et al. Prospects of remission in medullary thyroid carcinoma according to basal calcitonin level. J Clin Endocrinol Metab 2005;90(4):2029–34 [Epub 05 Jan 5].
14. Rendl LM, Manzl M, Hitzl W, et al. Long-term prognosis of medullary thyroid carcinoma. Clin Endocrinol (Oxf) 2008;69(3):497–505.
15. Machens A, Niccoli-Sire P, Hoegel J, et al. Early malignant progression of hereditary medullary thyroid cancer. N Engl J Med 2003;349(16):1517–25.
16. Machens A, Hauptmann S, Dralle H. Prediction of lateral lymph node metastases in medullary thyroid cancer. Br J Surg 2008;95(5):586–91.
17. Moley JF, Fialkowski EA. Evidence-based approach to the management of sporadic medullary thyroid carcinoma. World J Surg 2007;31(5):946–56.
18. Miyauchi A, Matsuzuka F, Hirai K, et al. Prospective trial of unilateral surgery for nonhereditary medullary thyroid carcinoma in patients without germline RET mutations. World J Surg 2002;26(8):1023–8 [Epub 2002 May 21].

19. Fialkowski E, DeBenedetti M, Moley J. Long-term outcome of reoperations for medullary thyroid carcinoma. World J Surg 2008;32(5):754–65.
20. Moley JF, Lairmore TC, Doherty GM, et al. Preservation of the recurrent laryngeal nerves in thyroid and parathyroid reoperations. Surgery 1999;126(4):673–7 [discussion: 7–9].
21. Brierley J, Tsang R, Simpson WJ, et al. Medullary thyroid cancer: analyses of survival and prognostic factors and the role of radiation therapy in local control. Thyroid 1996;6(4):305–10.
22. Stein R, Goldenberg DM. A humanized monoclonal antibody to carcinoembryonic antigen, labetuzumab, inhibits tumor growth and sensitizes human medullary thyroid cancer xenografts to dacarbazine chemotherapy. Mol Cancer Ther 2004;3(12):1559–64.
23. Cohen MS, Hussain HB, Moley JF. Inhibition of medullary thyroid carcinoma cell proliferation and RET phosphorylation by tyrosine kinase inhibitors. Surgery 2002; 132(6):960–6 [discussion: 6–7].
24. Carlomagno F, Vitagliano D, Guida T, et al. ZD6474, an orally available inhibitor of KDR tyrosine kinase activity, efficiently blocks oncogenic RET kinases. Cancer Res 2002;62(24):7284–90.
25. Carlomagno F, Anaganti S, Guida T, et al. BAY 43-9006 inhibition of oncogenic RET mutants. J Natl Cancer Inst 2006;98(5):326–34.
26. Chow LQ, Eckhardt SG. Sunitinib: from rational design to clinical efficacy. J Clin Oncol 2007;25(7):884–96.
27. Hong D, Ye L, Gagel R, et al. Medullary thyroid cancer: targeting the RET kinase pathway with sorafenib/tipifarnib. Mol Cancer Ther 2008;7(5):1001–6.
28. Dottorini ME, Assi A, Sironi M, et al. Multivariate analysis of patients with medullary thyroid carcinoma. Prognostic significance and impact on treatment of clinical and pathologic variables. Cancer 1996;77(8):1556–65.
29. Kebebew E, Ituarte PH, Siperstein AE, et al. Medullary thyroid carcinoma: clinical characteristics, treatment, prognostic factors, and a comparison of staging systems. Cancer 2000;88(5):1139–48.
30. Quayle FJ, Fialkowski EA, Benveniste R, et al. Pheochromocytoma penetrance varies by RET mutation in MEN 2A. Surgery 2007;142(6):800–5 [discussion: 805 e1].
31. Raue F, Frank-Raue K. Genotype-phenotype relationship in multiple endocrine neoplasia type 2. Implications for clinical management. Hormones (Athens) 2009;8(1):23–8.
32. Brandi ML, Gagel RF, Angeli A, et al. Guidelines for diagnosis and therapy of MEN type 1 and type 2. J Clin Endocrinol Metab 2001;86(12):5658–71.
33. Skinner MA, Moley JA, Dilley WG, et al. Prophylactic thyroidectomy in multiple endocrine neoplasia type 2A. N Engl J Med 2005;353(11):1105–13.
34. Eng C, Mulligan LM, Smith DP, et al. Mutation of the RET protooncogene in sporadic medullary thyroid carcinoma. Genes Chromosomes Cancer 1995; 12(3):209–12.
35. Zedenius J, Larsson C, Bergholm U, et al. Mutations of codon 918 in the RET proto-oncogene correlate to poor prognosis in sporadic medullary thyroid carcinomas. J Clin Endocrinol Metab 1995;80(10):3088–90.
36. Elisei R, Cosci B, Romei C, et al. Prognostic significance of somatic RET oncogene mutations in sporadic medullary thyroid cancer: a 10-year follow-up study. J Clin Endocrinol Metab 2008;93(3):682–7.

Surgical Management of Primary Hyperparathyroidism: State of the Art

John I. Lew, MD, FACS*, Carmen C. Solorzano, MD, FACS

KEYWORDS

- Primary hyperparathyroidism • Parathyroid hormone
- Preoperative localization
- Intraoperative parathyroid hormone monitoring
- Focused parathyroidectomy • Bilateral neck exploration

HISTORY OF PARATHYROID SURGERY

...It seems hardly credible that the loss of bodies so tiny as the parathyroids should be followed by a result so disastrous.

—*William S. Halsted, 1907*[1]

Discovery of the Parathyroid Glands

The parathyroid glands were first identified by Sir Richard Owen in 1850 during an autopsy of an Indian Rhinoceros acquired by the Zoological Society of London.[2] In the 1880s, a Swedish medical student from Uppsala, Ivor Sandstrom, first described the *glandulae parathyroideae* in humans including their gross anatomic and microscopic features.[3] It is remarkable that the elusive function of the parathyroid glands was appreciated before the anatomic discovery of these glands themselves; the association of postoperative tetany in patients after total thyroidectomy was first made by Anton Wolfer in 1879.[4] More than a decade later, Parisian physiologist Eugene Gley recognized the loss of parathyroid glands caused tetany in 1891 after conducting selective parathyroidectomy in dogs.[5] His observations, however, did not recognize the intimate association between the parathyroid glands and calcium homeostasis. In 1906, Jacob Erdheim identified enlarged parathyroid

Division of Endocrine Surgery, DeWitt Daughtry Family Department of Surgery, University of Miami Leonard M. Miller School of Medicine, 1475 NW 12th Avenue (M-875), Miami, FL 33136, USA
* Corresponding author.
E-mail address: jlew@med.miami.edu (J.I. Lew).

Surg Clin N Am 89 (2009) 1205–1225
doi:10.1016/j.suc.2009.06.014
0039-6109/09/$ – see front matter © 2009 Elsevier Inc. All rights reserved.

glands that he concluded compensatory in several patients with bone disease.[6] This relationship between the parathyroid glands and calcium was definitively demonstrated in 1909 by William MacCallum and Carl Voegtlin, who corrected clinical tetany in dogs by the administration of either parathyroid extract or exogenous calcium.[7] Although Max Askanazy first published the account of solitary parathyroid tumors in association with von Recklinghausen disease of bone in 1903 (osteitis fibrosa cystica), in 1915 Friedrich Schlagenhaufer unequivocally suggested that single parathyroid tumors were the primary cause of bone disease in 2 patients with osteomalacia, and recommended such tumors be surgically excised in similar patients with von Recklinghausen disease of bone.[8,9]

The First Operations for Hyperparathyroidism

Ten years would pass before Schalgenhaufer's treatment recommendations for hyperparathyroidism would be followed. Felix Mandl performed the first parathyroidectomy in 1925 on Albert Jahne, a 34-year old Viennese tram car conductor.[10] After Jahne had been unsuccessfully treated with parathyroid extract and tissue implantation, Mandl excised an enlarged parathyroid gland that in retrospect may have represented a parathyroid carcinoma. The operation was initially successful, and altered the practice dogma for treatment of hyperparathyroidism at that time. However, Jahne's condition recurred, and he died soon after a second unsuccessful operation. In 1926, EJ Lewis performed the first parathyroidectomy in the United States at Cook County Hospital in Chicago on a 29-year old woman with parathyroid carcinoma who required multiple reoperations.[11] A few months later, comprehensive surgical management of hyperparathyroidism would be learned through merchant marine captain Charles Martell, who underwent 7 operations by Oliver Cope and others in Boston and New York for his condition.[12] Martell was eventually found to have a mediastinal parathyroid adenoma, but unfortunately died 6 weeks later as a consequence of his disease and its treatment. In 1928, Issac Olch performed the first successful parathyroidectomy at Barnes Hospital in St. Louis on Elva Dawkins, who underwent excision of a solitary enlarged parathyroid gland. Physicians from this institution involved in the care of Dawkins would later define the term "hyperparathyroidism" in an article published in 1929, describing associated bone findings as well as muscle weakness, renal stones, high serum calcium, and elevated urine calcium excretion.[13]

Parathyroid Hormone and the Development of Immunoassays

To further elucidate the function of the parathyroid glands, and facilitate diagnosis and therapy, Adolf Hanson, a general surgeon from Faribault, Minnesota, and James Collip, a Canadian biochemist, separately purified parathyroid extract in 1923 and 1925, respectively, to treat tetany, hypoparathyroidism, and osteoporosis.[14,15] Furthermore, Collip also worked to make this parathyroid hormone (PTH) commercially available. In 1963, Solomon Berson and Rosalyn Yalow developed a radioimmunoassay for PTH.[16] In 1977, Yalow received the Nobel Prize for discovery of this PTH assay and its application to measuring other peptide hormones. In 1968, Eric Weiss and Janet Canterbury identified bovine crossover antibodies to human PTH, and they later developed a radioimmunoassay that measured the C-terminal and mid-molecule of the hormone.[17] In 1987, Samuel Nussbaum and colleagues developed a highly sensitive 2-site antibody immunoradiometric assay (IRMA) for measuring intact PTH.[18] Later the same year, Richard Brown and colleagues from Wales reported measuring circulating intact (1–84) PTH with a 2-site immunochemiluminometric assay (ICMA) that demonstrated the 5-minute half-life of intact PTH with a specificity to distinguish between patients with elevated PTH levels and hypercalcemia of malignancy.[19,20] From these scientific discoveries, George Irvin applied and refined such techniques to routine clinical practice in the surgical management of primary hyperparathyroidism at the University of Miami. In 1990, Irvin measured intraoperative PTH levels using IRMA to confirm complete removal of hypersecreting parathyroid glands and predict curative resection in a reoperative patient with an intrathyroidal parathyroid adenoma not appreciated at initial exploration.[21] With excellent results and applicability to the outpatient setting, Irvin popularized this approach of limited or "focused" parathyroidectomy by combining preoperative localization studies and rapid intraoperative PTH monitoring (IPM) for the treatment of patients with primary hyperparathyroidism.[22,23]

Evolution of Parathyroid Surgery

With recent advances that include preoperative parathyroid localization with Sestamibi ± single-photon emission computed tomography (SPECT) or ultrasound (US) with rapid IPM, limited or "focused" parathyroidectomy performed through a small cervical incision serves as an attractive alternative to conventional bilateral cervical exploration (BNE) for primary hyperparathyroidism. Parathyroid localization by imaging studies is an important prerequisite for successful focused neck exploration. Operative success rates are further improved by IPM before and after removal of all abnormal parathyroid glands. When intraoperative PTH levels are reduced by more than 50%, successful exploration is assured with a predictive cure of at least 95% or greater. Advantages of focused parathyroidectomy in the ambulatory setting include improved cosmetic results with smaller incisions, decreased postoperative pain, shorter operative time, decreased hospitalization, and rapid postoperative recovery with greater than 95% cure rate comparable to BNE. Other recent surgical options for the treatment of patients with primary hyperparathyroidism include radioguided, endoscopic, and video-assisted parathyroidectomy.

SURGICAL ANATOMY, EMBRYOLOGY, AND PATHOLOGY OF THE PARATHYROID GLANDS

Normal parathyroid glands present in varied shapes and sizes. When subscapular at the upper thyroid pole, parathyroid glands may appear flattened. At the cricothyroid junction or thymic tongue, such glands may resemble oval, spherical, or teardrop shapes. Most parathyroid glands are yellow-tan or reddish in color depending on fat content, number of oxyphilic cells, and degree of vascularity. The average parathyroid gland measures 5 mm at greatest dimension with an average weight ranging from 30 to 40 mg.[24] Composed of chief and oxyphilic cells, parathyroid glands also consist of adipose tissue and fibrovascular stroma.[25] Found in both children and adults, chief cells that predominantly contain lipids are usually involved in hypersecretory processes. In hyperparathyroidism, the amount of lipid within chief cells of the gland is significantly diminished. Oxyphilic cells that characteristically have granular cytoplasms are primarily found in adults.

Successful parathyroidectomy is inextricably related to the understanding of the anatomic and embryologic relationship of the parathyroid glands to the thyroid gland and thymus. Most humans typically have 4 parathyroid glands. Studies on human cadavers reveal 84% have 4 parathyroid glands, 13% have 5 or more (supernumerary) glands, and 3% of individuals have only 3 parathyroid glands.[26] Supernumerary glands that most often reside in the thymus are of clinical significance in patients with parathyroid hyperplasia associated with secondary, tertiary, and familial hyperparathyroidism. At 4 weeks of embryologic development, the superior parathyroid glands originate from the fourth branchial pouch undergoing very little migration, whereas the inferior parathyroid glands descend from the third branchial pouch to more varied locations along with the thymus.[27] The paired superior and inferior parathyroid glands are typically symmetric in location bilaterally. In about 80% of cases, the superior and inferior parathyroid glands receive their blood supply from the inferior thyroid artery.

The superior parathyroid glands are usually located on the posteromedial aspect of the superior poles of the thyroid gland about 1 cm above the intersection of the recurrent laryngeal nerve and inferior thyroid artery at the level of the cricoid cartilage. The superior glands are typically posterior and superior to the recurrent laryngeal nerve. Because they undergo less embryologic migration during development, the location of the superior glands is more constant and they are seldom found in ectopic positions. If ectopic, these glands are usually found in the tracheoesophageal groove, posterior mediastinal, retroesophageal, retropharyngeal, or intrathyroidal locations.

The inferior parathyroid glands are located on the posterolateral surface of the inferior poles of the thyroid gland below the intersection of the recurrent laryngeal nerve and inferior thyroid artery. Unlike the superior glands, the inferior glands are seldom subscapular and they are usually located anterior to the recurrent laryngeal nerve. Because these glands extensively migrate with the thymus during embryologic development, they may widely vary in distribution. About 80% of inferior parathyroid glands may reside anteriorly, inferiorly, or laterally within 2 cm of the inferior pole of the thyroid gland.[28] These glands may also be found in ectopic locations most commonly within the true sheath of the thymus (15%), and less frequently, in an intrathyroidal location (1%–4%), anterior mediastinum, submandibular location, tracheoesophageal groove, retroesophageal space, and carotid sheath.[28] The surgically excised thymus and these other sites should be examined carefully at the time of initial exploration when abnormal parathyroid glands are not found in orthotopic locations.

Primary hyperparathyroidism, resulting from the overproduction of PTH by one or more hyperfunctioning parathyroid glands, can be caused by 3 different pathologic lesions. Parathyroid adenoma is a benign encapsulated tumor that accounts for most cases (85%–96%) of primary hyperparathyroidism. Although most have a single affected gland, 2% to 5% of patients with primary hyperparathyroidism may have 2 affected glands ("double adenoma") with the remaining glands appearing normal. Parathyroid hyperplasia is caused by an increase of parenchymal mass within all the parathyroid glands, and it accounts for 4% to 15% of cases. The incidence of hyperplasia increases in patients with multiple endocrine neoplasia (MEN) type 1 and 2, and non-MEN familial isolated hyperparathyroidism (FIHPT). Parathyroid hyperplasia is treated either by subtotal (3.5) parathyroidectomy or total parathyroidectomy with autotransplantation. For patients with MEN, cervical thymectomy should also be performed. Parathyroid carcinoma is an indolent growing malignant tumor of parenchymal cells responsible for less than 5% of all primary hyperparathyroidism cases. Because this carcinoma is invasive, parathyroidectomy should be performed with en bloc resection of the ipsilateral thyroid lobe, avoiding parathyroid capsule violation.

CLINICAL PRESENTATION AND EVALUATION

Primary hyperparathyroidism results from PTH overproduction by one or more hyperfunctioning parathyroid glands that usually cause hypercalcemia. The widespread use of serum channel autoanalyzers since the 1970s has allowed for earlier diagnosis of primary hyperparathyroidism in patients before the manifestation of clinical symptoms.[29] This development along with the aging population in the United States has led to the reported increased incidence of primary hyperparathyroidism.[30,31] The most common cause of hypercalcemia in the outpatient setting, the incidence of primary hyperparathyroidism in the general population ranges from 0.1% to 0.3%, occurring more frequently in women than men with advanced age.[30–32] Known risk factors for primary hyperparathyroidism include abnormalities of the PRAD1, MEN1, and HRPT2 genes that encode for cyclin D1, menin, and parafibromin, respectively, and radiation exposure to the neck, especially during childhood.[33–36]

The clinical presentation of primary hyperparathyroidism has evolved throughout the years. The classic description of kidney "stones," painful "bones," abdominal "groans," lethargic "moans," and psychiatric "overtones" are now infrequently encountered in the United States. Today, patients with primary hyperparathyroidism present most commonly with abnormal biochemical results and do not have disease manifestations such as fatigue, musculoskeletal pain, weakness, polyuria, nocturia, memory loss, constipation, polydipsia, heartburn, and depression. Hypertension and nephrolithiasis are the most commonly associated preoperative conditions found in patients with primary hyperparathyroidism.[37] Nonetheless, when properly evaluated, up to 80% of patients currently present with nonspecific symptoms of depression, fatigue, and lethargy, and they often are considered asymptomatic.[38]

Once primary hyperparathyroidism is suspected or hypercalcemia is identified, biochemical confirmation is necessary. Oversecretion of PTH directly stimulates bone resorption, enhances intestinal absorption of calcium, inhibits renal calcium excretion, and indirectly stimulates the production of active vitamin D that also promotes intestinal calcium absorption. The negative feedback that controls PTH secretion is affected in primary hyperparathyroidism, resulting in inappropriate autonomous secretion of PTH concomitant with hypercalcemia. Diagnosis of primary hyperparathyroidism is made by demonstrating elevated total serum or ionized calcium levels, and high intact PTH levels in the setting of normal renal function. In primary hyperparathyroidism, vitamin D metabolism is typically characterized by low plasma levels of 25-hydroxyvitamin D, and high plasma levels of 1,25-dihydroxyvitamin D. Twenty-four-hour urine calcium collection is also helpful to exclude the diagnosis of benign familial hypocalciuric hypercalcemia (BFHH). A rare condition identified in patients with a family history of hypercalcemia and decreased urine calcium excretion since birth, BFHH biochemically mimics primary hyperparathyroidism with elevated calcium and PTH levels, but with low levels of urinary calcium (less than 100 mg/24 h). Similarly, the urinary calcium-to-creatinine (Ca/Cr) clearance ratio in BFHH is less than 0.01, whereas in patients with primary hyperparathyroidism the ratio is greater than 0.02. An autosomal dominant disease, BFHH is a benign condition that cannot be corrected by parathyroidectomy.

Patients may also present with normocalcemic hyperparathyroidism. Most of these patients have primary hyperparathyroidism with normal calcium and elevated PTH levels after appropriate diagnostic evaluation. This condition is generally recognized in patients being evaluated for osteoporosis.[39] In some individuals, this may be the earliest presentation of symptomatic primary hyperparathyroidism, whereas in others it may represent PTH elevation secondary to vitamin D deficiency or renal dysfunction.[40] Patients occasionally present with hypercalcemia and inappropriately normal PTH level, and many will have hyperparathyroidism after further workup. Nevertheless, surgeons treating hyperparathyroidism should be knowledgeable about these varied presentations to avoid poor surgical outcomes. Other causes of hypercalcemia that also need to be excluded include underlying malignancy, excessive thiazide diuretics, lithium, vitamin A or D excess, milk-alkali syndrome, sarcoidosis, Paget disease, or prolonged immobilization.

Although not required for diagnosis, dual-energy x-ray absorptiometry (DEXA) may be useful in the measurement of bone mineral density (BMD) in patients with primary hyperparathyroidism. Because many have decreased BMD secondary to this condition, most patients with primary hyperparathyroidism should undergo DEXA testing. If osteoporosis is documented (T-score less than –2.5), parathyroidectomy should be strongly considered. In primary hyperparathyroidism, bone density losses are greater in areas of cortical bone such as the femoral neck and radius, but can occur at all bony sites. The benefit of parathyroidectomy can be more pronounced at the hips because of the morbidity and mortality associated with bone fracture at these sites.

INDICATIONS FOR PARATHYROIDECTOMY

Although symptomatic primary hyperparathyroidism remains a clear indication for surgical treatment, there remains some controversy among clinicians regarding the indications for performing parathyroidectomy in asymptomatic patients. The efficacy of parathyroidectomy in asymptomatic patients has been questioned due to the indolent nature and less understood natural history of primary hyperparathyroidism. To address this issue, the National Institutes of Health (NIH) convened a consensus conference in 1990, and another workshop in 2002 to establish guidelines for the surgical management of asymptomatic patients that include: serum calcium level 1.0 mg/dL or greater above the accepted normal range; 24-h urinary calcium excretion greater than 400 mg/d; creatinine clearance reduced by 30%; T-score less than –2.5 at any site; and age younger than 50 years. Parathyroidectomy was also recommended in patients for whom medical surveillance is either undesirable or impossible.[41]

Many clinicians believe that the NIH criteria for asymptomatic patients are too conservative, with many experienced endocrine surgeons basing the operative decision not only on these objective criteria but on subjective complaints as well.[42] Others believe that these criteria fail to address the role of neurocognitive deficits in patients with primary hyperparathyroidism, with several studies showing improvements of depression, anxiety, sleep disturbances, poor memory, and cognitive impairment after parathyroidectomy.[43] Recent evidence from a long-term study of primary hyperparathyroidism over 15 years suggests the NIH guidelines for parathyroidectomy do not reliably predict worsening disease progression in asymptomatic patients.[44] Because meeting surgical NIH guidelines at the time of diagnosis did not predict a worse outcome of bone disease in patients who did not undergo parathyroidectomy, this report raises questions as to whether the guidelines for surgery in asymptomatic patients with primary hyperparathyroidism are appropriate for clinical decision making. Nonetheless, it is the opinion of the article authors (J.I.L., C.C.S.) that all "asymptomatic" patients with clear biochemical diagnosis of primary hyperparathyroidism should be offered a surgical consultation with an experienced parathyroid surgeon.

PREOPERATIVE PARATHYROID LOCALIZATION

The only localization that a patient needs who has primary hyperparathyroidism is the localization of an experienced surgeon!
—John L. Doppmann, 1991[45]

An important advancement in the surgical treatment of primary hyperparathyroidism has been the improved preoperative localization of hyperfunctioning parathyroid glands using a variety of imaging techniques including sestamibi-technetium 99m scintigraphy (sestamibi), ultrasonography (US), and 4-dimensional computed tomography(4D-CT). Sestamibi, especially combined with SPECT, is considered the best single study for preoperative parathyroid localization.[46,47] However, US has recently been used more frequently, and it has been shown to be accurate and cost-effective in distinguishing enlarged parathyroid glands from surrounding structures.[48–50] Although either study can adequately localize abnormal glands alone in many patients, both studies can be used concordantly, significantly improving preoperative localization for successful focused parathyroidectomy.[51–54] For patients undergoing reoperative exploration for recurrent or persistent parathyroid disease, 4D-CT may have an important role in preoperative gland localization.[55]

Sestamibi scintigraphy has played a key role in the acceptance of more limited approaches to the surgical treatment of primary hyperparathyroidism. Sestamibi is avidly retained by parathyroid adenomas thought to be secondarily related to the high mitochondrial content of this tissue. Sestamibi can localize 80% to 90% of single abnormal parathyroid glands, but it is less sensitive in the diagnosis of multiglandular disease (MGD).[56–58] The specificity of sestamibi scanning can be improved with delayed (2-hour) planar and multidimensional imaging obtained by SPECT.[59,60] Although there are no significant differences in the sensitivity of the varied types of sestamibi scanning used to identify abnormal gland(s), multidimensional imaging (ie, SPECT) provides additional information regarding the anatomic location of these glands in many patients.[61] Although its sensitivity for MGD is low, misdiagnosis can be avoided with supplemental preoperative imaging or intraoperative PTH measurements.[57,58,62] The coexistence of thyroid nodules or lymph nodes that can mimic abnormal parathyroid glands may also cause false-positive results on sestamibi scans. Such results can be minimized by combining sestamibi with neck US to distinguish between thyroid lesions and enlarged parathyroid glands or by the combined use of SPECT that can provide simultaneous 3-dimensional functional and anatomic information delineating thyroid and parathyroid lesions.[46,47] Sestamibi-SPECT is particularly useful in detecting smaller parathyroid lesions that may reside posterior the thyroid gland (**Fig. 1**).

In recent years, US has been more commonly used for preoperative parathyroid localization. This imaging modality can be very accurate by providing important anatomic information delineating an enlarged parathyroid gland from surrounding structures with 70% to 80% accuracy.[48–50] This noninvasive imaging modality is inexpensive, but has a varied sensitivity in the localization of abnormal parathyroid glands. Furthermore, US is operator dependent with limited application to the neck for parathyroid localization because it cannot identify glands in the mediastinum. At the authors' institution, US is routinely performed by endocrine surgeons (J.I.L., C.C.S.) in the clinical setting. Surgeon-performed ultrasound (SUS) enables clinicians who best appreciate neck anatomy to obtain real-time information regarding the anatomic location of enlarged parathyroid glands among several other structures, and allows for evaluation of thyroid abnormalities that may require surgical treatment (**Fig. 2**). Several studies demonstrate that preoperative SUS localizes enlarged parathyroid glands similar to sestamibi with improved sensitivity over radiologist-performed ultrasound.[48–50] Like sestamibi, US has a lower sensitivity for MGD. The overall sensitivity of dual-phase ^{99m}Tc sestamibi scintigraphy in comparison with US is 88% versus 79% for single adenomas, 30% versus 16% for double adenomas, and 44% versus 35% for multiple-gland hyperplasia.[63]

Combined sestamibi and US can increase accuracy of localization of a single adenoma from 94% to 99%. When concordant, sestamibi and US localization has been reported to have an operative success rate approaching 99%, obviating the need for IPM.[51–54] Although studies show excellent outcomes in this subgroup of

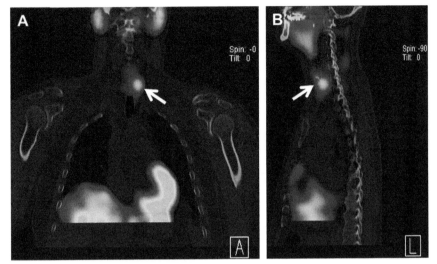

Fig. 1. (*A*) Coronal view of sestambi-SPECT scan demonstrating a left superior parathyroid gland (*arrow*). (*B*) Lateral view of the same left superior parathyroid gland (*arrow*) residing posterior to left thyroid lobe.

highly selected patients with concordant localizing studies, this selective approach significantly limits the number of eligible patients for focused parathyroidectomy. Preoperative sestamibi and US have been shown to be concordant only 50% to 60% of the time, leaving a great number of patients with no definitive or discordant localization.[64] Discordance between sestamibi and US has been reported as high as 38% in consecutive patients treated by parathyroidectomy with an 11% rate of MGD. Although sensitivity for MGD for both localizing studies is lower, missed abnormal glands can be minimized with additional IPM.[64]

In patients with recurrent or persistent disease, 4D-CT may have a useful role in the localization of abnormal parathyroid glands in conjunction with other imaging studies

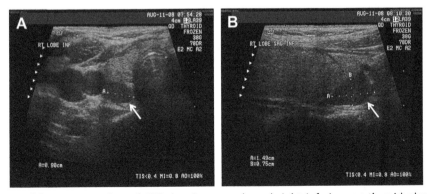

Fig. 2. (*A*) Transverse view of SUS showing an enlarged right inferior parathyroid gland (*arrow*) measuring 1.49 × 0.9 × 0.75 cm. (*B*) Longitudinal view of the same enlarged right inferior parathyroid gland (*arrow*) with typical ultrasound characteristics including hypoechogenicity and elliptical shape.

that may sometimes fail.[55] The wash-in and wash-out characteristics of parathyroid glands allow 4D-CT to identify hyperfunctioning glands with improved sensitivity (**Fig. 3**). Although under current investigation for routine preoperative parathyroid localization, 4D-CT nevertheless remains a useful imaging modality in reoperative patients.

INTRAOPERATIVE PARATHYROID HORMONE MONITORING

When surgeons have the ability to measure endocrine gland function intraoperatively, our dedication to chasing hormones will become a lot easier and much more fun.

—George L. Irvin, 1999 [21]

A significant innovation in the surgical treatment of primary hyperparathyroidism, IPM, serves as a surgical adjunct to quantitatively determine the excision of all hyperfunctioning parathyroid tissue. Refined and first implemented routinely by George Irvin at the University of Miami, IPM allows for more limited operations that minimize the need to identify all 4 parathyroid glands.[22,23] IPM can confirm adequate removal of all hyperfunctioning parathyroid glands and predict operative success with reduced operative time compared with BNE. IPM is possible due to the short half-life (3.5–5 minutes) of PTH. IPM involves the rapid assay measurement of preoperative, preexcision, and postexcision PTH levels at 5 and 10 minutes after removal of all hypersecreting parathyroid glands. Intraoperative criterion for successful and curative parathyroidectomy originally described by Irvin is defined by a decrease of intact PTH levels greater than 50% from the highest preincision or preexcision hormone level in a peripheral blood sample obtained 10 minutes after removal of all abnormal parathyroid tissue.[22,23,65] If this criterion is met, the operation is completed and the incision closed. If the 10-minute sample shows an insufficient decrease, further neck exploration is performed. With IPM, hypersecretory activity of parathyroid glands is determined exclusively by measured PTH levels, not by gland size or histology. Patients

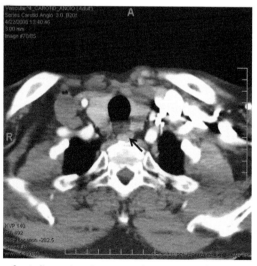

Fig. 3. An axial view of a 4-dimensional computed tomogram showing an enlarged parathyroid gland (*arrow*) located in the retroesophageal space of a patient who underwent 2 prior failed parathyroidectomies.

with more than one hypersecreting parathyroid gland by IPM measurement are determined to have MGD.

An example of IPM in a patient with primary hyperparathyroidism successfully treated following resection of a solitary hypersecreting parathyroid gland is illustrated in **Fig. 4.** This criterion has been designed to consider the half-life of PTH, and to avoid misleading results caused by spikes in PTH levels that may result from parathyroid gland mobilization. A decline of more than 50% in PTH level from the highest preincision or preexcision level indicates operative success with predictive cure in 97% of cases.[65] Other surgeons, however, use more stringent intraoperative criteria for operative cure of primary hyperparathyroidism. In addition to a greater than 50% reduction of intraoperative PTH level, these proponents additionally require that the final postexcision PTH level falls into normal range before concluding the surgical procedure to lower the incidence of operative failure or persistent hyperparathyroidism due to false-positive results.[66,67] Recent evidence, however, suggests that patients in whom intraoperative PTH levels decrease more than 50% and do not drop into normal range continue to be biochemically eucalcemic after parathyroidectomy, without an increased incidence of operative failure or recurrent hyperparathyroidism.[68] Each operating surgeon should validate the IPM criteria that maximizes cure and avoids excessive neck exploration at their respective institutions.

In patients with discordant or incorrect concordant preoperative localization studies, IPM remains a useful adjunct that limits exploration and prevents operative failure due to MGD.[64] The rapid P assay is additionally useful when surgeons and pathologists have difficulty distinguishing parathyroid, thyroid, and lymph node tissue. Aspirate of parathyroid tissue diluted in a syringe containing 1 mL saline, and measurement of its contents by rapid assay yields PTH values greater than 1500 pg/mL that confirm diagnosis.[69] When both sestambi and US studies are negative, differential venous PTH sampling measured by rapid assay can be performed to lateralize the hypersecreting gland to one side of the neck.[70,71] If this test is indeterminate, one side is randomly chosen to be explored first. Operative failure and BNE rates have decreased significantly for initial and reoperative parathyroidectomy with IPM. Failure

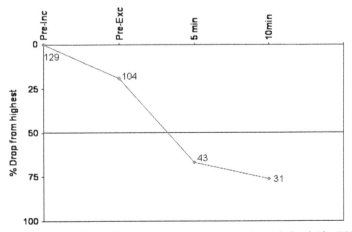

Fig. 4. IPM in a patient with a solitary hyperfunctioning parathyroid gland. The 76% drop in PTH level from 129 pg/mL to 31 pg/mL confirms that all abnormal parathyroid tissue has been surgically removed.

rates from initial parathyroidectomy have reportedly decreased by 4.5% after the implementation of IPM.[72] Although variable, IPM has been reported to increase success rates by 10% at initial operation, and by 18% in reoperative patients for failed parathyroidectomy.[73,74]

FOCUSED PARATHYROIDECTOMY

With the advent of improved preoperative localization techniques, increased availability of IPM, and the predominance of single gland disease in 85% to 96% of patients with primary hyperparathyroidism, limited or focused parathyroidectomy has replaced traditional BNE as the standard approach at many specialized centers worldwide.[75–79] Attractive advantages of focused parathyroidectomy include improved cosmetic results with smaller incisions, decreased pain, shorter operative time, ambulatory surgery, decreased hospitalization, rapid postoperative recovery, less injury to the recurrent laryngeal nerve, decreased postoperative hypocalcemia, and comparable success rates to conventional BNE.[76–79] In a survey among members of the International Association of Endocrine Surgeons (IAES), 92% of responding surgeons performed focused parathyroidectomy with small incisions, highlighting the profound worldwide shift in the surgical management of primary hyperparathyroidism over the last decade.[75]

Many techniques of focused parathyroidectomy have been described that incorporate and share common aspects and principles of minimally invasive surgery that result in less dissection, decreased operative time, less morbidity, and comparable reported operative success to BNE ranging from 97% to 99%.[73,76–79] In general terms, the procedure is performed in patients with a single parathyroid adenoma localized by preoperative sestamibi or US through a central or lateral incision measuring from 2 to 4 cm. Only the abnormal parathyroid gland is identified and excised. IPM is used by most to confirm that no additional hypersecreting parathyroid tissue remains. When IPM levels decrease by more than 50%, the limited operation is completed. Performed under general or local anesthesia, focused parathyroidectomy can be offered to most patients in the outpatient setting. Patients with known MGD preoperatively are not offered this focused approach.

At the institution where the authors practice (J.I.L., C.C.S.), focused parathyroidectomy is usually performed under general or local anesthesia in the ambulatory setting. Before limited exploration performed through a cervical incision measuring between 2 and 4 cm, a peripheral blood sample for a baseline (preincision) PTH level is obtained. After identification of the abnormal parathyroid gland, and just before clamping of its vascular pedicle, a preexcision PTH hormone level is measured followed by subsequent 5- and 10-minute blood samples. Intraoperative criterion for successful parathyroidectomy is defined by a decrease of intact PTH level more than 50% from the highest preincision or preexcision hormone level in a peripheral blood sample obtained 10 minutes after removal of all abnormal parathyroid tissue. If this criterion is met, the neck exploration is completed and the incision closed. If the 10-minute sample shows an insufficient decrease, further neck exploration is performed.[80] Secretory activity of parathyroid glands is determined exclusively by measured PTH levels, and not by gland size or histology. Patients with more than one hypersecreting parathyroid gland measured by IPM are determined to have MGD. Patients are carefully followed in the outpatient setting, with serum calcium, PTH, and vitamin D levels measured at 2 months, 6 months, and yearly thereafter to determine operative outcome. At this institution, operative success is defined as continuous eucalcemia lasting 6 months or longer whereas recurrent hyperparathyroidism is defined as elevated calcium and PTH levels more than 6 months after successful parathyroidectomy. Operative failure is defined as elevated calcium and PTH levels within 6 months after parathyroidectomy.

Outcomes

The success of focused parathyroidectomy has been confirmed by several studies with cure and complication rates that are comparable to traditional BNE.[73,76–79] In one study of 656 consecutive patients older than 11 years in which 255 underwent focused parathyroidectomy and 401 conventional BNE, the cure rates were 99% and 97% with complication rates of 1.2% and 3%, respectively.[76] Focused parathyroidectomy also had a reduced operating time of 1.3 hours compared with 2.4 hours for BNE, and a reduction in length of hospitalization of 0.24 days compared with 1.64 days, respectively. In another subsequent study of 718 patients older than 34 years, the cure rates for focused parathyroidectomy and BNE were 97% and 94% with operative failure rates of 3% and 6%, respectively.[78] Patients who underwent focused parathyroidectomy had a 7% lower incidence of MGD compared with BNE group. Finally, in a 5-year follow-up of a randomized controlled trial, focused parathyroidectomy provided the same long-term results as traditional BNE in patients with primary hyperparathyroidism.[81] The aforementioned studies all concluded that focused parathyroidectomy was a valid and attractive alternative to BNE for most patients with primary hyperparathyroidism.

At present there are minimal long-term data to confirm the durability of operative success from focused parathyroidectomy compared with conventional BNE. Critics of the focused approach predict that the combined use of preoperative localization and IPM lead to a high failure rate due to missed abnormal glands or MGD, risking future disease recurrence. What remains unknown is whether these enlarged parathyroid glands judged to be abnormal by the surgeon that might otherwise have been left alone and never seen during focused operations later become hyperfunctioning glands. In one study of simulated focused parathyroidectomy in 916 patients with primary hyperparathyroidism, preoperative sestamibi and US were used for parathyroid localization and IPM was performed in all patients.[82] Routine BNE was then performed in all these patients, revealing 16% of patients with additional enlarged glands, and raising the concern that the longer-term failure or recurrence rate for focused parathyroidectomy may be higher than reported in early results.[82]

Other reports, however, suggest otherwise, and indicate that focused parathyroidectomy has long-term durability of operative success comparable to BNE. In one study with a mean follow-up of almost 5 years, none of 181 patients cured by image-guided parathyroidectomy developed recurrent disease.[83] In a randomized clinical trial with a 5 year follow-up, the recurrence rates for focused parathyroidectomy and BNE were 5% and 3%, respectively.[81] In yet another analysis from the authors' institution, only a 3% rate of disease recurrence developed in 164 patients with a mean follow-up of almost 7 years after successful focused parathyroidectomy (John I. Lew and George L. Irvin III, 2009; unpublished results). Many other studies demonstrate that parathyroid size or histopathology do not necessarily correlate with PTH secretion and, therefore, may not be reliable indices in determining abnormal hypersecreting parathyroid glands.[84–86] These findings together indicate that the focused approach has a durable rate of operative success and does not fail to identify MGD as a cause of recurrent hyperparathyroidism, and strongly suggest that normal secreting, variously sized parathyroid glands left in situ do not contribute to higher long-term failure or recurrence rates.

BILATERAL NECK EXPLORATION

The traditional standard approach in the surgical treatment of primary hyperparathy-roidism, BNE requires the identification and careful examination of usually 4 parathyroid glands. When performed by experienced surgeons, the operative cure rate for BNE is more than 95% with a complication rate ranging from 1% to 4%.[87,88] There are certain clinical conditions in which BNE is preferred over focused parathyroidectomy. BNE is indicated for cases of MEN and non-MEN FIHPT wherein there is a higher incidence of MGD than single-gland disease. Lithium-associated hyperparathyroidism is another condition in which BNE is preferable due to its higher incidence of MGD. When patients have more than one gland localized on preoperative studies or no localization, BNE should be considered. BNE is also indicated in patients with secondary or tertiary hyperparathyroidism in whom parathyroid hyperplasia is most common. In patients with concomitant thyroid disease requiring both parathyroidectomy and thyroidec-tomy, and in cases of parathyroid cancer, the traditional open cervical approach is performed.

BNE is performed through a 3- to 5-cm cervical incision under general anesthesia. The procedure involves identification of usually 4 parathyroid glands, removal of the abnormal glands, and biopsy of one or more normal parathyroid glands. In cases in which more than one parathyroid gland appears abnormal, only the involved glands are excised. IPM can be used as a surgical adjunct to confirm removal of all hyperse-creting parathyroid tissue. When not identified initially during BNE, a diligent search for the ectopic abnormal parathyroid gland(s) is performed, involving exploration of the upper mediastinum, retroesophageal area, carotid sheaths, and thyroid gland. If the gland is still not found, the procedure is ended. A planned cervical reexploration, ster-notomy, or video-assisted mediastinal parathyroid exploration may be performed at a later date after reevaluation of initial diagnosis and further imaging to localize a possible unidentified mediastinal gland. In conditions of hyperplasia in which all 4 parathyroid glands appear abnormal, subtotal parathyroidectomy (3.5-gland resec-tion) or total parathyroidectomy with autotransplantation is performed. For subtotal parathyroidectomy, the one gland closest to appearing normal is biopsied and subto-tally resected first, leaving a tissue remnant of approximately 50 mg. The remaining glands are removed. In cases of total parathyroidectomy, remnant parathyroid tissue is autotransplanted preferably into the brachioradialis muscle of the nondominant forearm with cryopreservation of remaining parathyroid tissue. Bilateral thymectomy is recommended in both surgical approaches due to a high incidence of supernu-merary parathyroid glands within this structure.

RADIOGUIDED PARATHYROIDECTOMY

Radioguided parathyroidectomy is another more recent surgical approach used in the treatment of primary hyperparathyroidism. Patients are injected with Tc-99m sestamibi isotope about 2 hours before surgery, and then taken to the operating room where a gamma probe is used to direct the incision site and localize the abnormal parathyroid glands for excision. After the suspected adenoma is removed, the gamma probe is used to measure the radioactivity of the excised tissue, which is compared with the radioactivity of the surgical bed. Radioguided parathyroidec-tomy may also be useful in reoperative cases, patients who have undergone total thyroidectomy, or cases of ectopic parathyroid tissue. IPM can be used as an adjunct to this technique to increase its operative success rate.[89,90]

Radioguided parathyroidectomy is usually performed in the ambulatory setting under local anesthesia and sedation. A 2- to 4-cm incision is made at the site of highest radioactivity that corresponds to the location of the abnormal gland shown by preoperative sestamibi. Investigators report that radioguided parathyroidectomy with the gamma probe achieves 93% sensitivity, 88% positive predictive value, and 83% overall accuracy of parathyroid localization, with a conversion rate to BNE of 10% for single gland disease, 50% for MGD, and 50% for hyperplasia.[89,90] Some investigators report that the gamma probe is not helpful in up to 48% of patients who undergo parathyroidectomy due to confusing radioactivity counts, easily identified abnormal glands, equipment problems, and logistical timing problems of isotope administration before surgery.[91] The routine use of radioguided parathyroidectomy has not been widely adopted and most parathyroid surgeons do not use this approach, arguing that the gamma probe does not provide additional useful information that can otherwise be obtained with preoperative localization studies and IPM.[90–92]

ENDOSCOPIC AND VIDEO-ASSISTED PARATHYROIDECTOMY

Recent interest has revolved around the development of minimal access surgical techniques that include endoscopic and video-assisted parathyroidectomy performed with clear preoperative localization, and IPM used to verify the adequacy of abnormal parathyroid gland resection. For the endoscopic approach as described by Gagner, a 5-mm trocar for a 30° laparoscope is first placed at the cervical midline superior to the sternal notch, and carbon dioxide is insufflated to create the work space.[93] Another 5-mm port is placed in the right neck about 2 to 3 cm anterior to the sternocleidomastoid muscle. Two additional 5-mm ports are placed for the procedure, one in the right neck and another in the left neck. The strap muscles are divided at midline and the thyroid lobe is mobilized anteromedially to allow for visualization of the ipsilateral parathyroid glands. Many other variations to this technique have been described including axillary, anterior wall, and lateral neck approaches.[94–96] Although the technique reportedly has cure rates approaching 100% with excellent cosmetic results, less postoperative pain, fewer analgesic requirements, and increased patient satisfaction, endoscopic parathyroidectomy is associated with the longest learning curve and potential difficulties already described that include parathyroid capsule violation, suboptimal recurrent laryngeal nerve visualization, tachycardia, hypercapnia, respiratory acidosis, subcutaneous emphysema, and air embolism. In contrast, video-assisted parathyroidectomy does not require carbon dioxide insufflation and allows for tactile assessment by the surgeon. Special retractors are used to create the working space. First described by Miccoli, the video-assisted technique is performed using a 5-mm 30° endoscope inserted through a 1.5- to 2-cm transverse incision in the neck.[97] The dissection is performed with video magnification that enables easier identification of the recurrent laryngeal nerve and abnormal parathyroid gland. Although this technique has reported cure rates ranging from 96% to 100% with reduced operative time, decreased postoperative pain, and higher patient satisfaction, video-assisted parathyroidectomy requires 2 additional assistants, and may also be associated with a long learning curve.[98]

Both surgical approaches have not been widely adopted, and most parathyroid surgeons do not consider the techniques more efficacious than the current surgical treatment of primary hyperparathyroidism with focused parathyroidectomy or BNE.[99] In addition to the long learning curve necessary to gain proficiency in these techniques, these surgical approaches are contraindicated in patients with large thyroid goiters, previous neck surgery, MGD, MEN or non-MEN familial hyperparathyroidism, equivocal or negative preoperative localization studies, or parathyroid carcinoma. Nevertheless, despite these drawbacks it is the opinion of the chapter authors that surgeons keen on performing endoscopic or video-assisted parathyroidectomy should have considerable experience with the conventional approaches of focused parathyroidectomy and BNE before attempting these minimal access procedures.

REOPERATIVE PARATHYROIDECTOMY

Reoperative neck exploration for persistent or recurrent disease can be very difficult to perform due to loss of normal tissue planes and replacement by scar tissue. Such operations are associated with higher rates of injury to the recurrent laryngeal nerves as well as permanent hypoparathyroidism.[100] It is therefore paramount that the surgeon review all operative and pathology reports from previous neck operations to determine which parathyroid glands have been removed and remain. Biochemical tests should be repeated to confirm the correct diagnosis of primary hyperparathyroidism. Preoperative laryngoscopy should also be performed for vocal cord assessment before all reexplorations. Furthermore, imaging studies such as sestambi, US, and 4D-CT should be obtained in an attempt to localize the abnormal gland. Parathyroid localization before reoperative parathyroidectomy may minimize unnecessary dissection and reduce potential complications. If such imaging studies fail to localize the abnormal gland, jugular venous sampling in the clinic or selective venous PTH sampling by the radiologist can be performed at medical centers with such experience.[101] At time of reexploration, intraoperative adjuncts such as the radioguided probe or IPM may help localize the abnormal gland and confirm excision and cure.[74,91,92] Nerve monitoring may also be useful to the surgeon during reoperative cases.

The most important determinant of success in reoperative parathyroidectomy is an experienced parathyroid surgeon. These procedures, for instance, may require a partial or complete median sternotomy or video-assisted procedure for removal of a mediastinal parathyroid gland. Most of the time, however, the majority of missed parathyroid glands are found in the cervical region. The lateral or "back-door" approach for parathyroidectomy that involves the dissection between the anterior border of the sternocleidomastoid muscle and posterior border of the strap muscles may be implemented.[102] This maneuver is particularly useful in reoperative parathyroidectomy because it provides direct access to the posterior surface of the thyroid gland free of scar tissue from previous operations, performed through the conventional anterior approach. In such initial reoperations, experienced parathyroid surgeons can achieve success rates of up to 94%.[74,103]

SUMMARY

With the advent of improved preoperative parathyroid localization studies, increased availability of IPM, and the predominance of single-gland disease in most patients with primary hyperparathyroidism, focused parathyroidectomy has become the alternative to conventional BNE. The focused approach has durable cure rates of more than 95%, comparable to BNE, and it can be performed in an ambulatory setting with minimal morbidity. The additional advantages of focused parathyroidectomy include improved cosmetic results with smaller incisions, decreased postoperative pain, shorter operative time, decreased hospitalization, and rapid postoperative recovery, all most beneficial to patients treated for primary hyperparathyroidism. The focused approach has also served as an impetus for further investigation and development of more minimally invasive parathyroidectomy through endoscopic and video-enhanced methods, challenging the current methods of surgical therapy for parathyroid disease. Although some controversy continues to exist as to which operative approach should be considered the standard surgical treatment for primary hyperparathyroidism, nothing can replace the success of these operations performed by experienced parathyroid surgeons.

REFERENCES

1. Halsted WS. Hypoparathyreosis, status parathyreoprivus, and transplantation of the parathyroid glands. Am J Med Sci 1907;134:1–12.
2. Owen R. On the anatomy of the Indian rhinoceros (*Rh. unicornis*, L). Tran Zool Soc Lon 1862;4:31–58.
3. Sandstrom IV. On new gland in man and several mammals. Bull Hist Med 1938;6:192–222. English translation of "Glandulae Parathyreoidae," with biographical notes by Professor J. August Hammar [Carl M. Seipel]. Bull Ins Hist Med 1938;6:179–222.
4. Weiss N. Ueber Tetanie. Samml Klin Vortr, 189. Inn Med 1881;63:1675–704 [in German].
5. Gley ME. Sur les fonctions du corps thyroide. C R Seances Soc Biol Fil 1891;43:841–3 [in French].
6. Erdheim J. Tetania parathyreopriva. Mitt Grenzgeb Med Chir 1906;16:632–744 [in German].
7. MacCallum WJ, Voegtlin C. On the relation of the parathyroid to calcium metabolism and the nature of tetany. Bull Johns Hopkins Hosp 1908;19:91–2.
8. Askanazy M. Ueber ostitis deformans ohne osteides Gewebe. Arb Pathol Inst Tubingen (Leipzig) 1904;4:398–422 [in German].
9. Schlagenhaufer F. Zwei falle von parathyreoideatumoren. Wien Kiln Wochenschr 1915;28:1362 [in German].
10. Mandl F. Therapeutischer versuch bein einem falls von otitis fibrosa generalisata mittles. Exstirpation eines epithelkorperchentumors. Wien Klin Wochenschr Zentral 1926;53:260–4 [in German].
11. Guy CC. Tumors of the parathyroid glands. Surg Gynecol Obstet 1929;48:557–65.
12. Cope O. The story of hyperparathyroidism at the Massachusetts General Hospital. N Engl J Med 1966;274:1174–82.
13. Barr DP, Bulger HA, Dixon HH. Hyperparathyroidism. JAMA 1929;92:951–2.
14. Hanson AM. An elementary chemical study of the parathyroid glands of cattle. Mil Surgeon 1923;52:280–4.
15. Collip JP. Extraction of a parathyroid hormone which will prevent or control parathyroid tetany and which regulates the levels of blood calcium. J Biol Chem 1925;63:395–438.
16. Berson SA, Yalow RS, Auerbauch GD, et al. Immunoassay of bovine and human parathyroid hormone. Proc Natl Acad Sci U S A 1963;49:613–7.
17. Reiss E, Canterbury JM. A radioimmunoassay for parathyroid hormone in man. Proc Soc Exp Biol Med 1968;128:501–4.
18. Nussbaum SR, Zahrachnik RJ, Lavigne JR, et al. Highly sensitive two-site immunoradiometric assay of parathyrin, and its clinical utility in evaluating patients with hypercalcemia. Clin Chem 1987;33:1364–7.
19. Brown RC, Aston JP, Weeks I, et al. Circulating intact parathyroid hormone measured by a two-site immunochemiluminometric assay. J Clin Endocrinol Metab 1987;65:407–14.
20. Curley IR, Wheeler MH, Aston JP, et al. Studies in patients with hyperparathyroidism using a new two-site immunochemiluminometric assay for circulating intact (1–84) parathyroid hormone. Surgery 1987;102:926–31.
21. Irvin GL. Presidental address: chasin' hormones. Surgery 1999;126(6):993–7.

22. Irvin GL, Prudhomme DL, Deriso GT, et al. A new approach to parathyroidectomy. Ann Surg 1994;219(5):574–81.
23. Irvin GL, Sfakianakis G, Yeung L, et al. Ambulatory parathyroidectomy for primary hyperparathyroidism. Arch Surg 1996;131:1074–8.
24. Gilmour JR, Martin WJ. The weight of the parathyroid glands. J Pathol Bacteriol 1937;44:431–62.
25. Gilmour JR. The normal histology of the parathyroid glands. J Pathol Bacteriol 1937;48:187–222.
26. Akerstrom G, Malmaeus J, Bergstrom R. Surgical anatomy of human parathyroid glands. Surgery 1984;95(1):14–21.
27. Gilmour JR. The embryology of the parathyroid glands, the thymus and certain associated rudiments. J Pathol Bacteriol 1937;45:507–22.
28. Thompson NW, Eckhauser FE, Harness JK. The anatomy of the primary hyperparathyroidism. Surgery 1982;92:814–21.
29. Wermers RA, Khosla S, Atkinson EJ, et al. Incidence of primary hyperparathyroidism in Rochester, Minnesota, 1993–2001: an update on the changing epidemiology of the disease. J Bone Miner Res 2006;21(1):171–7.
30. Heath HW III, Hodgson SF, Kennedy MA. Primary hyperparathyroidism: incidence, morbidity and potential economic impact on the community. N Engl J Med 1980;302:189–93.
31. Chen H, Parkerson S, Udelsman R. Parathyroidectomy in the elderly: do the benefits outweigh the risks? World J Surg 1998;22:531–6.
32. Uden P, Chan A, Duh QY, et al. Primary hyperparathyroidism in younger and older patients: symptoms and outcome of surgery. World J Surg 1992;16:791–7.
33. Arnold A, Kim HG, Gaz RD, et al. Molecular cloning and chromosomal mapping of DNA rearranged with the parathyroid gene in a parathyroid adenomas. J Clin Invest 1989;83:2034–7.
34. Heppner C, Kester MB, Agarwal SK, et al. Somatic mutation of the MEN 1 gene in parathyroid tumours. Nat Genet 1997;16:375–8.
35. Carpten JD, Robbins CM, Villablanca, et al. HRPT2, encoding parafibromin, is mutated in hyperparathyroidism-jaw tumor syndrome. Nat Genet 2002;32:676–80.
36. Christensson T. Hyperparathyroidism and radiation therapy. Ann Intern Med 1978;89:216–7.
37. Eigelberger MS, Cheah WK, Ituarte PH, et al. The NIH criteria for parathyroidectomy in asymptomatic primary hyperparathyroidism: are they too limited? Ann Surg 2004;239(4):528–35.
38. Belezikian JP, Potts JP. Asymptomatic primary hyperparathyroidism: new issues and questions. J Bone Miner Res 2002;17(Suppl 2):N57–67.
39. Monchik JM, Gorgun E. Normocalcemic hyperparathyroidism in patients with osteoporosis. Surgery 2004;136(6):1242–6.
40. Tordjman KM, Greenman Y, Osher E. Characterization of normocalcemic primary hyperparathyroidism. Am J Med 2004;117(11):861–3.
41. Bilezikian JP, Potts JT Jr, Fuleihan Gel H, et al. Summary statement from a workshop on asymptomatic primary hyperparathyroidism: a perspective for the 21st century. J Clin Endocrinol Metab 2002;87(12):5353–61.
42. Kouvaraki MA, Greer M, Sharma S, et al. Indications for operative intervention in patients with asymptomatic primary hyperparathyroidism: practice patterns of endocrine surgery. Surgery 2006;139:527–34.
43. Pasieka JL, Parsons LL. Prospective surgical outcome study of relief of symptoms following surgery in patients with primary hyperparathyroidism. World J Surg 1998;22(6):513–9.

44. Rubin MR, Bilezikian JP, McMahon DJ, et al. The natural history of primary hyperparathyroidism with or without parathyroid surgery after 15 years. J Clin Endocrinol Metab 2008;93(9):3462–70.
45. Brennan MF. Lessons learned. Ann Surg Oncol 2006;13(10):1322–8.
46. Melton GB, Somervell H, Friedman KP, et al. Interpretation of 99mTc sestamibi parathyroid SPECT scan is improved when read by the surgeon and nuclear medicine physician together. Nucl Med Commun 2005;26(7):633–8.
47. Eslamy HK, Ziessman HA. Parathyroid scintigraphy in patients with primary hyperparathyroidism: 99mTc sestamibi SPECT and SPECT/CT. Radiographics 2008;28(5):1461–76.
48. Solorzano CC, Carneiro-Pla DM, Irvin GL. Surgeon performed ultrasound as the initial and only localizing study in sporadic primary hyperparathyroidism. J Am Coll Surg 2006;202(1):18–24.
49. Berri RN, Lloyd LR. Detection of parathyroid adenoma in patients with primary hyperparathyroidism: the use of office-based ultrasound in preoperative localization. Am J Surg 2006;191:311–4.
50. Kairys JC, Daskalakis C, Weigel RJ. Surgeon performed ultrasound for preoperative localization of abnormal parathyroid glands in patients with primary hyperparathyroidism. World J Surg 2006;30:1658–63.
51. Arici C, Cheah WK, Ituarte PHG, et al. Can localization studies be used to direct focused parathyroid operations? Surgery 2001;129(6):720–9.
52. Haber RS, Kim CK, Inabnet WB. Ultrasonography for preoperative localization of enlarged parathyroid glands in primary hyperparathyroidism: comparison with (99m) technetium sestamibi scintigraphy. Clin Endocrinol 2002;57:241–9.
53. Gawande AA, Monchik JM, Abbruzzese TA, et al. Reassessment of parathyroid hormone monitoring during parathyroidectomy for primary hyperparathyroidism after 2 preoperative localization studies. Arch Surg 2006;141(4):381–4.
54. Mihai R, Palazzo FF, Gleeson FV, et al. Minimally invasive parathyroidectomy without intraoperative parathyroid hormone monitoring in patients with primary hyperparathyroidism. Br J Surg 2007;94:42–7.
55. Rodgers SE, Hunter GJ, Hamberg LM, et al. Improved preoperative planning for directed parathyroidectomy with 4-dimensional computed tomography. Surgery 2006;140:932–40.
56. Chiu B, Sturgeon C, Angelos P. What is the link between nonlocalizing sestamibi scans, multigland disease and persistent hypercalcemia? A study of 401 consecutive patients undergoing parathyroidectomy. Surgery 2006;140:418–22.
57. Carniero-Pla DM, Solorzano CC, Irvin GL. Consequences of targeted parathyroidectomy guide by localizing studies without intraoperative parathyroid hormone monitoring. J Am Coll Surg 2006;202:715–22.
58. Yip L, Pryma DA, Yim JH, et al. Can a lightbulb sestamibi SPECT accurately predict single-gland disease in sporadic primary hyperparathyroidism. World J Surg 2008;32(5):784–92.
59. Casas A, Burke G, Sathyanarayana, et al. Prospective comparison of technetium-99m-sestamibi/iodine-123 radionuclide scan versus high-resolution ultrasonography for the preoperative localization of abnormal parathyroid glands in patients with previously unoperated primary hyperparathyroidism. Am J Surg 1993;166:369–73.
60. Caixas A, Berna L, Hernandez A, et al. Efficacy of preoperative diagnostic imaging localization of technetium 99m-sestamibi scintigraphy in hyperparathyroidism. Surgery 1997;121:535–41.

61. Sharma J, Mazzaglia P, Milas M, et al. Radionuclide imaging for hyperparathyroidism (HPT): which is the best technetium-99m sestamibi modality? Surgery 2006;140:856–63.
62. Anderson SR, Vaughn A, Karakla D, et al. Effectiveness of surgeon interpretation of technetium Tc 99m sestamibi scans in localizing parathyroid adenomas. Arch Otolaryngol Head Neck Surg 2008;134(9):953–7.
63. Ruda JM, Hollenbeak CS, Stack BC Jr. A systematic review of the diagnosis and treatment of primary hyperparathyroidism from 1995 to 2003. Otolaryngol Head Neck Surg 2005;132(3):359–72.
64. Lew JI, Solorzano CC, Montano RE, et al. Role of intraoperative parathormone monitoring during parathyroidectomy in patients with discordant localization studies. Surgery 2008;144(2):299–306.
65. Carneiro DM, Solorzano CC, Nader MC, et al. Comparison of intraoperative iPTH assay (QPTH) criteria in guiding parathyroidectomy: which criterion is the most accurate? Surgery 2003;134(6):973–81.
66. Clerici T, Brandle M, Lange J, et al. Impact of intraoperative parathyroid hormone monitoring on the prediction of multiglandular parathyroid disease. World J Surg 2004;28:187–92.
67. Chiu B, Sturgeon C, Angelos P. Which intraoperative parathyroid hormone assay criterion best predicts operative success? A study of 352 consecutive patients. Arch Surg 2006;141:483–8.
68. Carneiro-Pla DM, Solorzano CC, Lew JI, et al. Long term outcome of patients with intraoperative parathyroid hormone level remaining above the normal range during parathyroidectomy. Surgery 2008;144(6):989–94.
69. Perrier ND, Ituarte P, Kikuchi S, et al. Intraoperative parathyroid aspiration and parathyroid hormone assay as an alternative to frozen section for tissue identification. World J Surg 2000;24:1319–22.
70. Taylor J, Fraser W, Banaszkiewicz P, et al. Lateralization of parathyroid adenomas by intraoperative parathormone estimation. J R Coll Surg Edinb 1996;41:174–7.
71. Ito F, Sippel R, Lederman J, et al. The utility of intraoperative bilateral internal jugular venous sampling with rapid parathyroid hormone testing. Ann Surg 2007;245(6):959–63.
72. Boggs JE, Irvin GL, Carneiro DM, et al. The evolution of parathyroid failures. Surgery 1999;126(6):998–1003.
73. Chen H, Pruhs Z, Starling JR, et al. Intraoperative parathyroid hormone testing improves cure rates in patients undergoing minimally invasive parathyroidectomy. Surgery 2005;138(4):583–90.
74. Irvin GL, Molinari AS, Figueroa C, et al. Improved success rate in reoperative parathyroidectomy with intraoperative PTH assay. Ann Surg 1999;229(6):874–9.
75. Sackett WR, Barraclough B, Reeve TS, et al. World trends in the surgical treatment of primary hyperparathyroidism in the era of minimally invasive parathyroidectomy. Arch Surg 2002;137:1055–9.
76. Udelsman R. Six hundred fifty six consecutive explorations for primary hyperparathyroidism. Ann Surg 2002;235:665–72.
77. Westerdahl J, Lindblom P, Bergenfelz A. Measurement of intraoperative parathyroid hormone predicts long-term operative success. Arch Surg 2002;137(2):186–90.
78. Irvin GL, Carneiro DM, Solorzano CC. Progress in the operative management of sporadic primary hyperparathyroidism over 34 years. Ann Surg 2004;239(5):704–8.

79. Grant CS, Thompson G, Farley D, et al. Primary hyperparathyroidism surgical management since the introduction of minimally invasive parathyroidectomy: Mayo Clinic experience. Arch Surg 2005;140:472–8.
80. Irvin GL, Solorzano CC, Carneiro DM. Quick intraoperative parathyroid hormone assay: surgical adjunct to allow limited parathyroidectomy, improve success rate, and predict outcome. World J Surg 2004;28:1287–92.
81. Westerdahl J, Bergenfelz A. Unilateral versus bilateral neck exploration for primary hyperparathyroidism: five-year follow-up of a randomized controlled trial. Ann Surg 2007;246(6):976–81.
82. Siperstein A, Berber E, Barbosa GF, et al. Predicting the success of limited exploration for primary hyperparathyroidism using ultrasound, sestamibi and intraoperative parathyroid hormone: analysis of 1158 cases. Ann Surg 2008; 248(3):420–8.
83. Sidhu S, Neill AK, Russell CFJ. Long-term outcome of unilateral parathyroid exploration for primary hyperparathyroidism due to presumed solitary adenoma. World J Surg 2003;27(3):339–42.
84. Mun HC, Conigrave A, Wilkinson M, et al. Surgery for hyperparathyroidism: Does morphology or function matter most? Surgery 2005;138:758–65.
85. Elliott DD, Monroe DP, Perrier ND. Parathyroid histopathology: is it of any value today? J Am Coll Surg 2006;203(5):758–65.
86. Carneiro-Pla DM, Romaguera R, Nadji M, et al. Does histopathology predict parathyroid hypersecretion and influence correctly the extent of parathyroidectomy in patients with sporadic primary hyperparathyroidism? Surgery 2007; 142(6):930–5.
87. Kaplan EL, Yashiro T, Salti G. Primary hyperparathyroidism in the 1990s: choice of surgical procedures for this disease. Ann Surg 1992;215(4):300–17.
88. Allendorf J, DiGorgi M, Spanknebel K, et al. 1112 consecutive bilateral neck explorations for primary hyperparathyroidism. World J Surg 2007;31:2075–80.
89. Chen H, Mack E, Starling JR. Radioguided parathyroidectomy is equally effective for both adenomatous and hyperplastic glands. Ann Surg 2003;238(3): 332–8.
90. Chen H, Mack E, Starling JR. A comprehensive evaluation of perioperative adjuncts during minimally invasive parathyroidectomy: which is most reliable? Ann Surg 2005;242(3):375–80.
91. Inabnet WB, Dakin GF, Haber RS, et al. Targeted parathyroidectomy in the era of intraoperative parathormone monitoring. World J Surg 2002;26:921–5.
92. Jaskowiak NT, Sugg SL, Helke J, et al. Pitfalls of intraoperative quick parathyroid hormone monitoring and gamma probe localization in surgery for primary hyperparathyroidism. Arch Surg 2002;137(6):659–68.
93. Gagner M. Endoscopic subtotal parathyroidectomy in patients with primary hyperparathyroidism. Br J Surg 1996;83:875.
94. Ikeda Y, Takami H, Niimi M, et al. Endoscopic thyroidectomy and parathyroidectomy by the axillary approach. Surg Endosc 2002;16:92–5.
95. Ikeda Y, Takami H, Niimi M, et al. Endoscopic total parathyroidectomy by the anterior chest approach for renal hyperparathyroidism. Surg Endosc 2002; 16(2):320–2.
96. Henry JF, Defechereux T, Gramatica L, et al. Minimally invasive videoscopic parathyroidectomy by lateral approach. Langenbecks Arch Surg 1999;384(3): 298–301.
97. Miccoli P, Pinchera A, Cecchini G, et al. Minimally invasive video-assisted parathyroid surgery for hyperparathyroidism. J Endocrinol Invest 1997;20:429–30.

98. Miccoli P, Bendinelli C, Berti P, et al. Video-assisted versus conventional parathyroidectomy in primary hyperparathyroidism: a prospective randomized study. Surgery 1999;126:1117–22.
99. Duh QY. Presidential Address: minimally invasive endocrine surgery—standard of treatment or hype? Surgery 2003;134(6):849–57.
100. Jurhult J, Nordenstrom J, Perbeck L. Reoperation for suspected primary hyperparathyroidism. Br J Surg 1993;80:453–6.
101. Jones JJ, Brunaud L, Dowd CF, et al. Accuracy of selective venous sampling for intact parathyroid hormone in difficult patients with recurrent or persistent hyperparathyroidism. Surgery 2002;132:944–51.
102. Feind CR. Re-exploration for parathyroid adenoma. Am J Surg 1964;108:543–6.
103. Jaskowiak N, Norton JA, Alexander HR. A prospective trial evaluating a standard approach to reoperation for missed parathyroid adenoma. Ann Surg 1996; 224(3):308–22.

Secondary and Tertiary Hyperparathyroidism, State of the Art Surgical Management

Susan C. Pitt, MD, Rebecca S. Sippel, MD, Herbert Chen, MD*

KEYWORDS

- Secondary hyperparathyroidism
- Tertiary hyperparathyroidism • Radioguided
- Parathyroidectomy • Parathyroid hormone monitoring

Secondary and tertiary hyperparathyroidism (HPT) usually result from parathyroid gland hyperplasia that produces excess parathyroid hormone (PTH). Secondary and tertiary HPT comprise collectively a minority of the patients diagnosed with HPT. Due to the relative rarity of these conditions and common underlying disease pathology, they are frequently discussed and researched together. Although the disease processes are related, secondary and tertiary HPT are 2 distinct and separate entities.

ETIOLOGY

Secondary HPT occurs most commonly "secondary" to chronic renal failure (CRF). For this reason, secondary HPT is frequently referred to as renal HPT. Estimates report that as many as 90% of patients with CRF develop this disease by the time hemodialysis is initiated.[1] Other causes of secondary HPT include osteomalacia, rickets, and malabsorption. The pathophysiology of secondary HPT results from the relationship between CRF and parathyroid hyperplasia. Abnormalities in the renal tubular absorption of phosphate lead to reduced phosphate excretion and hyperphosphatemia. Impaired renal conversion of 25-hydroxycholecalciferal to 1,25-dihydroxycholecalciferol (vitamin D, calcitriol) also causes a decrease in the intestinal absorption of calcium. In combination, elevated serum phosphate levels and reduced vitamin D production result in decreases in serum calcium levels or hypocalcemia.

Susan Pitt's address will change in the next nine months, but is currently unknown. She is moving to St. Louis to Washington University in St. Louis.
Section of Endocrine Surgery, Department of Surgery, University of Wisconsin, 600 Highland Avenue, H4/722 CSC, Madison, WI 53792-3284, USA
* Corresponding author.
E-mail address: chen@surgery.wisc.edu (H. Chen).

Surg Clin N Am 89 (2009) 1227–1239
doi:10.1016/j.suc.2009.06.011
0039-6109/09/$ – see front matter © 2009 Elsevier Inc. All rights reserved.
surgical.theclinics.com

Hyperphosphatemia, and low vitamin D also cause elevated PTH levels. As a consequence of prolonged hypocalcemia, parathyroid chief cell hyperplasia occurs and PTH secretion increases. Skeletal resistance to PTH results in persistent and frequently extremely elevated PTH levels and renal osteopathy.

Tertiary HPT occurs most commonly in the setting of renal transplant whereby patients with secondary HPT continue to have elevated PTH levels after receiving a renal allograft. This disease is observed in up to 30% of kidney transplant recipients and was first described in the early 1960s.[2] After undergoing transplantation, these patients have persistent or recurrent (secondary) HPT after an initial period of resolution. However, tertiary HPT can develop after any long-standing period of hypocalcemia such as those seen with chronic dialysis or gastrointestinal malabsorption. In these patients, prolonged hypocalcemia also causes parathyroid chief cell hyperplasia and excess PTH. After correction of the primary disorder (CRF) by renal transplant, the hypertrophied parathyroid tissue fails to resolute and continues to oversecrete PTH. Serum calcium levels consequently are normal or even elevated in these patients because the hyperplastic glands function autonomously despite withdrawal of calcium and calcitriol therapy. Tertiary HPT is classically caused by hyperplasia of all 4 glands, though some reports indicate that more than 20% of patients may have single or double adenomas as the underlying pathology.[2,3] Whether these cases represent posttransplant patients in whom sporadic primary HPT (adenomas) has developed or resolution of autonomous function in all but 1 or 2 glands is unclear. Tertiary HPT in this subset of patients may also result from asymmetric hyperplasia.[2]

DIAGNOSIS

The diagnosis and workup of patients with secondary and tertiary HPT combine clinical and laboratory investigation. Many patients with these diseases are asymptomatic and will only have abnormalities detectable by laboratory and radiographic studies. In patients with secondary HPT, laboratory tests may reveal hypocalcemia or normocalcemia and hyperphosphatemia. In addition, patients with secondary HPT have extremely elevated intact PTH levels and decreased vitamin D levels. In contrast, patients with tertiary HPT will have normal or elevated serum calcium concentrations in combination with moderately elevated intact PTH levels. Laboratory tests in patients with tertiary HPT may also reveal decreased vitamin D (1,25-dihydroxycholecalciferol) and phosphate levels, and elevated alkaline phosphatase levels. Patients with both diseases also can become symptomatic. Untreated secondary HPT leads to progressive bone disease, osteitis fibrosa cystica, and soft tissue calcifications. Patients with tertiary HPT may experience bone pain or fractures, pruritus, nephrolithiasis, pancreatitis, soft tissue or vascular calcifications, and mental status changes. Plain radiography films or bone density studies can show changes consistent with osteopenia or osteoporosis. Imaging of the neck is normally unnecessary, because secondary and tertiary HPT primarily result from 4-gland hyperplasia. However, preoperative imaging may be useful in facilitating surgery, especially in the reoperative setting and if one of the glands is in an ectopic position.

MEDICAL TREATMENT OF SECONDARY AND TERTIARY HPT

Management of patients with secondary HPT is predominantly medical, whereas treatment of patients with tertiary HPT is surgical. Supplementation of calcium using oral calcitriol and vitamin D is usually sufficient to manage PTH levels in patients with CRF and secondary HPT. To treat patients with secondary HPT who become refractory to replacement of calcium and vitamin D, several alternative therapies have become available over the last 10 to 15 years. These treatment options include calcimimetics, such as cinacalcet, new phosphate binders, and vitamin D analogues that are less likely to result in hypercalcemia.[4–6] These agents are designed to bridge patients to renal transplant, the optimal treatment for secondary HPT.

In patients with tertiary HPT, medical treatment is not curative and, generally, not indicated. In contrast to patients with secondary HPT, these patients are not routinely given oral calcium and phosphate binders because they are typically normocalcemic or hypercalcemic and concurrently hypophosphatemic. Vitamin D (calcitriol) supplementation can be prescribed, but often only delays surgical intervention because patients typically become refractory to vitamin D replacement. Supplementing phosphate levels with oral agents can lead to nephrocalcinosis and hyperphosphaturia, and should be performed sparingly.

INDICATIONS FOR SURGICAL MANAGEMENT

Although novel methods for medically treating patients with secondary HPT have been introduced, surgical intervention is still necessary at times. About 1% to 2% of patients with secondary HPT require parathyroidectomy each year.[7] In the early 1960s the first operations for patients with renal HPT were performed. The indications for parathyroidectomy in secondary HPT are listed in **Box 1**. The most life-threatening indication for parathyroidectomy in patients with secondary HPT is calciphylaxis, which occurs in only 4% of patients undergoing surgery.[8] Calciphylaxis results in expanding, painful, cutaneous, purpuritic lesions that cause tissue calcification and ischemic necrosis, which lead to dry gangrene if untreated (**Fig. 1**). Overwhelming sepsis and wound breakdown cause significant mortality, as high as 87% in one report.[9] In patients with calciphylaxis who are urgently treated with total parathyroidectomy, wound healing is enhanced and median survival is prolonged.[10] In addition, surgery has been shown to help avoid amputation, decrease pain, and reduce the use of narcotics.[11]

Unlike patients with secondary HPT, the mainstay of treatment of tertiary HPT is surgery. The development of tertiary HPT requiring surgical intervention occurs in 1% to 5% of patients with HPT after undergoing kidney transplant.[3,7,12] Indications for parathyroidectomy in patients with tertiary HPT are listed in **Box 2**. Additional minor

---

Box 1
Indications for parathyroidectomy in patients with secondary HPT

Calciphylaxis

Patient preference

Medical observation not possible

Failure of maximal medical management with:

Hypercalcemia

Hypercalcuria

PTH >800 pg/mL

Hyperphosphatemia (with calcium × phosphorus >70)

Osteoporosis

Symptoms: pruritus, pathologic bone fracture, ectopic soft tissue calcifications, severe vascular calcifications, bone pain

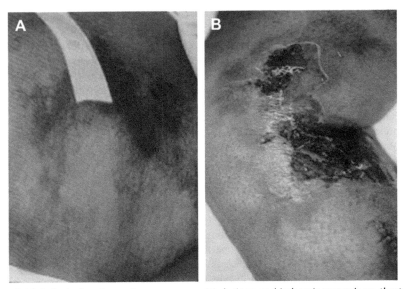

Fig. 1. Calciphylaxis showing cutaneous purpuritic lesions and ischemic necrosis on the torso (*A*) and medial leg (*B*) of a patient with secondary HPT.

indications that have been proposed include renal phosphorus wasting (including hypophosphatemia) and parathyroid gland weight >500 mg on ultrasound evaluation.[7] Unfortunately, evidence-based guidelines on the selection criteria for parathyroidectomy in patients with tertiary HPT are inconsistent.

PREOPERATIVE LOCALIZATION STUDIES

After the decision to proceed with surgery has been made, preoperative localization studies are not always routinely performed in patients with secondary or tertiary HPT for many reasons. However, localization is useful in terms of identifying otherwise

---

Box 2
Indications for parathyroidectomy in patients with tertiary HPT

Severe hypercalcemia (serum calcium >11.5 or 12 mg/dL)

Persistent hypercalcemia (serum calcium >10.2 mg/dL more than 3 months to 1 year after surgery)

Severe osteopenia (low bone mineral density)

Symptomatic HPT

    Fatigue

    Pruritis

    Bone pain or pathologic bone fracture

    Peptic ulcer disease

    Mental status changes

    History of renal calculi

unsuspected ectopic glands and facilitating the operation in reoperative cases. First, the diseases result in hyperplasia of all 4 parathyroid glands. The sensitivity of imaging modalities such as ^{99m}Tc-sestimibi scintigraphy and ultrasound is poor in patients with multiple gland disease, regardless of the cause of HPT.[13–15] In a study that examined patients with both secondary and tertiary HPT, ^{99m}Tc-sestamibi scintigraphy failed to identify all hyperfunctioning parathyroids in every case.[11] In another investigation, the reported sensitivities of preoperative localization with ^{99m}Tc-sestimibi and ultrasound in patients operated on for an initial diagnosis of tertiary HPT were 9% and 67%, respectively.[16] Other techniques such as computed tomography and magnetic resonance imaging (MRI) have been described, but in few cases.[16]

In patients with primary HPT and single adenomas, localizing studies are advantageous because they allow identification of parathyroid glands in ectopic locations. In patients with secondary and tertiary HPT, the ability of imaging techniques to identify ectopic parathyroids is limited. Ectopic mediastinal glands were identified in only 38% of patients with secondary and tertiary HPT who were discovered to harbor mediastinal parathyroids at surgery.[11] In an analysis of patients with only tertiary HPT, localization of ectopic glands with ^{99m}Tc-sestimibi scintigraphy, ultrasound, or MRI was not demonstrated in any case despite 32% of the study subjects having ectopic parathyroids at the time of surgery.[16] Another rationale for not performing preoperative imaging is that the surgical approach is unlikely to change; bilateral neck exploration is the standard of care for all patients with secondary and tertiary HPT. Even in series that have investigated single and double adenomas as the underlying cause of tertiary HPT, thorough exploration of the neck is still the recommended procedure.[3,12,16,17] As a result, routine preoperative imaging is not recommended before a primary resection for secondary or tertiary HPT. The use of imaging in cases of recurrent or persistent HPT before a reexploration is strongly encouraged and is discussed later in this review.

OPERATIVE APPROACHES

The surgical approaches described for patients with secondary and tertiary HPT are similar. For patients with secondary HPT who meet the indications for operative management, 3 different surgical procedures utilizing a bilateral neck exploration have been described. These surgeries include subtotal parathyroidectomy (removal of 3 and one-half glands leaving a remnant in situ), total parathyroidectomy (4-gland resection) with autotransplantation, and total parathyroidectomy without autotransplantation. Surgical management of tertiary HPT can be performed using either one of two accepted approaches: subtotal parathyroidectomy or total parathyroidectomy with autotransplantation. In all cases, cryopreservation of resected tissue is important to address possible complications of postoperative hypoparathyroidism wherein the autograft or remnant fails to function. The surgical procedure performed is often due to surgeon's preference. At their institution the authors favor total parathyroidectomy with autotransplantation and cryopreservation of the remaining parathyroid tissue for treatment of patients with secondary HPT (**Fig. 2**). When performing this procedure, marking the reimplanted tissue in the forearm with nonabsorbable silk suture and a hemoclip is important. If persistent or recurrent HPT occurs after total parathyroidectomy with autotransplantation, reoperation in these patients can be performed under local anesthesia only, unless the persistence or recurrence is due to missed parathyroid glands at the initial operation. In patients with tertiary HPT, the authors prefer subtotal parathyroidectomy that leaves the native blood supply to half of a parathyroid intact and, theoretically, is associated with a reduced risk of

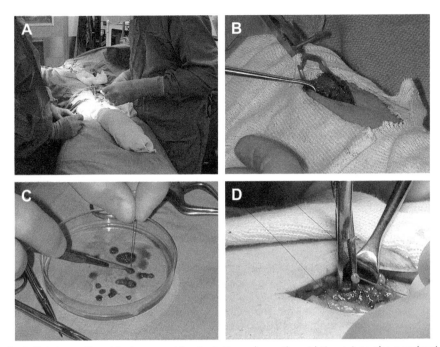

Fig. 2. Total parathyroidectomy and implantation of parathyroid tissue into the nondominant forearm. Before surgery the nondominant forearm should be prepped (*A*). After a small incision is made (*B*) and 50 to 100 mg of parathyroid tissue is dissected from a gland (*C*), the parathyroid tissue is transplanted into the brachioradialis muscle (*D*).

hypocalcemia. Advocates of this procedure recommend carrying out a biopsy and marking (with a clip or suture) the most normal-appearing gland first. If the tissue remains viable, the remaining 3 glands can be excised, and the biopsied parathyroid is left in situ. In the event that reoperation in the neck is necessary after subtotal parathyroidectomy, marking the parathyroid remnant is very important to facilitate dissection.

For patients with tertiary HPT, simultaneous thymectomy can be performed with either subtotal or total parathyroidectomy. Some surgeons routinely resect the thymus bilaterally to reduce the risk of recurrence, because ectopic glands are frequently found within the thymic tissue. However, the authors' approach is to only resect the thymus if an inferior gland cannot be found or when the radioguided probe suggests increased activity within an area of the thymus. Data on thymectomy in these patients are lacking.

In addition to these traditional surgical approaches, limited or less-than-subtotal parathyroid resection in select patients with only 1 or 2 diseased glands has been described in patients with tertiary HPT, but remains controversial.[2,3,16,18–21] Traditionally caused by hyperplasia of all 4 glands, tertiary HPT also can result from a single or double adenoma, asymmetric hyperplasia, or incomplete resolution of all hyperplastic glands in up to 30% of patients.[2,3] Of note, bilateral neck exploration should still be performed in all of these cases with resection of only the diseased glands. Intraoperative PTH (ioPTH) measurement can aid in identifying these cases with the goal being more than a 50% drop at 10 minutes.[18] Studies have shown equivalent (more than 95%) success rates using a limited approach compared with subtotal or total parathyroidectomy based on normocalcemia and symptom improvement postoperatively.[3,20] However, Triponez and colleagues reported a 5.2 times greater risk of persistent or recurrent HPT after limited resection for tertiary HPT.[21] The difference between the results of these reports may result from the indications for performing a less-than-subtotal resection. If only 1 or 2 glands were resected in a patient with tertiary HPT because other glands could not be located, and the patient has 4 hyperplastic parathyroids, the rate of persistent or recurrent disease should be 100% because an inadequate resection has been performed.

OUTCOMES AFTER PARATHYROIDECTOMY

Surgeon preference is often the main driving force behind the type of operation performed in patients with secondary and tertiary HPT. Overall, the success rates after any form of parathyroidectomy discussed are high. The differences between procedures are related more to risks of recurrence and complications. To date, several retrospective analyses and one randomized trial have attempted to identify the superiority of one surgical approach over another in patients with secondary HPT. However, direct comparisons between surgical approaches have not been made in patients with tertiary HPT.

In a study that randomized 40 patients with secondary HPT to either subtotal parathyroidectomy or total parathyroidectomy with autografting, the cure rate was higher and the recurrence rate lower after total parathyroidectomy.[22] Patients undergoing total parathyroidectomy with implantation had significantly better calcium level normalization, improved bone mineral density, and less pruritus and muscle weakness.[22] Because reoperation is simpler in the forearm, these investigators favor total parathyroidectomy with autotransplantation over subtotal surgery in patients with secondary HPT. Despite these findings, a retrospective review of the same 2 procedures performed for secondary HPT found no difference in the rates of failure or recurrence.[23] The results of this review do support the findings that patients treated with total parathyroidectomy and autotransplantation have significantly higher calcium levels and bone remineralization after surgery.[23] In these 2 studies, 100% of patients with secondary HPT who underwent total parathyroidectomy and autotransplantation were considered cured compared with 90% of patients after subtotal parathyroidectomy.[22,23] A variation of subtotal surgery described as "near-total" parathyroidectomy, in which the parathyroid remnant is made more precisely, has a cure rate of 96%.[11]

Although subtotal parathyroidectomy or total parathyroidectomy with autotransplantation have been the standard procedures of choice for patients with secondary HPT, more recently total parathyroidectomy without autotransplantation has been proposed. In a retrospective analysis of total parathyroidectomy with and without autotransplantation, one group showed a significantly higher rate of recurrence in patients with autografts in the forearm tissue versus those without autografts (45% vs 0%).[24] Lorenz and colleagues also revealed a recurrence rate of 0% after total parathyroidectomy without autotransplantation.[25] Therefore, these studies favor total parathyroidectomy without autotransplantation because omission of the forearm autograft seems to prevent recurrence.

In patients with tertiary HPT, success rates after surgery also are high. Furthermore, similar outcomes are observed after subtotal parathyroidectomy when compared with total parathyroidectomy with autotransplantation. In several reviews, many with long-term follow-up, more than 94% of patients with tertiary HPT achieved biochemical cure on the basis of total serum calcium levels after subtotal parathyroidectomy,[3,11,14,16] although one study reported that only 71% of patients also had normalized PTH levels.[16] In addition, symptoms are improved in more than 90% of patients with tertiary HPT treated by subtotal parathyroidectomy.[3,14]

PERSISTENT OR RECURRENT HPT

After operation for secondary or tertiary HPT, management of persistent or recurrent disease is challenging to the surgeon and radiologist alike. Persistent secondary and tertiary HPT generally results from an inadequate initial resection or a missed fifth or ectopic gland and requires reoperation. In patients with secondary HPT, the risk of developing recurrent HPT increases over time and can occur after any of the surgical procedures. Subtotal and total parathyroidectomy with autotransplantation have higher rates of recurrence in patients with secondary HPT (reported range 5%–80%) compared with total parathyroidectomy without autotransplantation (reported range 0%–4%) due to hyperplasia of the parathyroid remnant.[17,24,26] However, in patients with tertiary HPT, recurrence rates are equivalent among the surgical approaches discussed. Rates of recurrence after operation for tertiary HPT range from 0% to 8% and are increased in patients with a nodular variety of hyperplasia, an elevated proliferative index, or redevelopment of CRF.[3,14,16,20]

In patients with persistent or recurrent HPT due to residual functioning parathyroid tissue, reoperation is facilitated by preoperative localization. ^{99m}Tc-sestamibi scintigraphy of the neck, mediastinum, or forearm is advantageous in these cases because only a single hyperfunctioning focus remains. Chou and colleagues demonstrated that ^{99m}Tc-sestamibi scanning successfully identified the parathyroid remnant in 85% of patients with persistent or recurrent secondary HPT.[27] The locations of these remaining glands were in the normal anatomic position, carotid sheath, and mediastinum, indicating the usefulness of this test in identifying ectopic parathyroids.[27] Patients with persistent or recurrent tertiary HPT benefit from preoperative localization studies as well. The true positive rates of localization for ^{99m}Tc-sestimibi scans, ultrasound, and MRI were 100% for each of these modalities in this population.[16] If imaging of the neck and forearm fails to identify the location of the active parathyroid, differential PTH sampling of the arms can be performed, with a gradient of 20:1 suggesting forearm graft hyperplasia. On rare occasions transplanted tissue is placed into the sternocleidomastoid muscles.

Surgical treatment of persistent or recurrent secondary or tertiary HPT in patients who have undergone total parathyroidectomy with autotransplantation can be performed under local anesthesia and avoids the risks associated with reexploration of the neck, such as recurrent laryngeal nerve injury. Success rates for reoperation in secondary HPT patients with persistent disease range from 89% to 100%, whereas patients with recurrent secondary HPT have success 70% to 100% of the time.[27,28] One study found that the success rate of reoperation for recurrent secondary HPT was significantly better in patients undergoing initial subtotal resection compared with total resection with autotransplantation (87% vs 70%, $P = .02$).[28] This finding is counterintuitive because reoperation on the forearm is theoretically easier compared with the neck. However, the recurrence was located in the neck or mediastinum in more than 50% of the patients initially treated with total parathyroidectomy and forearm grafting.[28]

IOPTH MONITORING

Surgical adjuncts that have revolutionized the treatment of patients with primary HPT have been applied to patients with secondary and tertiary HPT as well. In particular, ioPTH measurement is now being used in patients with both secondary and tertiary HPT. However, unlike patients with primary disease, surgery for either disease still requires bilateral exploration to remove all 4 parathyroid glands. IoPTH monitoring is complicated in this patient population because of impaired renal function and delayed renal clearance of PTH. Conflicting results regarding the usefulness of ioPTH monitoring for secondary HPT have been published.[29–32] Studies have shown that ioPTH testing depends on renal function and PTH assay specificity.[29,30,32] However, studies differ in their definition of successful parathyroidectomy. When a 50% drop from the baseline ioPTH is considered predictive of sufficient parathyroid tissue resection, these investigations support the utility of ioPTH monitoring in patients with secondary HPT. Depending on the specificity of the assay, an adequate drop in ioPTH levels (>50%) may not be seen for up to 30 minutes after curative resection because of CRF and delayed PTH clearance.[29,30,32]

For both initial and reoperative treatment of patients with tertiary HPT, ioPTH testing also has been shown to be beneficial.[11,18,31,33,34] However, the ioPTH criteria that are predictive of cure in these patients are debated. Applying the traditional Miami criteria proposed for patients with primary HPT (>50% ioPTH drop at 10 minutes) affords a 94% or greater sensitivity in patients with tertiary HPT.[18,33] In patients with primary HPT from hyperplasia, a final ioPTH level of less than 35 pg/mL or a greater than 90% drop from baseline is predictive of cure about 90% of the time, suggesting that a cutoff ioPTH value should be utilized in patients with multigland disease of any cause.[34] In patients with tertiary HPT, Milas and Weber have proposed that a target ioPTH level less than 200 pg/mL predicts curative resections, whereas others support an ioPTH level less than 65 pg/mL.[11,31,34] Lack of consensus guidelines for ioPTH monitoring in patients with tertiary HPT and skepticism over the potential impact on the overall success rate of parathyroidectomy has led some groups to abandon the routine use of this adjunct.[33] However, one investigation did report that ioPTH impacted operative management in 16% of cases.[18]

RADIOGUIDED PARATHYROIDECTOMY

Another state of the art advance that some believe facilitates intraoperative management of patients with secondary and tertiary HPT is application of radioguided techniques. Patients are injected with 10 mCi of ^{99m}Tc-sestamibi approximately 1 to 2 hours before surgery. A gamma probe is then utilized in the same manner as in primary HPT except that all 4 glands are explored.[35] Therefore, this technique should be applicable to patients with secondary or tertiary HPT.

The authors have previously shown that radioguidance reduces operative time, length of stay, and the need for frozen section in patients with secondary and tertiary HPT.[19] Other reports also support the use of radioguided parathyroidectomy in this patient population.[36–38] The ability of the gamma probe to locate supernumerary and ectopic parathyroid glands decreases the risk of persistent or recurrent disease and is an advantage associated with using this technology in patients with secondary and tertiary HPT.[19] The radioguided probe also is advantageous in patients with recurrent HPT from forearm graft hyperplasia, especially if the parathyroid fragment is unmarked.[39] Another benefit of the gamma probe is that it can confirm the presence of parathyroid tissue and omit the need for frozen section or ioPTH of tissue aspirate.[12,19] Thus, radioguided surgery can be a useful adjunct in patient with secondary and tertiary HPT.

CRYOPRESERVATION

In any patient undergoing subtotal or total parathyroidectomy, regardless of HPT etiology, cryopreservation of parathyroid tissue should be obligatory. The success rates of cryopreserved autografts are variable throughout the literature, but are always lower than immediate, fresh autografts. In a study of long-term functionality of cryopreserved tissue, about 60% of autografts are functional to some degree; however, less than 50% of patients had fully functioning tissue.[40] These data also suggested that the duration of cryopreservation predicted graft failure, and no functioning autografts occurred after 2 years of cryopreservation.[40]

COMPLICATIONS

When performing any of these operations, the risks of postoperative hypocalcemia must be considered. Accelerated bone remineralization ("hungry bone syndrome") and delayed forearm graft or cervical remnant function increase the risk of transient hypocalcemia. Thus, supplementation with calcium and vitamin D immediately after surgery helps to prevent hypocalcemia during the postoperative period. Oral calcium carbonate (2–3 g) is recommended with or without calcitriol initiated immediately following parathyroidectomy. Patients with secondary HPT are typically already on calcium and calcitriol and are continued postoperatively.

Because the procedures performed for secondary and tertiary HPT are the same, complications after subtotal or total parathyroidectomy are common to both diseases. The most frequently reported minor complication after subtotal or total parathyroidectomy is transient hypocalcemia, which varies widely but generally is observed in 15% to 30% of patients.[3,16,20] Severe or permanent hypocalcemia requiring prolonged admission or readmission for intravenous calcium, or lifelong calcium and vitamin D supplementation also is seen, but much less frequently (0% to 7%).[3,11,16,20] In addition, hypoparathyroidism requiring reimplantation of cryopreserved tissue has been reported in up to 7% of patients.[2,10,14,32] Recurrent laryngeal nerve injuries are frequently discussed, but typically are transient neuropraxias, and permanent injuries occur in only about 1% of cases.[3,7,16,20] Other complications such as wound infection, hematomas, dehiscence, and death have been described, but are rarely seen. Cardiac dysrhythmias, gout or pseudogout, pancreatitis, and renal failure may develop secondary to hypocalcemia or hypoparathyroidism, though these complications are exceedingly rare.

SUMMARY

Despite advances in medical and surgical treatment, the incidence of secondary and tertiary HPT is on the rise in the United States and elsewhere because of the increasing incidence and prevalence of CRF.[41] From 1990 to 2001, according to the United States Renal Data System (USRDS), the prevalence of CRF increased more than 100%. Because of earlier diagnosis of secondary HPT and new medical treatment options, the incidence of parathyroidectomy in this population has been constant or decreasing throughout the world even though the incidence of secondary HPT has increased.[37,41] Nonetheless, cutting-edge innovations including ioPTH testing using rapid PTH assays and the use of radioguided gamma probe have kept the surgical treatment of secondary HPT current with the times.

In the face of medical and surgical advances, ongoing controversy remains concerning the optimal surgical management of patients with secondary HPT, largely due to the relatively small number of patients to study. A multi-institutional randomized controlled trial of all 3 procedures would be ideal, but challenging to organize and conduct. At present a trial comparing total parathyroidectomy without autotransplantation or thymectomy to total parathyroidectomy with autotransplantation and thymectomy in patients with secondary HPT is under way.[28]

Surgical management of secondary and tertiary HPT is safe and effective at correcting bone mineralization and metabolic disturbances. Improved neuropsychiatric symptoms, survival, and quality of life with reduced cardiovascular events also are benefits of parathyroidectomy. The most commonly accepted approaches in these patients are subtotal parathyroidectomy or total parathyroidectomy with autotransplantation of parathyroid tissue into the nondominant forearm. Techniques such as intraoperative PTH monitoring and radioguided surgery have advanced these surgical procedures by eliminating the need for frozen section and decreasing operative times. Whereas surgery remains the only cure for patients with tertiary HPT, the treatment of secondary HPT is predominantly medical, using newer calcimimetics, phosphate binders, and vitamin D analogues. Future advances in the surgical management of these patients will likely require the creation of consensus guidelines and multi-institutional collaborative studies.

REFERENCES

1. Memmos D, Williams G, Eastwood J, et al. The role of parathyroidectomy in the management of hyperparathyroidism in patients on maintenance haemodialysis and after renal transplantation. Nephron 1982;30:143–8.
2. Kerby J, Rue L, Blair H, et al. Operative treatment of tertiary hyperparathyroidism: a single-center experience. Ann Surg 1998;227:878–86.
3. Kilgo M, Pirsch J, Warner T, et al. Tertiary hyperparathyroidism after renal transplantation: surgical strategy. Surgery 1998;124:677–83 [discussion: 83–4].
4. Block G, Martin K, de Francisco A, et al. Cinacalcet for secondary hyperparathyroidism in patients receiving hemodialysis. N Engl J Med 2004;350: 1516–25.
5. Martin K, González E, Gellens M, et al. 19-Nor-1-alpha-25-dihydroxyvitamin D2 (Paricalcitol) safely and effectively reduces the levels of intact parathyroid hormone in patients on hemodialysis. J Am Soc Nephrol 1998;9:1427–32.
6. Slatopolsky E, Burke S, Dillon M. RenaGel, a nonabsorbed calcium- and aluminum-free phosphate binder, lowers serum phosphorus and parathyroid hormone. The RenaGel Study Group. Kidney Int 1999;55:299–307.
7. Triponez F, Clark O, Vanrenthergem Y, et al. Surgical treatment of persistent hyperparathyroidism after renal transplantation. Ann Surg 2008;248:18–30.
8. Angelis M, Wong L, Myers S, et al. Calciphylaxis in patients on hemodialysis: a prevalence study. Surgery 1997;122:1083–9 [discussion: 9–90].
9. Coates T, Kirkland G, Dymock R, et al. Cutaneous necrosis from calcific uremic arteriolopathy. Am J Kidney Dis 1998;32:384–91.
10. Girotto J, Harmon J, Ratner L, et al. Parathyroidectomy promotes wound healing and prolongs survival in patients with calciphylaxis from secondary hyperparathyroidism. Surgery 2001;130:645–50 [discussion: 50–1].
11. Milas M, Weber C. Near-total parathyroidectomy is beneficial for patients with secondary and tertiary hyperparathyroidism. Surgery 2004;136:1252–60.
12. Jorna F, Jager P, Lemstra C, et al. Utility of an intraoperative gamma probe in the surgical management of secondary or tertiary hyperparathyroidism. Am J Surg 2008;196:13–8.

13. Haciyanli M, Lal G, Morita E, et al. Accuracy of preoperative localization studies and intraoperative parathyroid hormone assay in patients with primary hyperparathyroidism and double adenoma. J Am Coll Surg 2003;197:739–46.

14. Punch J, Thompson N, Merion R. Subtotal parathyroidectomy in dialysis-dependent and post-renal transplant patients. A 25-year single-center experience. Arch Surg 1995;130:538–42 [discussion: 42–3].

15. Sebag F, Hubbard J, Maweja S, et al. Negative preoperative localization studies are highly predictive of multiglandular disease in sporadic primary hyperparathyroidism. Surgery 2003;134:1038–41 [discussion: 41–2].

16. Kebebew E, Duh Q, Clark O. Tertiary hyperparathyroidism: histologic patterns of disease and results of parathyroidectomy. Arch Surg 2004;139:974–7.

17. Zou Q, Wang H, Zhou J, et al. Total parathyroidectomy combined with partial auto-transplantation for the treatment of secondary hyperparathyroidism. Chin Med J (Engl) 2007;120:1777–82.

18. Haustein S, Mack E, Starling J, et al. The role of intraoperative parathyroid hormone testing in patients with tertiary hyperparathyroidism after renal transplantation. Surgery 2005;138:1066–71 [discussion: 71].

19. Nichol P, Mack E, Bianco J, et al. Radioguided parathyroidectomy in patients with secondary and tertiary hyperparathyroidism. Surgery 2003;134:713–7 [discussion: 7–9].

20. Nichol P, Starling J, Mack E, et al. Long-term follow-up of patients with tertiary hyperparathyroidism treated by resection of a single or double adenoma. Ann Surg 2002;235:673–8 [discussion: 8–80].

21. Triponez F, Kebebew E, Dosseh D, et al. Less-than-subtotal parathyroidectomy increases the risk of persistent/recurrent hyperparathyroidism after parathyroidectomy in tertiary hyperparathyroidism after renal transplantation. Surgery 2006;140:990–7 [discussion: 7–9].

22. Rothmund M, Wagner P, Schark C. Subtotal parathyroidectomy versus total parathyroidectomy and autotransplantation in secondary hyperparathyroidism: a randomized trial. World J Surg 1991;15:745–50.

23. Gagné E, Ureña P, Leite-Silva S, et al. Short- and long-term efficacy of total parathyroidectomy with immediate autografting compared with subtotal parathyroidectomy in hemodialysis patients. J Am Soc Nephrol 1992;3:1008–17.

24. Ockert S, Willeke F, Richter A, et al. Total parathyroidectomy without autotransplantation as a standard procedure in the treatment of secondary hyperparathyroidism. Langenbecks Arch Surg 2002;387:204–9.

25. Lorenz K, Ukkat J, Sekulla C, et al. Total parathyroidectomy without autotransplantation for renal hyperparathyroidism: experience with a qPTH-controlled protocol. World J Surg 2006;30:743–51.

26. Skinner K, Zuckerbraun L. Recurrent secondary hyperparathyroidism. An argument for total parathyroidectomy. Arch Surg 1996;131:724–7.

27. Chou F, Lee C, Chen H, et al. Persistent and recurrent hyperparathyroidism after total parathyroidectomy with autotransplantation. Ann Surg 2002;235:99–104.

28. Schlosser K, Veit J, Witte S, et al. Comparison of total parathyroidectomy without autotransplantation and without thymectomy versus total parathyroidectomy with autotransplantation and with thymectomy for secondary hyperparathyroidism: TOPAR PILOT-Trial. Trial 2007;8:22.

29. Bieglmayer C, Kaczirek K, Prager G, et al. Parathyroid hormone monitoring during total parathyroidectomy for renal hyperparathyroidism: pilot study of the impact of renal function and assay specificity. Clin Chem 2006;52:1112–9.

30. Chou F, Lee C, Chen J, et al. Intraoperative parathyroid hormone measurement in patients with secondary hyperparathyroidism. Arch Surg 2002;137:341–5.
31. Kaczirek K, Prager G, Riss P, et al. Novel parathyroid hormone (1-84) assay as basis for parathyroid hormone monitoring in renal hyperparathyroidism. Arch Surg 2006;141:129–34 [discussion: 34].
32. Kaczirek K, Riss P, Wunderer G, et al. Quick PTH assay cannot predict incomplete parathyroidectomy in patients with renal hyperparathyroidism. Surgery 2005;137:431–5.
33. Triponez F, Dosseh D, Hazzan M, et al. Accuracy of intra-operative PTH measurement during subtotal parathyroidectomy for tertiary hyperparathyroidism after renal transplantation. Langenbecks Arch Surg 2006;391:561–5.
34. Weber K, Misra S, Lee J, et al. Intraoperative PTH monitoring in parathyroid hyperplasia requires stricter criteria for success. Surgery 2004;136:1154–9.
35. Chen H, Mack E, Starling J. Radioguided parathyroidectomy is equally effective for both adenomatous and hyperplastic glands. Ann Surg 2003;238:332–7 [discussion: 7–8].
36. Kitagawa W, Shimizu K, Akasu H, et al. Radioguided parathyroidectomy for renal hyperparathyroidism. Med Sci Monit 2003;9:CS9–12.
37. Malberti F, Marcelli D, Conte F, et al. Parathyroidectomy in patients on renal replacement therapy: an epidemiologic study. J Am Soc Nephrol 2001;12: 1242–8.
38. Oyama Y, Kazama J, Maruyama H, et al. Combined radioguided parathyroidectomy and intravenous vitamin D therapy for the treatment of uraemic hyperparathyroidism. Nephrol Dial Transplant 2003;18(Suppl 3):iii76–8.
39. Sippel R, Bianco J, Chen H. Radioguided parathyroidectomy for recurrent hyperparathyroidism caused by forearm graft hyperplasia. J Bone Miner Res 2003;18: 939–42.
40. Cohen M, Dilley W, Wells SJ, et al. Long-term functionality of cryopreserved parathyroid autografts: a 13-year prospective analysis. Surgery 2005;138:1033–40 [discussion: 40–1].
41. Cohen E, Moulder J. Parathyroidectomy in chronic renal failure: has medical care reduced the need for surgery? Nephron 2001;89:271–3.

Aldosteronomas—State of the Art

Travis J. McKenzie, MD[a], Joseph B. Lillegard, MD, PhD[a],
William F. Young Jr, MD[b], Geoffrey B. Thompson, MD[a],*

KEYWORDS

- Primary aldosteronism • Aldosterone-producing adenoma
- Aldosteronoma • Idiopathic hyperplasia
- Adrenal vein sampling

Primary aldosteronism (PA), first described by Conn in 1955,[1] is characterized by hypertension, suppressed plasma renin activity (PRA), and increased aldosterone secretion. Original estimates suggested that PA occurred with a frequency of 0.1% to 1.5% of all patients with hypertension,[2–4] but with simplified case detection methodology, using the plasma aldosterone concentration (PAC) to PRA ratio (PAC/PRA), the prevalence of PA in the hypertensive population may actually be as high as 8% to 15%.[5–12] Patients with PA have high PAC and suppressed PRA. With routine use of the PAC/PRA ratio in patients with hypertension at Mayo Clinic, there has been a ten-fold increased annual detection rate of PA.[13] Two thirds of these patients have bilateral idiopathic hyperaldosteronism (IHA), and approximately one third have aldosterone-producing adenomas (APA) (**Figs. 1** and **2**) amenable to surgical cure. Up to two thirds of these patients may be normokalemic at presentation with treatment-resistant hypertension as their only manifestation.[5,13–16]

Other rare causes of PA include primary (unilateral) adrenal hyperplasia, pure aldosterone-secreting adrenocortical carcinoma, familial hyperaldosteronism (FH) (see below).[17–19] Primary unilateral adrenal hyperplasia is an important entity as its proper recognition can lead to surgical cure. These variations demonstrate a continuum between adenoma and hyperplasia, increasing the importance of adrenal venous sampling for subtype evaluation.[20–22]

Pure aldosterone-secreting adrenocortical carcinomas are exceedingly rare with the only curative treatment being early surgical intervention.

FH can either be type II, the familial occurrence of APA or IHA, or type I, glucocorticoid-remediable aldosteronism (GRA).[23–25] GRA is inherited in an autosomal dominant fashion and is caused by a chimeric gene consisting of the regulatory regions of the gene coding for the enzyme 11β-hydroxylase (CYP11B1), corticotropin (ACTH), and

[a] Department of Surgery, Mayo Clinic, 200 First Street SW, Rochester, MN 55905, USA
[b] Division of Endocrinology, Department of Medicine, Mayo Clinic, 200 First Street SW, Rochester, MN 55905, USA
* Corresponding author.
E-mail address: thompson.geoffrey@mayo.edu (G.B. Thompson).

Surg Clin N Am 89 (2009) 1241–1253
doi:10.1016/j.suc.2009.06.017
0039-6109/09/$ – see front matter © 2009 Elsevier Inc. All rights reserved.

surgical.theclinics.com

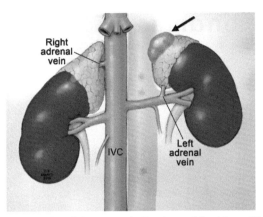

Fig. 1. Left adrenal adenoma (APA) (see *arrow*). *Courtesy of* the Mayo Clinic, Rochester, MN; with permission.

the coding region of the gene for aldosterone synthesis (CYP11B2).[23–26] Aldosterone synthesis, in these patients, is primarily regulated by ACTH (as opposed to the renin-angiotensin system), resulting in excess aldosterone production. This entity should be suspected based on family history of PA, onset of PA at a young age, or a family history of strokes at a young age. GRA can be confirmed with genetic testing. Treatment is with glucocorticoid administration and ACTH suppression.[23–25]

CLINICAL FEATURES

PA is most commonly diagnosed between the ages of 30 and 60, with a range of 2 to 75 (mean 47) years. Females predominate 1 to 1.5 in most series.[27–33]

The hypertension seen in PA is moderate to severe and can be indistinguishable from essential hypertension. The duration of hypertension can vary from a few months to several decades, with a median of 100 months reported in one series.[27,32,33] Treatment resistant hypertension (defined as uncontrolled hypertension despite treatment with an adrenergic inhibitor, a vasodilator, and a diuretic) and spontaneous hypokalemia (<3.5 mEq/L) are consistent with more severe hyperaldosteronism and suggestive of APA. Muscle cramping and weakness, headaches, intermittent or periodic paralysis, polydipsia, polyuria, and nocturia are less common and generally attributable to the degree of hypokalemia.[31,34] One percent of adrenal incidentalomas are associated with autonomous aldosterone production.[35]

PATHOLOGY

APA are usually solitary but, on rare occasions, can be bilateral or even associated with primary medullary tumors (pheochromocytoma). They are most often less than

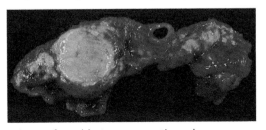

Fig. 2. Pathologic specimen of an aldosterone secreting adenoma.

2 cm in greatest diameter with a mean diameter between 1.5 and 2.0 cm.[36] The cut surface is characteristically a uniform bright golden yellow, without the pigmentation that is often seen in cortisol-secreting tumors (see **Fig. 2**). IHA is typically characterized by micronodular or macronodular hyperplasia. Nonfunctioning adrenal cortical adenomas occur with increasing frequency as patients age, thus complicating the clinical, radiographic, and pathologic diagnosis in patients more than 40 years of age.

CASE DETECTION OF PA

PA should be suspected in patients with treatment-resistant hypertension, hypertension and hypokalemia, poorly controlled hypertension, a family history of PA, an adrenal incidentaloma and hypertension, and whenever considering a secondary hypertension evaluation (**Fig. 3**). Screening of large populations of hypertensive patients is being performed with increasing frequency. The prevalence of PA in these cohorts ranges anywhere from 2% to 15%.[5–12] Most patients with PA have normal serum potassium levels at diagnosis of PA, thus normokalemia in and of itself should not be an exclusion criteria for case detection testing.[37–39] At Mayo Clinic, up to two thirds of patients are normokalemic at presentation (APA and IHA patients combined).[17]

The PAC/PRA ratio has become the accepted case detection modality for PA.[14,17,40–48] Cut-off values from 20:1 to 50:1 have been advocated. The addition of a PAC at least above the mid-reference range has increased the specificity of PAC/PRA ratio for PA.[43–45] One study found that a PAC/PRA ratio more than 30 with a PAC value greater than 20 ng/dL had a sensitivity and specificity of 90% and

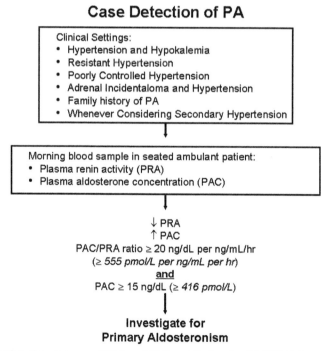

Case Detection of PA

Clinical Settings:
- Hypertension and Hypokalemia
- Resistant Hypertension
- Poorly Controlled Hypertension
- Adrenal Incidentaloma and Hypertension
- Family history of PA
- Whenever Considering Secondary Hypertension

↓

Morning blood sample in seated ambulant patient:
- Plasma renin activity (PRA)
- Plasma aldosterone concentration (PAC)

↓

↓ PRA
↑ PAC
PAC/PRA ratio ≥ 20 ng/dL per ng/mL/hr
(≥ 555 pmol/L per ng/mL per hr)
and
PAC ≥ 15 ng/dL (≥ 416 pmol/L)

↓

**Investigate for
Primary Aldosteronism**

Fig. 3. Algorithm showing use of PRA and PAC and their ratio (PAC/PRA) for case finding in hyperaldosteronism in patients with resistant hypertension, hypokalemia, or both.

91%, respectively.[42] Young at Mayo Clinic found that a PAC/PRA ratio greater than 20 with a PAC greater than 15 ng/dL was highly sensitive.[43–45] Reported ratios are all laboratory dependent. No special preparation is necessary with the exception of withholding spironolactone and eplerenone (mineralocorticoid receptor [MR] antagonists), high-dose amiloride, and direct renin inhibitors. In addition, hypokalemia, if present, should be corrected before case detection testing (see **Fig. 3**). Although other drugs may alter the accuracy of the PAC/PRA ratio, they are not usually an issue in patients with APA. Thiazide diuretics, calcium channel blockers, angiotensin converting enzyme inhibitors, and angiotensin receptor blockers can actually improve the diagnostic discriminatory power of the PAC/PRA ratio, while beta-adrenergic blockers and central alpha-2 agonists (eg, clonidine) suppress PRA and have the potential to give false positive results, especially if an absolute PAC cutoff is not used. Blood samples are best obtained in the morning in an ambulatory seated patient.

CONFIRMATION OF PA

Four confirmatory tests for PA have been validated and include: captopril stimulation test, fludrocortisone suppression test, saline infusion test, and oral sodium loading test .[6,14,36,38] PA is usually confirmed by demonstrating lack of suppressibility of aldosterone after sodium loading. This can be performed in one of two ways:

1. The saline suppression test: 2L of isotonic saline is infused over 4 hours (with caution in severe hypertension or heart failure). PAC is measured at the conclusion of the infusion. Nonsuppression of PAC (>10 ng/dL) is confirmatory of PA.[17]
2. Oral sodium loading test: Mayo Clinic patients are instructed to liberally salt their food and to consume high sodium content foods for 3 to 4 days. A 24-hour urine is collected from the morning of day 3 to the morning of day 4. Aldosterone, sodium, and creatinine are measured. Adequate sodium-loading is confirmed with a 24-hour urinary sodium excretion of more than 200 mEq. Failure to suppress urinary aldosterone levels to less than 12 mcg is confirmatory of PA and one should then proceed on to imaging and subtype evaluation.[14,17,43,44,46–48] The oral sodium loading test is not without risks. Blood pressure and serum potassium concentration must be monitored daily.

Information on Captopril stimulation and fludrocortisone suppression tests can be found elsewhere.[49,50]

SUBTYPE EVALUATION

In patients who want to pursue a surgical resolution or amelioration of their hypertension and PA, the accurate distinction between APA and IHA is critical (**Fig. 4**). These two entities account for over 95% of all cases of PA (ie, one third APA, two thirds IHA). The distinction is critical as APA is often successfully managed surgically (unilateral laparoscopic adrenalectomy), whereas IHA is best managed medically with MR antagonists. This distinction, however, is clouded by a physiologic and pathologic continuum that includes solitary unilateral APA, bilateral or double APA, primary unilateral hyperplasia, bilateral micronodular or macronodular hyperplasia, and PA in conjunction with one or more nonfunctioning adrenal incidentalomas.[14,17,46–48]

Patients with APA are often younger with more severe hypertension and hypokalemia in addition to demonstrating higher PAC and urinary aldosterone levels.[14,17,46–48] Patients with APA often respond better to spironolactone than those

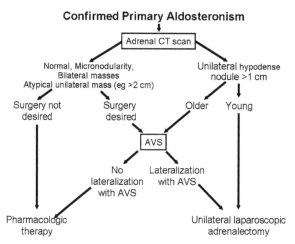

Fig. 4. Confirmed PA. Subtype evaluation.

with IHA. Unfortunately, none of these observations are specific enough for confident subtype assignment.

Of historic interest are three studies previously used for subtype evaluation: posture stimulation test, plasma 18-hydroxycorticosterone (18-OHB) concentration, and iodocholesterol scintigraphy with [6β-131I]iodomethyl-19-norcholesterol (NP-59).

APA are unresponsive to the renin-angiotensin-aldosterone system but are affected by the ACTH circadian rhythm. On the other hand, patients with IHA are sensitive to slight increases in angiotensin II seen with the upright posture.[51] Thus, in patients with IHA, PAC may rise after standing for four hours, whereas in patients with an APA, PAC levels will generally decrease in accordance with normal circadian rhythms. Many patients demonstrate an anomalous response (43% in one study) along with many false negatives.[28,36,52–54] In one study of 246 patients with verified APAs, the accuracy of this test was only 85%.[36]

A plasma 18-hydrocorticosterone concentration greater than 100 ng/dL is suggestive of APA. The assay showed a cumulative diagnostic accuracy of only 82% in four separate studies and is not readily available.[36,55]

NP-59 scintigraphy during dexamethasone suppression (to avoid uptake by the zona fasciculata and reticularis) has been used by some in an attempt to differentiate APA from IHA.[56–58] Laterality, unfortunately, depends on adenoma size and iodocholesterol scanning falls short where you need the most help, (ie, small tumors). The agent is not readily available in the United States. Iodine must be administered to prevent thyroid uptake of the isotope and the test takes from five to seven days to complete.[56–58]

Imaging and Localization (Subtype Evaluation Continued)

The ability to image a unilateral adrenal cortical adenoma or lateralize the site of aldosterone excess greatly facilitates our ability to select patients for surgery who have the greatest likelihood for cure. The sensitivity of locating adenomas with newer generation high-resolution CT scanners ranges from 82% to 90% (**Fig. 5**).[28,36,59,60] The problem is that the scanners are so sensitive that they are now picking up smaller and smaller nodules and adrenal limb thickening, which may or may not be clinically relevant. Although enhanced CT imaging reduces the number of false negative studies, it clearly increases the number of false positive studies that could lead to

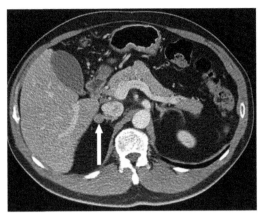

Fig. 5. Computed tomography image demonstrating an aldosterone secreting adenoma (*arrow*).

inappropriate withholding of surgical intervention or worse yet surgical removal of the wrong gland. This becomes increasingly more important with age as the incidence of adrenal incidentalomas increases. A young patient, less than 40 years, with PA with a solitary cortical macroadenoma (>1 cm) that is uniform, low density, and has fast contrast washout in concert with a morphologically normal contralateral gland needs no further imaging or evaluation and should be referred for surgery. Older patients, patients with bilateral morphologically normal or abnormal glands, or a unilateral microadenoma should be sent for bilateral adrenal venous sampling to optimize patient selection for those who wish to consider a surgical approach. Patients too infirm for surgery, those with a limited life expectancy, and those comfortable with medical therapy using MR antagonists need go no further.[14,17,46–48]

The success of adrenal venous sampling is dependent on experience and dedication and should be relegated to centers with an interventional radiologist dedicated to this particular procedure.[20–22,61] Cannulation of the small right adrenal vein is formidable (**Fig. 6**). Morbidity, including minor bleeding, hematoma, dissection, and infarction are exceedingly rare occurrences. In over 200 patients with PA recently treated (1990–2003) at Mayo Clinic, the success of bilateral adrenal venous catheterization, as demonstrated by high adrenal vein cortisol to systemic cortisol levels under continuous cosyntropin infusion was 95%. Cosyntropin infusion also augments the aldosterone secretion from APA. Aldosterone/cortisol ratios are compared to account for the dilutional effect on the left side caused by mixing of blood from the inferior phrenic vein. Corrected aldosterone/cortisol ratios of greater than 4:1 are indicative of a unilateral source of aldosterone excess, likely to be responsive to unilateral adrenalectomy. If adrenal venous sampling had not been used and CT alone used to determine laterality in this cohort of 203 patients, 42 patients or 22% would have been inappropriately excluded as candidates for adrenalectomy and 25% might have had an unnecessary or inappropriate adrenalectomy. Thus, selective adrenal venous sampling should be considered as an essential step in differentiating APA and primary unilateral hyperplasia from IHA.[21,61]

DEFINITIVE THERAPY

Definitive therapy is essential for patients with PA. Excess aldosterone is deleterious even when hypertension and hypokalemia are adequately controlled. If left untreated

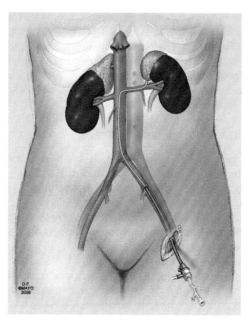

Fig. 6. Adrenal venous sampling. *Courtesy of* the Mayo Clinic, Rochester, MN; with permission.

or unblocked, aldosterone excess can lead to myocardial fibrosis, worsening left ventricular hypertrophy, increased mortality from congestive heart failure, more ischemic events, and increased vascular and clotting abnormalities.[62–74] Patients too old or too sick, those with IHA, and those not wanting surgery should be treated with a MR antagonist (eg, spironolactone or eplerenone) and other classes of antihypertensives as needed.[14,17,46–48] Unlike spironolactone, eplerenone has little androgen receptor antagonist or progesterone receptor agonists activities, which can lead to untoward side effects in men (gynecomastia and impotence) and menstrual irregularities in women.[46,75–79]

In patients with solid evidence of unilateral source of aldosterone excess and PA, unilateral (laparoscopic) adrenalectomy is the treatment of choice. The laparoscopic approach is well-suited to patients with PA, as the tumors are most often small and benign.[80–85] Although cortical-sparing or partial adrenalectomy has been performed successfully in select cases, this should be exercised with caution in patients with a unilateral source of aldosterone excess. Pathologic specimens often demonstrate additional nodules in the same gland of patients with a dominant nodule. Theoretically, the dominant nodule may be nonfunctioning; leaving the other nodules behind could result in a surgical failure. Little long-term morbidity has been seen in patients undergoing total unilateral adrenalectomy for PA.

Laparoscopic adrenalectomy has advantages over open posterior and anterior adrenalectomy in terms of shorter operative times, recovery, postoperative pain, blood loss, and overall long-term morbidity (T12 nerve injury, hernias).[82,83,86–88] When laparoscopic transperitoneal adrenalectomy cannot be accomplished because of extensive prior upper abdominal surgery (a rarity), a posterior endoscopic or open approach can be used[89]; the former being preferable when expertise with this technique is available. The first laparoscopic adrenalectomy was performed transperitoneally by Gagner and colleagues[90] in 1992. Mercan and colleagues[91] developed a technique for endoscopic retroperitoneal adrenalectomy (ERA) a year later, which they described in 1995. While most surgeons prefer the transperitoneal approach given its familiarity, ERA offers an alternative technique with more direct access to the adrenal gland. This can be beneficial in minimizing the amount of dissection necessary in a patient with previous abdominal surgery. Both procedures are acceptable for small tumors. Large aldosterone-secreting tumors (>4–6 cm) should raise suspicion of malignancy and should be managed accordingly.

PREPARATION FOR SURGERY AND POSTOPERATIVE CARE

In preparation for surgery, patients are placed on an MR antagonist along with other necessary antihypertensive and cardiac medications. Potassium stores are repleted cautiously in patients on MR antagonists. Postoperatively, potassium chloride replacement is continued cautiously until normokalemia is established. MR antagonists are stopped and antihypertensives are withheld unless blood pressure values remain elevated. Antihypertensive medications are added back or weaned in accordance with blood pressure measurements. Normotension off all medications may take weeks to months to achieve, if at all.[14,17,46–48] β-adrenergic blockers should not be abruptly stopped in the perioperative period and may require continued use in patients on long-term therapy for ischemic heart disease. Patients leaving the hospital requiring oral potassium need to be monitored twice weekly to avoid serious hyperkalemia when postoperative suppression of aldosterone levels occurs. We routinely obtain a PAC on the day of dismissal (24–48 hours postoperative). A suppressed PAC level is a good indication of an appropriate response to unilateral adrenalectomy. PRA remains suppressed for longer periods of time.

OUTCOMES

Physiologic outcomes are identical whether laparoscopic or open adrenalectomy is performed.[13] Patients with a unilateral source of aldosterone excess as determined by AVS can expect a 100% cure of hypokalemia. Over 90% will show marked improvement in hypertension as evidenced by a decrease in the number and dosing of antihypertensive medications. Approximately 30% to 60% of patients will achieve normotension without the aid of medications; these most often being younger patients that have a shorter clinical course and lack a family history of hypertension.[13,14,17,29,46–48] Renal insufficiency may be masked preoperatively because of the increased filtration associated with aldosterone excess. Thus, in addition to weekly serum potassium checks, serum creatinine should also be monitored during the first postoperative month. Patients with an excellent response to spironolactone often fare best with adrenalectomy.[22,29,92,93]

SUMMARY

PA is the most common cause of secondary hypertension in nonsmokers. Widespread screening of unselected hypertensives has identified PA in as many as 15% of patients. With such screening efforts using the PAC/PRA ratio and PAC, the widespread prevalence of the disease has become apparent while the relative percentage of APA has decreased. PA is confirmed by demonstrating lack of aldosterone suppressibility with sodium loading. Subtype evaluation is best achieved with high resolution CT scanning and AVS in the appropriate setting. In PA patients with a unilateral source of aldosterone excess, laparoscopic adrenalectomy is the treatment of choice with excellent outcomes and low morbidity as compared with older open approaches. Patients with IHA or those not amenable or agreeable to surgery are best managed with a MR antagonist.

REFERENCES

1. Conn JW. Presidential address. Part I, painting background. Part II, primary aldosteronism, a new clinical syndrome. J Lab Clin Med 1955;45(1):3–17.
2. AACE Hypertension Task Force. American Association of Clinical Endocrinologists medical guidelines for clinical practice for the diagnosis and treatment of hypertension. Endocr Pract 2006;12(2):193–222.
3. Tucker RM, Labarth DR. Frequency of surgical treatment for hypertension in adults at the Mayo clinic from 1973 through 1975. Mayo Clin Proc 1977;52(9): 549–55.
4. Anderson GH Jr, Blakeman N, Streeten DH. The effect of age on prevalence of secondary forms of hypertension in 4429 consecutively referred patients. J Hypertens 1994;12(5):609–15.
5. Rossi E, Regolisti G, Negro A, et al. High prevalence of primary aldosteronism using postcaptopril plasma aldosterone to renin ratio as a screening test among Italian hypertensives. Am J Hypertens 2002;15(10 Pt 1):896–902.
6. Gordon RD, Stowasser M, Tunny TJ, et al. High incidence of primary aldosteronism in 199 patients referred with hypertension. Clin Exp Pharmacol Physiol 1994;21(14):315–8.
7. Kumar A, Lall SB, Ammini A, et al. Screening of a population of young hypertensives for primary hyperaldosteronism. J Hum Hypertens 1994;8(9):731–2.
8. Kreze A Jr, Okalova D, Vanuga P, et al. Occurrence of primary aldosteronism in a group of ambulatory hypertensive patients. Vnitr Lek 1999;45(1):17–21.
9. Lim PO, Dow E, Brennan G, et al. High prevalence of primary aldosteronism in the Tayside hypertension clinic population. J Hum Hypertens 2000;14(5):311–5.
10. Loh KC, Koay ES, Khaw MC, et al. Prevalence of primary aldosteronism among Asian hypertensive patients in Singapore. J Clin Endocrinol Metab 2000;85(8): 2854–9.
11. Fardella CE, Mosso L, Gomez-Sanchez C, et al. Primary hyperaldosteronism in essential hypertensives: prevalence, biochemical profile, and molecular biology. J Clin Endocrinol Metab 2000;85(5):1863–7.
12. Schwartz GL, Turner ST. Prevalence of unrecognized primary aldosteronism in essential hypertension [abstract]. Am J Hypertens 2002;15:18A.
13. Sawka AM, Young WF Jr, Thompson GB, et al. Primary aldosteronism: factors associated with normalization of blood pressure after surgery. Ann Intern Med 2001;135(4):258–61.
14. Young WF Jr. Primary aldosteronism: management issues. Ann N Y Acad Sci 2002;970:61–76.
15. Calhoun DA, Nishizaka MK, Zaman MA, et al. Hyperaldosteronism among black and white subjects with resistant hypertension. Hypertension 2002;40(6):892–6.
16. Mulatero P, Rabbai F, Milan A, et al. Drug effects on aldosterone/plasma renin activity ration in primary hyperaldosteronism. Hypertension 2002;40(6): 897–902.
17. Young WF Jr. Minireview: primary aldosteronism—changing concepts in diagnosis and treatment. Endocrinology 2003;144(6):2208–13.
18. Ganguly A, Zager P, Luetscher J. Primary aldosteronism due to unilateral adrenal hyperplasia. J Clin Endocrinol Metab 1980;51(5):1190–4.

19. Irony I, Kater C, Biglieri E, et al. Correctable subsets of primary aldosteronism. Am J Hypertens 1990;3(7):576–82.
20. Doppman JL, Gill JR Jr. Hyperaldosteronism: sampling the adrenal veins. Radiology 1996;198(2):309–12.
21. Young WF Jr, Stanson AW, Grant CS, et al. Primary aldosteronism: adrenal venous sampling. Surgery 1996;120(6):913–20.
22. Rossi GP, Sacchetto A, Chiesura-Corona M, et al. Identification of the etiology of primary aldosteronism with adrenal vein sampling in patients with equivocal computed tomography and magnetic resonance findings: results in 104 consecutive cases. J Clin Endocrinol Metab 2001;86(3):1083–90.
23. McMahon GT, Dluhy RG. Glucocorticoid-remediable aldosteronism. Cardiol Rev 2004;12(1):44–8.
24. Lifton RP, Dluhy RG, Powers M, et al. A chimeric 11β-hydroxylase/aldosterone synthase gene causes glucocorticoid-remedial aldosteronism and human hypertension. Nature 1992;355(6357):262–5.
25. Jackson RV, Lafferty A, Torpy DJ, et al. New genetic insights in familial hyperaldosteronism. Ann N Y Acad Sci 2002;970:77–88.
26. Lifton RP, Dluhy RG, Powers M, et al. Hereditary hypertension caused by chimaeric gene duplication and ectopic expression of aldosterone synthase. Nat Genet 1992;2(1):66–74.
27. Lins P, Adamson U. Primary aldosteronism: a follow-up study of 28 cases of surgically treated aldosterone-producing adenomas. Acta Med Scand 1987;221(3): 275–82.
28. Vetter H, Fischer M, Galanski M, et al. Primary aldosteronism: diagnosis and noninvasive lateralization procedures. Cardiology 1985;72(Suppl 1):57–63.
29. Celen O, O'Brien MJ, Melby JC, et al. Factors influencing outcome of surgery for primary aldosteronism. Arch Surg 1996;131(6):646–50.
30. Favia G, Lumachi F, Scarpa V, et al. Adrenalectomy in primary aldosteronism: a long-term follow-up study in 52 patients. World J Surg 1992;16(4):680–3.
31. Lo CY, Tam PC, Kung AW, et al. Primary aldosteronism. Results of surgical treatment. Ann Surg 1996;224(2):125–30.
32. Milsom SR, Espiner EA, Nicholls MO, et al. The blood pressure response to unilateral adrenalectomy in primary aldosteronism. Q J Med 1986;61(236):1141–51.
33. Proye CA, Mulliez EA, Carnaille BM, et al. Essential hypertension: first reason for persistent hypertension after unilateral adrenalectomy for primary aldosteronism? Surgery 1998;124(6):1128–33.
34. Huang YY, Hsu BR, Tsai JS. Paralytic myopathy—a leading clinical presentation for primary aldosteronism in Taiwan. J Clin Endocrinol Metab 1996;81(11): 4038–41.
35. Obara T, Ito Y, Iihara M. Hyperaldosteronism. In: Clark OH, Duh Q-Y, Kebebew E, editors. Textbook of endocrine surgery. 2nd edition. Philadelphia: Elsevier Saunders; 2005. p. 595–603.
36. Young WF Jr, Klee G. Primary aldosteronism. Diagnostic evaluation. Endocrinol Metab Clin North Am 1988;17(2):367–95.
37. Streeten DH, Tomycz N, Anderson GH. Reliability of screening methods for the diagnosis of primary aldosteronism. Am J Med 1979;67(3):403–13.
38. Bravo EL. Primary aldosteronism. Issues in diagnosis and management. Endocrinol Metab Clin North Am 1994;23(2):271–83.
39. Melby JC. Clinical review 1: endocrine hypertension. J Clin Endocrinol Metab 1989;69(4):697–703.

40. Hiramatsu K, Yamada T, Yukimura Y, et al. A screening test to identify aldoste-rone-producing adenoma by measuring plasma renin activity. Arch Intern Med 1981;141(12):1589–93.
41. Hamlet SM, Tunny TJ, Woodland E, et al. Is aldosterone/renin ratio useful to screen a hypertensive population for primary aldosteronism? Clin Exp Pharmacol Physiol 1985;12(3):249–52.
42. Weinberger MH, Fineberg NS. The diagnosis of primary aldosteronism and sepa-ration of two major subtypes. Arch Intern Med 1993;153(18):2125–9.
43. Young WF Jr. Primary aldosteronism: a common and curable form of hyperten-sion. Cardiol Rev 1999;7(4):207–14.
44. Young WF Jr. Primary aldosteronism: update on diagnosis and treatment. Endo-crinologist 1997;7(4):213–21.
45. Young WF Jr. Management approaches to adrenal incidentaloma. A view from Rochester, Minnesota. Endocrinol Metab Clin North Am 2000;29(1):159–85.
46. Lim PO, Young WF, MacDonald TM. A review of the medical treatment of primary aldosteronism. J Hypertens 2001;19(3):353–61.
47. Montori VM, Young WF Jr. Use of plasma aldosterone concentration-to-plasma renin activity ratio as a screening test for primary aldosteronism: a systematic review of the literature. Endocrinol Metab Clin North Am 2002;31(3):619–32.
48. Young WF Jr. Primary aldosteronism – treatment options. Growth Horm IGF Res 2003;13(Suppl A):S102–8.
49. Gordon RD, Ziesak MD, Tunny TJ, et al. Evidence that primary aldosteronism may not be uncommon: 12% incidence among antihypertensive drug trial volunteers. Clin Exp Pharmacol Physiol 1993;20(5):296–8.
50. Lyons DF, Kemn DC, Brown RD, et al. Single dose captopril as a diagnostic test for primary aldosteronism. J Clin Endocrinol Metab 1983;57(5):892–6.
51. Ganguly A, Melada GA, Luetscher JA, et al. Control of plasma aldosterone in primary aldosteronism: distinction between adenoma and hyperplasia. J Clin Endocrinol Metab 1973;37(5):765–75.
52. Obara T, Ito Y, Okamoto T, et al. Risk factors associated with postoperative persistent hypertension in patients with primary aldosteronism. Surgery 1992; 112(6):987–93.
53. McLeod M, Thompson N, Gross M, et al. Idiopathic aldosteronism masquerading as discrete aldosterone-secreting adrenal cortical neoplasms among patients with primary aldosteronism. Surgery 1989;106(6):1161–7.
54. Nomura K, Toraya S, Horiba N, et al. Plasma aldosterone response to upright posture and angiotensin II infusion in aldosterone-producing adenoma. J Clin Endocrinol Metab 1992;75(1):323–6.
55. Kem DC, Tang K, Hanson CS, et al. The prediction of anatomical morphology of primary aldosteronism using serum 18-hydroxycorticosterone. J Clin Endocrinol Metab 1985;60(1):67–73.
56. Gross M, Shapiro B. Scintigraphic studies in adrenal hypertension. Semin Nucl Med 1989;19(2):122–43.
57. Hollak CE, Prummel MF, Tiel-van Buul MM. Bilateral adrenal tumours in primary aldosteronism: localization of a unilateral aldosteronoma by dexamethasone suppression scan. J Intern Med 1991;229(6):545–8.
58. Nomura K, Kusakabe K, Maki M, et al. Iodomethylnorcholesterol uptake in an al-dosteronoma shown by dexamethasone-suppression scintigraphy: relationship to adenoma size and functional activity. J Clin Endocrinol Metab 1990;71(4): 825–30.

59. Gleason PE, Weinberger MH, Pratt JH, et al. Evaluation of diagnostic tests in the differential diagnosis of primary aldosteronism: unilateral adenoma versus bilateral micronodular hyperplasia. J Urol 1993;150(5 Pt 1):1365–8.

60. Weigel RJ, Wells SA, Gunnells JC, et al. Surgical treatment of primary hyperaldosteronism. Ann Surg 1994;219(4):347–52.

61. Young WF Jr, Stanson AW, Thompson GB, et al. Role for adrenal venous sampling in primary aldosteronism. Surgery 2004;136(12):1227–35.

62. Rocha R, Rudolph AE, Frierdich GE, et al. Aldosterone induces a vascular inflammatory phenotype in the rat heart. Am J Physiol Heart Circ Physiol 2002;283(5): H1802–10.

63. Rocha R, Funder JW. The pathophysiology of aldosterone in the cardiovascular system. Ann N Y Acad Sci 2002;970:89–100.

64. Stier CT Jr, Chander PN, Rocha R. Aldosterone as a mediator in cardiovascular injury. Cardiol Rev 2002;10(2):97–107.

65. Martinez DV, Rocha R, Mastumura M, et al. Cardiac damage prevention by eplerenone: comparison with low sodium diet or potassium loading. Hypertension 2002;39(2 Pt 2):614–8.

66. Brilla CG, Pick R, Tan LB, et al. Remodeling of the rat right and left ventricles in experimental hypertension. Circ Res 1990;67(6):1355–64.

67. Pitt B, Zannad F, Remme WJ, et al. The effect of spironolactone on morbidity and mortality in patients with severe heart failure. N Engl J Med 1999;341(10):709–17.

68. Rocha R, Williams GH. Rationale for the use of aldosterone antagonists in congestive heart failure. Drugs 2002;62(5):723–31.

69. Alderman MH, Madhavan S, Ooi WL, et al. Association of the renin-sodium profile with the risk of myocardial infarction in patients with hypertension. N Engl J Med 1991;324(16):1098–104.

70. Vaughan DE, Lazos SA, Tong K. Angiotensin II regulates the expression of plasminogen activator inhibitor-1 in cultured endothelial cells. A potential link between the renin-angiotensin system and thrombosis. J Clin Invest 1995;95(3):995–1001.

71. Kerins DM, Hao Q, Vaughan DE. Angiotensin induction of PAI-1 expression in endothelial cells is mediated by the hexapeptide angiotensin IV. J Clin Invest 1995;96(5):2515–20.

72. Brown NJ, Kim KS, Chen YQ, et al. Synergistic effect of adrenal steroids and angiotensin II on plasminogen activator inhibitor-1 production. J Clin Endocrinol Metab 2000;85(1):336–44.

73. Brown NJ, Agirbasli MA, Williams GH, et al. Effect of activation and inhibition of renin angiotensin system on plasma PAI-1. Hypertension 1998;32(6):965–71.

74. Sawathiparnich P, Kumar S, Vaughan DE, et al. Spironolactone abolishes the relationship between aldosterone and plasminogen activator inhibitor-a in humans. J Clin Endocrinol Metab 2002;87(2):448–52.

75. Jeunemaitre X, Chatellier G, Kreft-Jais C, et al. Efficacy and tolerance of spironolactone in essential hypertension. Am J Cardiol 1987;60(10):820–5.

76. Zillich AJ, Carter BL. Eplerenone: a novel selective aldosterone blocker. Ann Pharmacother 2002;36(10):1567–76.

77. de Gasparo M, Joss U, Ramjoue HP, et al. Three new epoxy-spirolactone derivatives: characterization in vivo and in vitro. J Pharmacol Exp Ther 1987;240(2): 650–6.

78. Weinberger MH, Roniker B, Krause SL, et al. Eplerenone, a selective aldosterone blocker, in mild-to-moderate hypertension. Am J Hypertens 2002;15(8):709–16.

79. Krum H, Nolly H, Workman D, et al. Efficacy of eplerenone added to renin-angiotensin blockade in hypertensive patients. Hypertension 2002;40(2):117–23.

80. Gagner M. Laparoscopic adrenalectomy. Surg Clin North Am 1996;76(3):523–37.
81. Kebebew E, Siperstein AE, Duh QY. Laparoscopic adrenalectomy: the optimal surgical approach. J Laparoendosc Adv Surg Tech A 2001;11(6):409–13.
82. Marescaux J, Mutter D, Wheeler MH. Laparoscopic right and left adrenalectomies. Surgical procedures. Surg Endosc 1996;10(9):912–5.
83. Gagner M, Lacroix A, Prinz RA, et al. Early experience with laparoscopic approach for adrenalectomy. Surgery 1993;114(6):1120–4.
84. Higashihara E, Tanaka Y, Hori S, et al. Laparoscopic adrenalectomy: the initial three cases. J Urol 1993;149(5):973–6.
85. Suzuki K, Kageyama S, Ueda D, et al. Laparoscopic adrenalectomy: clinical, experience with 12 cases. J Urol 1993;150(4):1099–102.
86. Linos DA, Stylopoulos N, Boukis M, et al. Anterior, posterior, or laparoscopic approach for the management of adrenal diseases? Am J Surg 1997;173(2):120–5.
87. Prinz RA. A comparison of laparoscopic and open adrenalectomies. Arch Surg 1995;130(5):489–92.
88. Thompson GB, Grant CS, van Heerden JA, et al. Laparoscopic versus open posterior adrenalectomy: a case-control study of 100 patients. Surgery 1997;122(6):1132–6.
89. Walz MK, Alesina RF, Wenger A, et al. Posterior retroperitoneoscopic adrenalectomy—results of more than 500 procedures. Surgery 2006;140(6):943–8.
90. Gagner M, Lacroix A, Bolte E. Laparoscopic adrenalectomy in Cushing's syndrome and pheochromocytoma. N Engl J Med 1992;327(14):1033.
91. Mercan S, Seven R, Ozarmagan S, et al. Endoscopic retroperitoneal adrenalectomy. Surgery 1995;118(6):1071–5.
92. Ferriss JB, Brown JJ, Fraser R, et al. Results of adrenal surgery in patients with hypertension, aldosterone excess, and low plasma renin concentration. Br Med J 1975;1(5950):135–8.
93. Hunt T, Schambelan M, Biglieri E. Selection of patients and operative approach in aldosteronism. Ann Surg 1975;182(4):353–61.

Adrenocortical Cancer

Melissa Wandoloski, BS[a], Kimberly J. Bussey, PhD[a],
Michael J. Demeure, MD, MBA[a,b],*

KEYWORDS

- Adrenal • Adrenocortical cancer • Molecular oncogenesis
- Surgery • Endocrine tumors

INCIDENCE AND PRESENTATION

Adrenocortical carcinoma (ACC) is a rare endocrine malignancy causing up to 0.2% of all cancer deaths. Its annual incidence is 1 to 2 per million people. ACC typically is diagnosed during one's fourth and fifth decade of life, but it can also be seen in childhood.[1] Women are afflicted more often than men, at a ratio reported at 1.5:1.[2,3] In southern Brazil, the incidence of ACC increases up to 12 per million per year where childhood ACC is more prevalent due to the frequent occurrence of the associated germ-line p53 mutation.[1–6] Benign adrenocortical adenomas are discovered in a much higher proportion of the population, typically through diagnostic imaging for nonadrenal-related reasons. Unfortunately, it can be difficult to ascertain whether some of these "adrenal incidentalomas" will ultimately develop into a malignant tumor or remain a benign mass.[2–4,6–8]

Many ACC patients have no symptoms until their tumors reach a large size and cause symptoms due to a mass effect and compression of nearby structures. Symptoms in these cases are typically vague and include abdominal fullness, nausea, obstipation or early satiety, weight loss, weakness, fatigue, or fever.[1] In about 40% to 60% of patients, increased hormone production results in symptoms that lead to the diagnosis of an adrenal tumor.[1,2] Malignant adrenal tumors can secrete a variety of steroids, steroid precursors, and mineralocorticoids.[1,3,7] As many as 75% of ACC are associated with occult hypercortisolism demonstrable with hormone testing only. A lesser proportion of patients will present with overt Cushing syndrome. The behavior of benign adrenal tumors may be distinguishable from malignant ACC based on their profile of cortico steroid and androgen production. Cosecretion of androgens and cortico steroids by an adrenal tumor is suggestive of malignancy. Benign, functional adrenal tumors normally secrete only one class of steroids. This distinction is of only limited clinical utility, as patients with ACC may harbor nonfunctioning tumors.[3] At the time of diagnosis most ACC patients

This work supported by a grant from the ATAC fund.
[a] Translational Genomics Research Institute, Clinical Translational Research Division, TGEN 445 N. Fifth Street, Phoenix, AZ 85004, USA
[b] Scottsdale Healthcare Shea Medical Center, Virginia G. Piper Cancer Center, 10460 N. 92nd Street, Suite 200, Scottsdale, AZ 85260, USA
* Corresponding author. Scottsdale Healthcare Shea Medical Center, Virginia G. Piper Cancer Center, 10460 N. 92nd Street, Suite 200, Scottsdale, AZ 85260.
E-mail address: mdemeure@tgen.org (M.J. Demeure).

surgical.theclinics.com

have become symptomatic, but this is not until relatively late into the course of their disease. At diagnosis most patients present with a large tumor and disease advancement. Metastases are present in more than half of the patients with ACC.[2,3,7]

EVALUATION OF ADRENAL TUMORS INCLUDING INCIDENTALOMAS

Adrenal masses discovered by imaging such as ultrasound, magnetic resonance imaging (MRI), and computed tomography (CT) done for nonadrenal reasons are considered to be "adrenal incidentalomas." Adrenal incidentalomas have been detected for 20 years, but their incidence is increasing rapidly due to a more frequent use of diagnostic imaging techniques.[9–13] The incidence of incidentalomas of the adrenal gland is approaching 3% in middle-aged adults and 10% in the elderly. The overall occurrence rate is about 4% to 6% in those patients who undergo abdominal imaging studies with CT or MRI.[9,14] Although most of these adrenal masses prove to be nonfunctioning adenomas, it has been reported that approximately 6% of adrenal incidentalomas are functional tumors; 5% cortisol secreting, and 1% sex hormone or aldosterone producing.[14] As a result, evaluation of hormone activity and an assessment of the potential for malignancy are important in diagnosing the nature of the mass.[10,12–14] Although rare, pheochromocytomas and aldosterone-producing tumors can also present in patients with no overt symptoms.[10]

To examine tumors that are clinically asymptomatic but might be hormonally active, the authors use an overnight dexamethasone (1 mg) suppression test to assess cortisol production.[11,12] Plasma cortisol levels less than 5 µg/dL are normal and levels more than 5 to 10 µg/dL are abnormal, with a 15% false positive rate.[11] It has been reported that up to 12% of subjects with adrenal incidentalomas have had tumors with pathologic cortisol production. It is also possible that a functional tumor would not produce sufficient cortisol to cause Cushing syndrome but could produce enough cortisol to cause hypertension, diabetes mellitus, or obesity. These patients should be further assessed for adrenalectomy. "Pre Cushing syndrome" and "Subclinical Cushing syndrome" are terms used for healthy patients with cortical-producing tumors, but without the overt signs or symptoms allowing for a diagnosis of Cushing syndrome.[12] Particularly in hypertensive patients, plasma aldosterone concentration and plasma renin activity should be assessed.[11] An increased aldosterone to renin ratio suggests primary hyperaldosteronism, although the optimal cutoff value is not yet established.

Tumor size is the most significant factor in distinguishing benign and malignant adrenal incidentalomas.[11,13,14] ACC has been identified in 2% of tumors smaller than 4 cm, 6% of tumors of 4.1 to 6 cm, and 25% of tumors larger than 6 cm.[11,13] Consequently, tumors 4.0 cm and greater have the highest risk for malignancy and should therefore be considered for removal.[11,13,14] Moreover, any patients whose tumors increase in size over a 6-month period should be considered for surgery because this finding is also suggestive of the presence of a malignant adrenal tumor.[14]

Although characteristics such as an irregular border or heterogeneity seen on more common imaging techniques can be useful tools in characterizing adrenal masses, [18F]fluorodeoxyglucose positron emission tomography (FDG-PET) may become a valuable technique in discriminating between benign and malignant lesions. FDG is taken up by active metabolic cells and is used to recognize metastasis. FDG-PET has been shown to be up to 100% sensitive in identification of lesions. However, FDG-PET should not substitute for other imaging but should be used in combination with other common imaging techniques.[11] [123I]Iodometomidate (IMTO) has been identified as a highly specific radiotracer that can be used for adrenal imaging. IMTO binds to Cyp11B enzymes that are highly expressed in adrenocortical originating tissue only. The uptake has been shown in both animals and humans at a faster rate and lower dosage, with a longer half-life than with other imaging. The specificity of this tracer is therefore a potentially useful tool for the diagnosis of adrenal lesions. The reliability and cost-effectiveness of FDG uptake warrant further study in the evaluation of potentially malignant adrenal masses.[10–12] Close serial observation of a patient's adrenal tumor over time with advanced imaging remains the best current method of accurately diagnosing adrenal incidentalomas.[14]

PATHOLOGY

ACC typically present as a large heterogeneous mass with an average size of 10 cm, irregular margins, and areas of necrosis, and may exhibit vascular, local, or capsular invasion. The tumor may also extend into the renal vein or vena cava (**Fig. 1**).[1,3,5] In general, the benign tumors weigh up to 50 g whereas malignant tumors weigh more than 100 g.[1]

Due to the significant difference in the prognosis of adrenocortical adenomas and carcinomas, an accurate pathologic diagnosis is paramount. Although this distinction is often straightforward, as is the case when one has proven metastases, there are times when the diagnosis of these tumors can be difficult. Pathologists rely on the various pathologic features of the tumor as detailed in the Weiss criteria.[2–4,7,8] The Weiss score catalogs 9 different histologic features: high mitotic rate, atypical mitoses, high nuclear grade, low percentage of clear cells, necrosis, diffuse architecture of the tumor, capsular invasion, sinusoidal invasion, and venous invasion.[1,3,4,6] A Weiss score of 1 is given to features that are present and a score of 0 is given to absent features.[3,6] A total score less than or equal to 2 is classified as an adrenocortical adenoma, and a score of 3 or more is suggestive of an ACC.[4,6] However, a score of 2 or 3 is commonly considered ambiguous, requiring other criteria to classify the tumor, and others believe some of the 9 criteria are not reliable measurements.[2–4,6,7] More recently, some investigators have advocated the use of adjunct pathologic diagnostic tools to facilitate a more accurate diagnosis. Suggested markers of a malignant adrenal tumor include insulinlike growth factor 2 (IGF-2) overexpression, allelic loss at 17p13, increased Ki-67, and cyclin E expression via immunohistochemistry.[1,3,4,6] Other investigators, including most recently Giordano and colleagues and de Reyniès and colleagues, have shown gene sets identified by expression array that

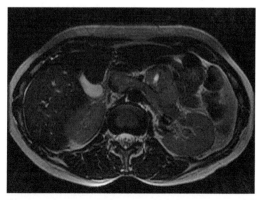

Fig. 1. CT scan depicting an adrenocortical cancer with invasion into left renal vein.

purport to distinguish malignant from benign adrenal tumors.[4,15] Furthermore, some gene sets, particularly those related to cell cycle regulation, have been associated with high-grade ACC and a poor prognosis.[3,5–7]

MOLECULAR ONCOGENESIS
Genomics

The changes that underpin the development of benign and malignant adrenal tumors are still relatively undefined. From a classic cytogenetics perspective, adenomas are almost always diploid with a loss of a sex chromosome and potential rearrangement of chromosome 7, whereas carcinomas can be diploid with single chromosomal gains, or have highly aneuploid DNA content due to complex numerical and structural rearrangements.[16] Comparative genomic hybridization (CGH) studies have revealed that adenomas in adults generally have few if any changes, and the number of aberrations accumulates as a function of tumor size. No specific changes have been identified, however, that reliably distinguish adenomas from ACC. Five studies report the results of applying conventional CGH to ACC.[17–21] The abnormalities detected are present in 50% to 60% or less of the tumors examined in each series, and no single aberration has been reported in higher prevalence. There is also a great deal of heterogeneity within tumors and between studies. However, taken as a whole ACC demonstrate gains of 4p16, 5p15, 5q12-13, 5q32-qter, 9q34, 12q13, 12q24, and 19p. Regions of loss include 1p21-31, 2cen-q21, 9p, and 11q24-qter. Similar data emerge from array CGH studies in which instead of metaphase chromosomes as the hybridization target, the samples and controls are hybridized to DNA microarrays. This method permits a resolution that is limited only by the genomic distance between 2 probes on the array. The authors' group reported that among 25 tumors there were overall gains within chromosomes 5, 6q, 7, 8q, 12, 16q, and 20. Losses were found within chromosomes 1, 2q, 3, 6p, 7p, 8p, 9, 10, 11, 13q, 14q, 15q, 16, 17, 19q, and 22q.[22] It was also demonstrated that amplifications of 6q, 7q, 12q, and 19p and losses of 3, 8, 10p, 16q, 17q, and 19q were significantly associated with poor survival.[22]

Expression Microarrays

Recent studies have shown gene expression patterns that can be used to distinguish adenomas from carcinomas.[4,5,7,15,23,24] Giordano and colleagues demonstrated that genes showing differential expression in ACC compared with adenoma or normal adrenal are enriched for cell cycle progression. This study also identified 12q and 5q as chromosomal regions with evidence of enrichment for overexpressed genes in ACC, whereas 11q, 1p, and 17p had evidence of enrichment for underexpressed genes. Both Giordano and colleagues and de Reyniès and colleagues reported that amongst ACC, hierarchical clustering revealed 2 clusters that corresponded to better and worse prognosis.[4,15] In the Giordano group study, the clustering was associated with mitotic index, suggesting an approximate grouping by grade. In addition, the genes differentially expressed in the poor prognosis cluster were enriched for the G2/M transition. Given the enrichment for cell cycle genes, and mitosis in particular, and because the mitotic index is one component of tumor grade, one might expect that the approximation of grade by gene expression data was due to the mitotic index component. To check for this, the study employed a Cox proportional hazards model incorporating tumor grade, log of the mitotic index, and the gene expression data from the first principal component. Mitotic index was not significant whereas grade and the principal component were significant. This result suggests that the gene expression data contain information beyond what is captured by grade.[15] De Reyniès and colleagues identified a 2-gene signature, PINK1 and BUB1B, as being predictive of overall survival. A patient was predicted to have a poor prognosis if analysis of their tumor sample by quantitative polymerase chain reaction showed the delta crossover threshold of BUB1B minus the delta crossover threshold of PINK1 to be less than 6.32.[4]

Inherited Syndromes: Li-Fraumeni

Further clues to the molecular oncogenesis arise from the observation that ACC occurs in the context of two inherited syndromes, Li-Fraumeni and Beckwith-Wiedemann. Li-Fraumeni syndrome is caused by a germ-line defect in the tumor suppressor gene, TP53, which encodes p53. Patients with Li-Fraumeni syndrome have a higher susceptibility to breast carcinoma, soft tissue sarcomas, brain tumors, osteosarcoma, leukemia, and ACC. Some argue that diagnosis of ACC, particularly in a child, is sufficient to warrant testing to determine the patient's p53 mutation status.[25] The spectrum of germ-line mutation for Li-Fraumeni families with one or more cases of ACC shows a shift outside of the normal hot spots in the DNA-binding domain. Sixty percent of kindreds with ACC have mutations that cluster in a region of the p53 protein within non-DNA binding loops, the b-sheet skeleton, and the oligomerization domain.[26] TP53 has been reported to be mutated in approximately 25% of sporadic ACC cases.[3] Loss of heterogeneity (LOH) for 17p has been reported in 85% or more of ACC,[27] further supporting the role of p53 aberrations in the pathogenesis of ACC. In Brazil, a unique germ-line mutation at R337H has resulted in an increased incidence of ACC of 4 to 6 per million but does not result in Li-Fraumeni syndrome in most patients, giving rise to 1 in 10 carriers developing ACC. In keeping with the distribution of ACC-associated mutations in Li-Fraumeni, R337H is a pH-sensitive mutation localized to the oligomerization domain.[28] Polymorphisms in TP53 may play a role in the development of ACC as well. In a study of Polish ACC patients, the proline allele of the R72P polymorphism was more prevalent in patients with ACC than in normal controls, suggesting that it may contribute to ACC susceptibility.[29]

Inherited Syndromes: Beckwith-Wiedemann

ACC also occurs as part of the constellation of tumor types seen in the overgrowth syndrome, Beckwith-Wiedemann. The disease arises from the misexpression of genes from an imprinted domain on 11p15.5, usually due to paternal uniparental disomy (2 copies of 11p15.5 from the father without any contribution of the region from the mother) or an imprinting defect that silences the genes on the maternal chromosome. Patients generally have overexpression of IGF-2 and a lack of maternally expressed genes such as H19, KCQN1, and CDK1N, which encodes p57^{kip}. Two regions in the imprinted domain have been implicated in the variation of the tumor spectrum (ie, the types of tumors associated with the disease) of this disease. The telomeric region encompasses paternally expressed IGF-2 and maternally expressed H19. Abnormalities that lead to the lack of H19 expression and overexpression of IGF-2, such as paternal uniparental disomy or aberrant methylation of H19, give rise to Beckwith-Wiedemann syndrome with a preponderance of Wilms tumor. The centromeric region of the 11p15 imprinted domain includes the LIT1 transcript of the KCQN1 gene and CDKN1C, the gene that encodes p57^{kip}. Hypomethylation of LIT1 or mutations in CDKN1C have been implicated in Beckwith-Wiedemann syndrome with a tumor spectrum that is skewed toward embryonal tumors such as rhabdomyosarcoma, hepatoblastoma, gonadoblastoma, and ACC.[30] p57^{kip} is a known negative regulator of cell cycle progression, making it a prime candidate for a tumor suppressor in this region.

Insulinlike growth factor 2

One of the most common features of ACC is an overexpression, either at the RNA or protein level, of IGF-2. Approximately 90% of ACC demonstrate overexpression of IGF-2 and LOH for the IGF-2 locus has been found in 95% or more of ACC.[3] In microarray studies of gene expression, IGF-2 and associated binding proteins are consistently identified as differentially expressed in ACC compared with normal adrenal tissue or adenomas, with most studies identifying IGF-2 as upregulated. It is hypothesized that overexpression of IGF-2 forms a positive autocrine loop that promotes cell proliferation, which is selected for in the ACC. However, the role of IGF-2 overexpression in tumorigenesis is unclear. Targeted knockouts of H19 that when maternally inherited lack H19 expression and overexpress IGF-2 do not demonstrate evidence of increased cancer incidence unless crossed into a background that confers an increased risk in and of itself.[31,32] For example, in the APC[min] background, IGF-2 overexpression as a consequence of maternally inherited H19 knockout results in twice as many tumors as the APC[min] background alone.[33] In contrast, targeted overexpression of IGF-2 by transgene insertion (ie, inserting an exogenous copy of IGF-2 while leaving the endogenous imprinted domain intact and maintaining normal expression of the genes in the region) does lead to an increase in tumors in mice. The diversity of the tumor sites, including tissues that express the transgene as well as those that do not, coupled with a long latency (most tumors are seen after 18 months), suggests that IGF-2 overexpression may be tumor promoting but not tumor initiating.[34] It is worth noting that none of these models include ACC as a tumor type to which the mice are prone. That said, inhibition of IGF1R, the primary receptor for IGF-2, has been shown to reduce cell proliferation and viability in preclinical studies.[35,36]

OPERATIONS FOR ADRENOCORTICAL CANCER

The major predictor of long-term survival is presentation with either stage I or II disease, and the ability to undergo complete resection of tumor (**Fig. 2**). Adrenalectomy can be conducted in the supine or decubitus position. In the era before laparoscopic adrenalectomy, retrospective studies showed a flank approach was associated with a shorter hospital stay and quicker recovery than was associated

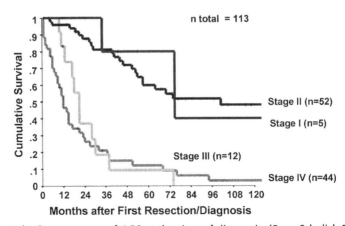

Fig. 2. Survival relates to stage of ACC at the time of diagnosis. (*From* Schulick R, Brennan MF. Long-term survival after complete resection and repeat resection in patients with adrenocortical cancer. Ann Surg Oncol 1999;6:719–26; with permission.)

with a transabdominal approach. For potentially malignant tumors, however, a transabdominal approach is favored because one can fully stage the abdomen, and one has better exposure for control of major vessels and for resection of adjacent organs when needed. The transabdominal approach can be conducted via a midline, paramedian, or extended subcostal incision. For very large tumors, a thoracoabdominal incision may be necessary. A multidisciplinary team of surgeons may be required for a cancer with intracaval tumor thrombus that on occasion can extend all the way into the right atrium. Before operation one should assess for subclinical excess of cortisol production and administer exogenous steroid replacement as appropriate. Postoperatively, one should taper hydrocortisone slowly, guided by recovery of the pituitary-adrenal axis, which can take up to 6 months.[37]

On the right side, care is taken to fully mobilize the duodenum by a Kocher maneuver and hepatic flexure of the colon by division of its retroperitoneal attachments. One then must fully divide the ligamentous attachments of the right lobe of the liver and identify the vena cava behind the liver, and the site of the junction of the right adrenal vein and the inferior vena cava. The adrenal vein typically enters the vena cava directly from the medial aspect of the tumor but may enter the vena cava on its posterior aspect. One should also be aware of potential accessory adrenal veins that may drain into the right renal vein. Routine nephrectomy is not required, but the tumor may directly invade the kidney or involve its vascular supply, making complete or partial nephrectomy necessary. On occasion, a right adrenal cancer may directly invade the right lobe of the liver. In this setting, a liver-hanging maneuver or transection of the liver has been described as a technique to fully obtain vascular control of the adrenal tumor and facilitate en bloc resection.[38]

On the left side, the splenic flexure of the colon is reflected inferiorly by dividing its attachments to the retroperitoneum and the spleen. The omentum is divided to allow entry into the lesser sac. If the tumor is relatively small, one may prefer to leave the spleen attached to the diaphragm and divide the retroperitoneum along the inferior aspect of the body and tail of the pancreas to expose the left adrenal gland. Downward retraction on the left kidney helps expose the adrenal gland, allowing for division of its superior and posterior attachments. Although typically the vascular supply is derived medially, extensive and large collateral vessels may form in this area, requiring one to proceed cautiously. If the adrenal tumor is large one may choose to divide the leinophrenic attachments to allow one to rotate the spleen and tail of the pancreas medially. If there is direct invasion of the pancreas, a distal pancreatectomy and splenectomy may be required for en bloc complete tumor resection. One then seeks exposure of the left adrenal vein as it enters the left renal vein to ligate this vessel. The posterior attachments and the attachments to the left kidney are then divided. Again, nephrectomy is not required unless there is direct invasion of the kidney or its vasculature by the tumor. On either side, one should resect enlarged regional lymph nodes, as lymphatic metastases portend a poor prognosis.

The best prognostic indicators for adrenocortical cancer are complete resection of tumor and an early stage at diagnosis (**Table 1**). Although anecdotal complete remissions have been observed with chemotherapy, a complete surgical resection is the only modality that offers a realistic prospect for cure. Overall 5-year survival for patients who undergo a complete resection is 32% to 48%. Given that laparoscopic approaches to the adrenal gland have become routine in the resection of benign functional adrenal adenomas, the optimal surgical approach to cancerous adrenal tumors has been debated. Admittedly, prospective randomized comparative trials of open and laparoscopic approaches have not been done. Caution is urged, stemming from the potential for tumor dissemination and a concern for tumor fracture, and

Table 1
Staging of adrenocortical cancer (Macfarlane)

Stage	T, N, M Staging	Criteria
1	T1, N0, M0	Tumor <5 cm Node negative No local invasion No metastases
2	T2, N0, M0	Tumor >5 cm Node negative No local invasion No metastases
3	T3, N0, M0 or T1–2, N1, M0	Presence of local invasion without involvement of adjacent organs or mobile, nodal metastases
4	T4, N0, M0 or T3, N1, M0 or T1–4, N0–1, M1	Invasion of adjacent organs, fixed positive lymph node metastases, or presence of distant metastases

this mitigates against the use of laparoscopic adrenalectomy if one suspects an adrenal tumor is malignant. Retrospective series suggest a higher risk of local recurrence and peritoneal carcinomatosis if a primary ACC had been resected via the laparoscope. The transabdominal open approach helps limit the risk of tumor fracture and therefore tumor spillage is reduced.

MITOTANE

No proven chemotherapeutic regimen exists for the treatment of ACC, and the toxicity of the only approved compound, mitotane (o,p'-DDD or 1,1-dichloro-2-(o-chlorophenyl)-2-(p-chlorophenyl)ethane), is often severe and dose limiting. An isomer of the pesticide DDT, mitotane is an agent that is directly toxic to adrenocortical cells. The biochemical mechanisms of action for mitotane are not well characterized, although it is thought to work after hydroxylation by a mitochondrial cytochrome P450 enzyme and subsequent conversion to an acyl chloride that is cytotoxic.[39] Cytotoxicity ultimately results in mitochondrial disruption and necrosis.[40] The primary metabolites of mitotane are o,p'-DDA and o,p'-DDE. Investigations of the localization of 3-methylsulfonyl-DDE, a metabolite of DDT, and mitotane demonstrated that both compounds accumulate in the zona fasciculata and the zona reticularis, but not in the zona glomerulosa.[41] The activity of mitotane is dependent on the 1,1-dichloro structure; conversion of this moiety to a methyl group significantly reduces activity.[42] Investigations of the protein profile of H295R cells and steroid production after mitotane exposure suggest that the cytochrome P450 enzyme involved in the initial activation step acts upstream of the steroidogenic cascade.[43]

The first report of mitotane use in patients with ACC was presented by Bergenstal and colleagues in 1959.[44] The therapeutic value of mitotane is dependent on achieving sufficiently high blood levels of the drug, but the therapeutic window is narrow.[45] Side effects of mitotane are predominantly gastrointestinal, neurologic, and cutaneous. Gastrointestinal disturbances occur in about 80% of patients and include anorexia, nausea and vomiting, and diarrhea. Central nervous system side effects occur in approximately 40% of patients. These side effects are often severe enough to require discontinuation of treatment.

Unfortunately, even after apparently curative operation, up to 85% of patients with ACC will eventually relapse. Repeated resections where possible have been recommended, as patients who are able to undergo complete resection of their recurrent disease or metastases fare better than those who do not, albeit in retrospective, nonrandomized series (**Fig. 3**). Because of the high rate of recurrence, there is a great need for effective adjuvant chemotherapy. The adjuvant use of mitotane remains controversial despite an article published in 2007. In this article from groups in Germany and Italy, the investigators studied a multi-institutional group of 177 patients. Forty-seven patients in Italy who received mitotane were compared with control groups in Italy and Germany who did not receive mitotane. In this series, the use of mitotane conferred a prolonged recurrence-free survival of 42 months compared with 10 and 25 months for the 2 control groups. Mitotane dosing was 3 to 5 g daily for 20 patients and 1 to 3 g daily for 27 patients, and both groups seemed to benefit. This article has been criticized because the patients were treated in 8 Italian centers and 47 German centers over a prolonged period of 20 years. Although this report is of a relatively large series in a rare disease, the fact remains that this is a nonrandomized, uncontrolled, retrospective analysis. Furthermore, there was no stratification based on surgical technique or status of surgical margins.

UNRESECTABLE DISEASE

In 20% of ACC cases, patients are unresectable due to disease advancement. The 5-year survival rate in patients with stage IV disease is between 16% and 38%.[1,3,4,6,7] Mitotane, alone or in combination with cytotoxic drugs, remains the standard therapy for nonresectable metastatic adrenocortical cancer. In a study led by the Eastern Cooperative Oncology Group, 22% of patients responded to mitotane treatment and experienced prolonged median survival of 50 months compared with 14 months for nonresponders.[46] These findings were confirmed in a later study by a group of investigators from MD Anderson Cancer Center (**Fig. 4**).[47] Van Slooten and colleagues showed an increase in survival or tumor regression in 57% of patients who had mitotane serum levels greater than 14 µg/mL, with complete remission in one patient.[48] However, no patient with a mitotane serum level less than 10 µg/mL had a significant response to chemotherapy. Other studies have failed to show

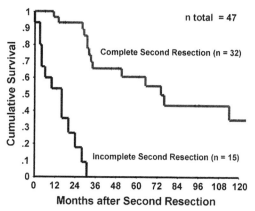

Fig. 3. Survival based on whether recurrent ACC was amenable to complete resection. (*From* Schulick R, Brennan MF. Long-term survival after complete resection and repeat resection in patients with adrenocortical cancer. Ann Surg Oncol 1999;6:719–26; with permission.)

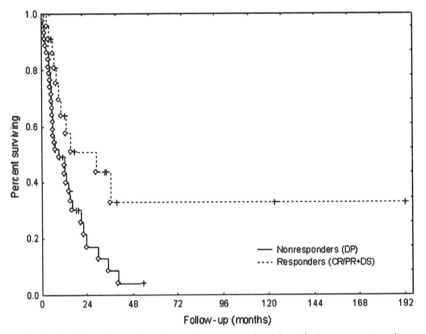

Fig. 4. Survival of 67 patients from date of recurrence based on their response to mitotane. (*From* Gonzales RJ, Tamm EP, Chaan N, et al. Response to mitotane predicts outcome in patients with recurrent adrenal cortical carcinoma. Surgery 2007;142:867–75; with permission.)

a response.[27,49] Chemotherapeutic strategies using mitotane in combination with other standard agents have been reported, with mixed results. In a study of 35 patients using mitotane in combination with doxorubicin, vincristine, and etoposide, a 22% response rate was reported and there was no evidence for improved survival over mitotane alone.[50] The most promising regimen thus far has been a combination of doxorubicin, etoposide, and cisplatin in conjunction with mitotane. The investigators reported that in 72 patients with metastatic disease, 5 responded completely and 30 had partial response, for an overall response rate of 48.6%. The median time to progression and overall survival of the entire cohort were 9.1 and 28.5 months, respectively, with responders having approximately double those values.[51] This regimen is currently under investigation in an international multicenter phase III trial comparing it to mitotane and streptocozin, known as the FIRM-ACT study.

REFERENCES

1. Allolio B, Hahner S, Weismann D, et al. Management of adrenocortical carcinoma. Clin Endocrinol 2004;60:273–87.
2. Bilimoria K, Shen W, Elaraj D, et al. Adrenocortical carcinoma in the United States: treatment utilization and prognostic factors. Cancer 2008;113:3130–6.
3. Libe R, Fratticci1 A, Bertherat J. Adrenocortical cancer: pathophysiology and clinical management. Endocr Relat Cancer 2007;14:13–28.

4. de Reynie's A, Assié G, Rickman D, et al. Gene expression profiling reveals a new classification of adrenocortical tumors and identifies molecular predictors of malignancy and survival. J Clin Oncol 2009;27:1108–15.

5. Giordano TJ, Thomas D, Kuick R, et al. Distinct transcriptional profiles of adrenocortical tumors uncovered by DNA microarray analysis. Am J Pathol 2003;162: 521–31.

6. Soon P, McDonald K, Robinson B, et al. Molecular markers and the pathogenesis of adrenocortical cancer. Oncologist 2008;5:548–61.

7. de Fraipont F, Atifi M, Cherradi MN, et al. Gene expression profiling of human adrenocortical tumors using complementary deoxyribonucleic acid microarrays identifies several candidate genes as markers of malignancy. J Clin Endocrinol Metab 2005;90:1819–29.

8. Herbet M, Feige J, Thomas M. Insights into the role of genetic alterations in adrenocortical tumorigenesis. Mol Cell Endocrinol 2009;300:169–74.

9. Bakthavathsalam G, Shanmugasundaram VP, Prabakaran J, et al. Nonfunctioning adrenocorticalcarcinoma. Int Surg 2008;93(2):81–7.

10. Brunt M, Moley J. Adrenal incidentaloma. World J Surg 2001;25:905–13.

11. Mitchell I, Nwariaku F. Adrenal masses in the cancer patient: surveillance or excision. Oncologist 2007;12:168–74.

12. Reincke M, Nieke J, Krestin G, et al. Preclinical Cushing's syndrome in adrenal "incidentalomas": comparison with adrenal Cushing's syndrome. J Clin Endocrinol Metab 1992;75(3):826–32.

13. Singh PK, Buch HN. Adrenal incidentaloma: evaluation and management. J Clin Pathol 2008;61:1168–73.

14. Michael B, Holalkere N, Boland G. Imaging techniques for adrenal lesion characterization. Radiol Clin North Am 2008;46:65–78.

15. Giordano TJ, Kuick R, Else T, et al. Molecular classification and prognostication of adrenocortical tumors by transcriptome profiling. Clin Cancer Res 2009;15: 668–76.

16. Mitelman F, Johansson B, Mertens F. Mitelman database of chromosome aberrations in cancer. 2009.

17. Dohna M, Reincke M, Mincheva A, et al. Adrenocortical carcinoma is characterized by a high frequency of chromosomal gains and high-level amplifications. Genes Chromosomes Cancer 2000;28:145–52.

18. Kjellman M, Kallioniemi OP, Karhu R, et al. Genetic aberrations in adrenocortical tumors detected using comparative genomic hybridization correlate with tumor size and malignancy. Cancer Res 1996;56:4219–23.

19. Sidhu S, Marsh DJ, Theodosopoulos G, et al. Comparative genomic hybridization analysis of adrenocortical tumors. J Clin Endocrinol Metab 2002;87:3467–74.

20. Zhao J, Roth J, Bode-Lesniewska B, et al. Combined comparative genomic hybridization and genomic microarray for detection of gene amplifications in pulmonary artery intimal sarcomas and adrenocortical tumors. Genes Chromosomes Cancer 2002;34:48–57.

21. Zhao J, Speel EJ, Muletta-Feurer S, et al. Analysis of genomic alterations in sporadic adrenocortical lesions. Gain of chromosome 17 is an early event in adrenocortical tumorigenesis. Am J Pathol 1999;155:1039–45.

22. Stephan EA, Chung TH, Grant CS, et al. Adrenocortical carcinoma survival rates correlated to genomic copy number variants. Mol Cancer Ther 2008;7:425–31.

23. Slater EP, Diehl SM, Langer P, et al. Analysis by cDNA microarrays of gene expression patterns of human adrenocortical tumors. Eur J Endocrinol 2006; 154:587–98.

24. Velazquez-Fernandez D, Laurell C, Geli J, et al. Expression profiling of adrenocortical neoplasms suggests a molecular signature of malignancy. Surgery 2005;138:1087–94.

25. Gonzalez KD, Noltner KA, Buzin CH, et al. Beyond Li Fraumeni Syndrome: clinical characteristics of families with p53 germline mutations. J Clin Oncol 2009;27:1250–6.

26. Olivier M, Goldgar DE, Sodha N, et al. Li-Fraumeni and related syndromes: correlation between tumor type, family structure, and TP53 genotype. Cancer Res 2003;63:6643–50.

27. Barzon L, Fallo F, Sonino N, et al. Comment—is there a role for low doses of mitotane (o, p′-DDD) as adjuvant therapy in adrenocortical carcinoma? J Clin Endocrinol Metab 1999;84:1488–9.

28. Zambetti GP. The p53 mutation "gradient effect" and its clinical implications. J Cell Physiol 2007;213:370–3.

29. Ignaszak-Szczepaniak M, Horst-Sikorska W, Sawicka J, et al. The TP53 codon 72 polymorphism and predisposition to adrenocortical cancer in Polish patients. Oncol Rep 2006;16:65–71.

30. Weksberg R, Nishikawa J, Caluseriu O, et al. Tumor development in the Beckwith-Wiedemann syndrome is associated with a variety of constitutional molecular 11p15 alterations including imprinting defects of KCNQ1OT1. Hum Mol Genet 2001;10:2989–3000.

31. Blake JA, Bult CJ, Eppig JT, et al. The mouse genome database genotypes::phenotypes. Nucleic Acids Res 2009;37:D712–9.

32. Bult CJ, Eppig JT, Kadin JA, et al. The Mouse Genome Database (MGD): mouse biology and model systems. Nucleic Acids Res 2008;36:D724–8.

33. Sakatani T, Kaneda A, Iacobuzio-Donahue CA, et al. Loss of imprinting of Igf2 alters intestinal maturation and tumorigenesis in mice. Science 2005;307:1976–8.

34. Moorehead RA, Fata JE, Johnson MB, et al. Inhibition of mammary epithelial apoptosis and sustained phosphorylation of Akt/PKB in MMTV-IGF-II transgenic mice. Cell Death Differ 2001;8:16–29.

35. Almeida MQ, Fragoso MC, Lotfi CF, et al. Expression of insulin-like growth factor-II and its receptor in pediatric and adult adrenocortical tumors. J Clin Endocrinol Metab 2008;93:3524–31.

36. Barlaskar FM, Spalding AC, Heaton JH, et al. Preclinical targeting of the type I insulin-like growth factor receptor in adrenocortical carcinoma. J Clin Endocrinol Metab 2009;94:204–12.

37. Doherty GM, Nieman LK, Cutler GB Jr, et al. Recover of the hypothalamic-pituitary-adrenal axis after curative resection of adrenal tumors in patients with Cushing's syndrome. Surgery 1990;108:1085–90.

38. Donadon M, Abdalla EK, Vauthey J-N. Liver hanging maneuver for large or recurrent right upper quadrant tumors. J Am Coll Surg 2006;204:329–33.

39. Martz F, Straw JA. The in vitro metabolism of 1-(o-chlorophenyl)-1-(p-chlorophenyl)-2,2-dichloroethane (o, p′-DDD) by dog adrenal mitochondria and metabolite covalent binding to mitochondrial macromolecules: a possible mechanism for the adrenocorticolytic effect. Drug Metab Dispos 1977;5:482–6.

40. Martz F, Straw JA. Metabolism and covalent binding of 1-(o-chlorophenyl)-1-(p-chlorophenyl)-2,2-dichloroethane (o, p′-DDD). Correlation between adrenocorticolytic activity and metabolic activation by adrenocortical mitochondria. Drug Metab Dispos 1980;8:127–30.

41. Lindhe O, Skogseid B. Brandt I cytochrome P450-catalyzed binding of 3-methylsulfonyl-DDE and o, p′-DDD in human adrenal zona fasciculata/reticularis. J Clin Endocrinol Metab 2002;87:1319–26.

42. Schteingart DE, Sinsheimer JE, Counsell RE, et al. Comparison of the adrenalytic activity of mitotane and a methylated homolog on normal adrenal cortex and adrenal cortical carcinoma. Cancer Chemother Pharmacol 1993;31:459–66.

43. Stigliano A, Cerquetti L, Borro M, et al. Modulation of proteomic profile in H295R adrenocortical cell line induced by mitotane. Endocr Relat Cancer 2008;15:1–10.

44. Bergenstal DM, Lipsett M, Moy RN, et al. Regression of adrenal cancer and suppression of adrenal function in man by o, p'-DDD. Trans Am Physicians 1959;72:341–50.

45. Haak HR, Hermans J, van de Velde CJ, et al. Optimal treatment of adrenocortical carcinoma with mitotane: results in a consecutive series of 96 patients. Br J Cancer 1994;69:947–51.

46. Decker RA, Elson P, Hogan TF, et al. Eastern Cooperative Oncology Group study 1879: mitotane and adriamycin in patients with advanced adrenocortical carcinoma. Surgery 1991;110:1006–13.

47. Gonzales RJ, Tamm EP, Chaan N, et al. Response to mitotane predicts outcome in patients with recurrent adrenal cortical carcinoma. Surgery 2007;142:867–75.

48. van Slooten H, Moolenaar AJ, van Seters AP, et al. The treatment of adrenocortical carcinoma with o, p'-DDD: prognostic implications of serum level monitoring. Eur J Cancer Clin Oncol 1984;20:47–53.

49. Vassilopoulou-Sellin R, Guinee VF, Klein MJ, et al. Impact of adjuvant mitotane on the clinical course of patients with adrenocortical cancer. Cancer 1993;71: 3119–23.

50. Abraham J, Bakke S, Rutt A, et al. A phase II trial of combination chemotherapy and surgical resection for the treatment of metastatic adrenocortical carcinoma: continuous infusion doxorubicin, vincristine, and etoposide with daily mitotane as a P-glycoprotein antagonist. Cancer 2002;94:2333–43.

51. Berruti A, Terzolo M, Sperone P, et al. Etoposide, doxorubicin and cisplatin plus mitotane in the treatment of advanced adrenocortical carcinoma: a large prospective phase II trial. Endocr Relat Cancer 2005;12:657–66.

Index

Note: Page numbers of article titles are in **boldface** type.

A

Ablation, for metastatic insulinoma, 1116–1117
Adrenal endocrinopathies, surgical management of, 1078–1082
    adrenocortical tumors, 1078–1079
    Beckwith-Wiedemann syndrome, 1078, 1082
    Carney complex, 1071, 1073, 1081–1082
    cortisol hypersecretion–related syndromes, 1081–1082
    Li-Fraumeni syndrome, 1078–1079
    neurofibromatosis 1, 1079–1080
    pheochromocytomas, 1079–1081
    Von Hippel-Lindau disease, 1080–1081
Adrenal tumors, evaluation of, 1256–1257
Adrenocortical cancer, **1255–1267**
    described, 1255
    evaluation of, 1256–1257
    expression microarrays in, 1258–1259
    genomics of, 1258
    IGF-2 in, 1260
    incidence of, 1255
    inherited syndromes, 1259
    management of
        mitotane in, 1262–1263
        surgical, 1260–1262
    molecular oncogenesis in, 1258–1260
    pathology of, 1257–1258
    presentation of, 1255–1256
    unresectable, 1263–1264
Adrenocortical tumors, surgical management of, 1078–1079
Aldosteronism, primary, **1241–1253.** See also *Primary aldosteronism (PA).*
Aldosteronoma(s), **1241–1253.** See also *Primary aldosteronism (PA).*
    described, 1241–1242
    pathology of, 1242–1243
American Thyroid Association (ATA), on thyroid cancer, 1171
Appendiceal carcinoids, 1132–1133
ATA. See *American Thyroid Association (ATA).*

B

Beckwith-Wiedemann syndrome, 1259
    surgical management of, 1078, 1082
Biotherapy, with ocreotide/interferon, for metastatic insulinoma, 1114
BRAF, in thyroid cancer diagnosis, 1142–1143

Surg Clin N Am 89 (2009) 1269–1278
doi:10.1016/S0039-6109(09)00135-2
0039-6109/09/$ – see front matter © 2009 Elsevier Inc. All rights reserved.

United States Postal Service

Statement of Ownership, Management, and Circulation
(All Periodicals Publications Except Requestor Publications)

1. Publication Title	2. Publication Number								3. Filing Date
Surgical Clinics of North America	5	2	9	-	8	0	0	0	9/15/09

4. Issue Frequency	5. Number of Issues Published Annually	6. Annual Subscription Price
Feb, Apr, Jun, Aug, Oct, Dec	6	$269.00

7. Complete Mailing Address of Known Office of Publication (Not printer) (Street, city, county, state, and ZIP+4®)

Elsevier Inc.
360 Park Avenue South
New York, NY 10010-1710

Contact Person
Stephen Bushing
Telephone (Include area code)
215-239-3688

8. Complete Mailing Address of Headquarters or General Business Office of Publisher (Not printer)

Elsevier Inc., 360 Park Avenue South, New York, NY 10010-1710

9. Full Names and Complete Mailing Addresses of Publisher, Editor, and Managing Editor (Do not leave blank)

Publisher (Name and complete mailing address)

John Schrefer , Elsevier, Inc., 1600 John F. Kennedy Blvd. Suite 1800, Philadelphia, PA 19103-2899

Editor (Name and complete mailing address)

Catherine Bewick, Elsevier, Inc., 1600 John F. Kennedy Blvd. Suite 1800, Philadelphia, PA 19103-2899

Managing Editor (Name and complete mailing address)

Catherine Bewick, Elsevier, Inc., 1600 John F. Kennedy Blvd. Suite 1800, Philadelphia, PA 19103-2899

10. Owner (Do not leave blank. If the publication is owned by a corporation, give the name and address of the corporation immediately followed by the names and addresses of all stockholders owning or holding 1 percent or more of the total amount of stock. If not owned by a corporation, give the names and addresses of the individual owners. If owned by a partnership or other unincorporated firm, give its name and address as well as those of each individual owner. If the publication is published by a nonprofit organization, give its name and address.)

Full Name	Complete Mailing Address
Wholly owned subsidiary of	4520 East-West Highway
Reed/Elsevier, US holdings	Bethesda, MD 20814

11. Known Bondholders, Mortgagees, and Other Security Holders Owning or Holding 1 Percent or More of Total Amount of Bonds, Mortgages, or Other Securities. If none, check box. ☐ None

Full Name	Complete Mailing Address
N/A	

12. Tax Status (For completion by nonprofit organizations authorized to mail at nonprofit rates) (Check one)

The purpose, function, and nonprofit status of this organization and the exempt status for federal income tax purposes:
☐ Has Not Changed During Preceding 12 Months
☐ Has Changed During Preceding 12 Months (Publisher must submit explanation of change with this statement)

PS Form 3526, September 2007 (Page 1 of 3 (Instructions Page 3)) PSN 7530-01-000-9931 PRIVACY NOTICE: See our Privacy policy in www.usps.com

---

13. Publication Title		14. Issue Date for Circulation Data Below
Surgical Clinics of North America		June 2009

15. Extent and Nature of Circulation			Average No. Copies Each Issue During Preceding 12 Months	No. Copies of Single Issue Published Nearest to Filing Date
a. Total Number of Copies (Net press run)			4583	4200
b. Paid Circulation (By Mail and Outside the Mail)	(1)	Mailed Outside-County Paid Subscriptions Stated on PS Form 3541. (Include paid distribution above nominal rate, advertiser's proof copies, and exchange copies)	1893	1728
	(2)	Mailed In-County Paid Subscriptions Stated on PS Form 3541 (Include paid distribution above nominal rate, advertiser's proof copies, and exchange copies)		
	(3)	Paid Distribution Outside the Mails Including Sales Through Dealers and Carriers, Street Vendors, Counter Sales, and Other Paid Distribution Outside USPS®	1641	1416
	(4)	Paid Distribution by Other Classes Mailed Through the USPS (e.g. First-Class Mail®)		
c. Total Paid Distribution (Sum of 15b (1), (2), (3), and (4))		▶	3534	3144
d. Free or Nominal Rate Distribution (By Mail and Outside the Mail)	(1)	Free or Nominal Rate Outside-County Copies Included on PS Form 3541	144	98
	(2)	Free or Nominal Rate In-County Copies Included on PS Form 3541		
	(3)	Free or Nominal Rate Copies Mailed at Other Classes Through the USPS (e.g. First-Class Mail)		
	(4)	Free or Nominal Rate Distribution Outside the Mail (Carriers or other means)		
e. Total Free or Nominal Rate Distribution (Sum of 15d (1), (2), (3) and (4))		▶	144	98
f. Total Distribution (Sum of 15c and 15e)		▶	3678	3242
g. Copies not Distributed (See instructions to publishers #4 (page 83))		▶	905	958
h. Total (Sum of 15f and g)		▶	4583	4200
i. Percent Paid (15c divided by 15f times 100)			96.08%	96.98%

16. Publication of Statement of Ownership

☐ If the publication is a general publication, publication of this statement is required. Will be printed
in the October 2009 issue of this publication. ☐ Publication not required.

17. Signature and Title of Editor, Publisher, Business Manager, or Owner

Stephen R. Bushing

Stephen R. Bushing – Subscription Services Coordinator

Date
September 15, 2009

I certify that all information furnished on this form is true and complete. I understand that anyone who furnishes false or misleading information on this form
or who omits material or information requested on the form may be subject to criminal sanctions (including fines and imprisonment) and/or civil sanctions
(including civil penalties).

PS Form 3526, September 2007 (Page 2 of 3)

Moving?

Make sure your subscription moves with you!

To notify us of your new address, find your **Clinics Account Number** (located on your mailing label above your name), and contact customer service at:

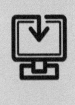

Email: journalscustomerservice-usa@elsevier.com

800-654-2452 (subscribers in the U.S. & Canada)
314-447-8871 (subscribers outside of the U.S. & Canada)

Fax number: 314-447-8029

**Elsevier Health Sciences Division
Subscription Customer Service
3251 Riverport Lane
Maryland Heights, MO 63043**

*To ensure uninterrupted delivery of your subscription, please notify us at least 4 weeks in advance of move.

Printed and bound by CPI Group (UK) Ltd, Croydon, CR0 4YY

03/10/2024

01040443-0006